CANCER ETIOLOGY, DIAGNOSIS AND TREATMENTS SERIES

MULTIPLE MYELOMA: SYMPTOMS, DIAGNOSIS AND TREATMENT

Cancer Etiology, Diagnosis and Treatments Series

Cell Apoptosis and Cancer
Albina W. Taylor (Editor)
2007. ISBN: 1-60021-506-8

Chronic Lymphocytic Leukemia Research Focus
Chadi Nabhan (Editor)
2007. ISBN: 1-60021-526-2

Cervical Cancer Research Trends
Eleanor P. Bankes (Editor)
2007. ISBN: 1-60021-648-x

Lung Cancer in Women
Varetta N. Torres (Editor)
2008. ISBN: 1-60021-659-5

Lung Cancer in Women
Varetta N. Torres (Editor)
2008. ISBN: 978-1-60692-765-6
(Online book)

Cancer Research at the Leading Edge
Ignatius K. Martakis (Editor)
2008. ISBN: 1-60021-728-1

Chronic Lymphocytic Leukemia: New Research
Inès B. Moreau (Editor)
2008. ISBN: 978-1-60456-081-7

Cancer and Stem Cells
Thomas Dittmar and Kurt S. Zander (Editors)
2008. ISBN: 978-1-60456-478-5

Cancer Prevention Research Trends
Louis Braun and Maximilian Lange (Editor)
2008. ISBN: 978-1-60456-639-0

Clinical, Genetic and Molecular Precursor Features in Colorectal Neoplasia
Kjetil Søreide and Håvard Søiland (Editors)
2008. ISBN: 978-1-60456-714-4

Human Polyomaviruses: Molecular Mechanisms for Transformation and Their Association with Cancers
Ugo Moens, Marijke Van Gheule and Mona Johannessen
2009. ISBN: 978-1-60692-812-7

Molecular Therapy of Breast Cancer: Classicism Meets Modernity
Marc Lacroix
2009. ISBN: 978-1-60741-593-0

Molecular Therapy of Breast Cancer: Classicism Meets Modernity
Marc Lacroix
2009. ISBN: 978-1-60876-726-7
(Online Book)

Aromatase Inhibitors: Types, Mode of Action and Indications
Jean R. Lamonte (Editor)
2009. ISBN: 978-1-60741-711-8

Anticancer Drugs: Design, Delivery and Pharmacology
Peter Spencer and Walter Holt (Editors)
2009. ISBN: 978-1-60741-004-1

Anticancer Drugs: Design, Delivery and Pharmacology
Peter Spencer and Walter Holt (Editors)
2009. ISBN: 978-1-60876-629-1
(Online Book)

Cancer Biology: An Updated Global Overview
Tarek H. EL-Metwally
2009. ISBN: 978-1-60876-193-7

Drug Resisant Neoplasms
Ethan G. Verrite (Editor)
2009. ISBN: 978-1-60741-255-7

Handbook of Prostate Cancer Cell Research: Growth, Signalling and Survival
Alan T. Meridith (Editor)
2009. ISBN: 978-1-60741-954-9

Multiple Myeloma: Symptoms, Diagnosis and Treatment
Milen Georgiev and Evgeni Bachev (Editors)
2009 ISBN: 978-1-60876-108-1

CANCER ETIOLOGY, DIAGNOSIS AND TREATMENTS SERIES

MULTIPLE MYELOMA: SYMPTOMS, DIAGNOSIS AND TREATMENT

MILEN GEORGIEV
AND
EVGENI BACHEV
EDITORS

Nova Biomedical Books
New York

For permission to use material from this book please contact us:
Telephone 631-231-7269; Fax 631-231-8175
Web Site: http://www.novapublishers.com

Library of Congress Cataloging-in-Publication Data

Multiple myeloma : symptoms, diagnosis and treatment / [edited by] Milen Georgiev and Evgeni Bachev.
p. ; cm.
Includes bibliographical references and index.
ISBN 978-1-60876-108-1 (hardcover : alk. paper)
1. Multiple myeloma. I. Georgiev, Milen. II. Bachev, Evgeni.
[DNLM: 1. Multiple Myeloma--diagnosis. 2. Multiple Myeloma--therapy. WH 540 M9637 2009]
RC280.B6M8515 2009
616.99'418--dc22 2009028849

Published by Nova Science Publishers, Inc. ✢ New York

Contents

Preface

Multiple myeloma (also known as myeloma or plasma cell myeloma) is a progressive hematologic disease. It is a cancer of the plasma cell, an important part of the immune system that produces immunoglobulins (antibodies) to help fight infection and disease. Multiple myeloma is characterized by excessive numbers of abnormal plasma cells in the bone marrow and overproduction of intact monoclonal immunoglobulin or Bence-Jones protein. Hypercalcemia, anemia, renal damage, increased susceptibility to bacterial infection, and impaired production of normal immunoglobulin are common clinical manifestations of multiple myeloma. It is often also characterized by diffuse osteoporosis, usually in the pelvis, spine, ribs, and skull. This new book gathers the latest research from around the globe on multiple myeloma research and related topics such as immune defects in multiple myeloma, surgical options in the treatment of spinal myeloma, the role of PBSC in multiple myeloma and allogeneic stem cell transplantation.

Chapter 1 - Multiple myeloma is a disease with a very heterogenous prognosis. Recent introduction of novel drugs with targeted mechanism of action has drawn the attention to those prognostic factors that have a close relation to internal properties of myeloma plasmocytes and reflect the behavior of the malignant clone.

This chapter summarizes the recent knowledge and clinical application of two biological parameters, proliferation and apoptosis of myeloma plasmocytes, which are regarded as the major factors of the tumor growth, accumulation and disease progression.

The authors' study presents a group of more than 300 patients with multiple myeloma (MM) and monoclonal gammopathy of undetermined significance (MGUS) in which the proliferative and apoptotic indices were measured at the time of diagnosis and in different phases of the disease course. The aim was to assess the prognostic significance of both of the parameters in patients treated not only with conventional chemotherapy, but also with high-dosed therapy with the support of autologous stem cell transplantation (HD-ASCT), and in patients treated with novel agents with biological mechanism of action (thalidomide, bortezomib). The authors also focused on longitudinal monitoring of proliferation and apoptosis in patients with MM with regard to the disease activity and the effect of chemotherapy. Finally the authors compared the behavior of both the indices in patients with long lasting stable MGUS and in a cohort of patients with the transformation of MGUS into overt symptomatic form of MM.

The results of their study revealed that the assessment of proliferative and apoptotic indices of myeloma plasmocytes has a prognostic significance in patients treated with conventional chemotherapy. HD-ASCT and the use of novel biological drugs overcome the adverse prognostic effects of unfavorable constellation of both of the indices, still maintaining certain differences in overall survival (OS) between groups of patients with different apoptosis. Both indices are useful for the evaluation of malignant transformation of MGUS into MM, detection of progression/relapse of MM and monitoring of the persistence of stable/plateau phase of the disease.

Chapter 2 - Multiple myeloma is a malignancy of terminally differentiated, antibody-secreting plasma cells frequently associated with osteolytic bone lesions. Wnt signaling is critical in normal bone development and homeostasis, and defects in Wnt signaling pathways have been associated with skeletal diseases. Recent identification of activated Wnt signaling and production of Wnt antagonists (e.g. Dkk1) in multiple myeloma (MM) has attracted attention to the importance of this signaling pathway in myeloma pathogenesis and osteolytic bone disease. Functional signaling through two distinct Wnt pathways (Wnt/β-catenin and Wnt/RhoA) has been characterized in MM plasma cells. Additionally, Wnt/β-catenin signaling plays a significant role in directly regulating osteoblast function responsible for bone formation and indirectly controlling osteoclast function leading to bone resorption. The disruption of this pathway by myeloma plasma cell-derived Dkk1 in the bone marrow microenvironment results in suppression of osteoblast differentiation and enhanced osteoclast function via inhibition of production of regulatory molecules, such as osteoprotegerin, normally produced by osteoblasts. Activation of Wnt/RhoA signaling is also associated with myeloma cell adhesion and drug resistance. Increase in Wnt/β-catenin signaling by Wnt ligands or blockage of Dkk1 via specific antibody prevents MM-induced bone disease and inhibits myeloma cell growth *in vivo*. Herein, the authors review the current understanding of Wnt signaling in myeloma pathogenesis and bone disease and discuss potential therapeutic implications of modulating this pathway in the treatment of MM.

Chapter 3 - Nuclear factor-kappaB (NF-κB) upregulates the transcription of proteins that promote cell survival, stimulate growth and reduce susceptibility to apoptosis. NF-κB signaling pathway is constitutively activated in multiple myeloma (MM). TNF (tumor necrosis factor) receptor associated factor 3 (TRAF3) mutation may account for many cases of constitutive NF-κB activation in MM. TRAF3 is a negative regulator of NF-κB signaling pathway. Three major mammalian inhibitors of NF-κB are IκB (α,β and ε). Two protein kinases with a high degree of sequence similarity, IKKα and IKKβ, mediate phosphorylation of IκB proteins and represent a convergence point for most signal transduction pathways leading to NF-κB activation. NF-κB regulates expression of many proteins that function as MM cell growth factors including interleukin-6 (IL-6), granulocyte-macrophage colony stimulation factor (GM-CSF), B-cell-activating factor (BAFF) and macrophage inflammatory protein-1α (MIP-1α). IL-6 is amajor growth and antiapoptotic cytokine in MM. GM-CSF activates the IL-6 signaling molecule STAT3 (signal transducer and activator of transcription 3) and synergizes with IL-6 to support MM growth. BAFF contributes to MM proliferation and survival. The chemokine MIP-1α mediates bone destruction in MM patients and contibutes to osteolytic bone lesions. MIP-1α acts also as a potential growth and survival factor in MM cells. NF-κB is also involved in transcriptional regulation of cyclin D and antiapoptotic proteins of the Bcl-2 family. Two members of vascular endothelial growth factor (VEGF) family (VEGF-C and placental growth factor /PLGF/), adhesion molecules (integrin /VLA-4/ and inter-cellular adhesion molecule 1 /ICAM-1/) and matrix metalloproteinases (MMP-1 and MMP-9) are transcriptionally regulated by NF-κB and correlate with bone disease. Upregulated expression of adhesion molecules is involved in the resistance of MM cells to drugs. Several drugs effective for the treatment of MM, including proteasome inhibitors, thalidomide, lenalidomide and arsenic trioxide, block NF-κB activation. These drugs inhibit survival and antiapoptotic pathways in MM cells. Therefore, the treated MM cells are more sensitive to cytotoxic stimuli including chemotherapy used at low doses. New agents with NF-κB inhibitory activity enhance the anti-MM effects of conventional chemotherapeutic agents and reduce different side-effects. Triptolide (diterpenoid triepoxyde), a purified component of a traditional Chinese medicine, extracted from a shrub-like vine named Trypterygium wilfordii Hook F (TWHF) inhibits transcriptional activation of NF-κB and downregulates the expression of various NF-κB-regulated genes, including IL-6, bcl-2, cIAP, XIAP,TNF, VEGF and the adhesion molecules. Triptolide (10-80 ng/ml) induces apoptosis of MM cells and effectively inhibits cell growth of MM cells. NF-κB activation can be also inhibited by IKK inhibitors, for example by PS-1145 dihydrochloride.

Chapter 4 - Multiple myeloma (MM) is the second most frequent hematological malignancy and remains fatal despite all available therapies, because of chemotherapeutic resistance. Novel targeted drugs for the treatment of MM are therefore needed to improve outcome of MM patients. Bortezomib (PS-341, Velcade; Millennium Pharmaceuticals, Cambridge MA), a dipeptidyl boronic acid that reversibly inhibits the chymotrypsin-like activity in the 20S core of the 26S mammalian proteasome, is the first proteasome inhibitor that was approved by the US Food amd Drug Administration (FDA) and the European Agency for the Evaluation of Medicinal Products (EMEA) for patients with relapsed and refractory MM who had received at least one prior therapy and who had already undergone or are unsuitable for the transplantation of bone marrow. Phase I-III trials based on previous preclinical studies showed very good antimyeloma activity. Bortezomib acts by disrupting various cell signaling pathways, thereby leading to cell cycle arrest, apoptosis, and inhibition of angiogenesis. The main action of bortezomib is the inhibition of the key transcription factor, nuclear factor-kappaB (NF-κB) activation. Activation of NF-κB has been noted in MM cells. Bortezomib interferes with NF-κB-mediated cell survival, tumor growth and angiogenesis. Several studies have shown that cancer cells are more sensitive than normal cells to the proapoptotic effects of bortezomib, perhaps due to their loss of checkpoint mechanisms for DNA repair. The accumulation of misfolded proteins in the endoplasmic reticulum (ER) leads to the induction of the unfolded protein response, provoking apoptosis. Proteasome inhibitors induce ER-mediated apoptosis. The increased susceptibility of MM cells to ER stress is caused by the large amounts of immunoglobulins produced by MM cells. The clinical success of bortezomib is encouraging. Bortezomib is relatively well tolerated, causing manageable nonhematologic and hematologic toxicity. However, the overall response rate was 40-50% and bortezomib resistance was also observed. Response rates may be improved with combination therapy (bortezomib with dexamethasone, thalidomide, lenalidomide, arsenic trioxide, cisplatin, doxorubicin, cyclophosphamide, etoposide or with melphalan and prednisone). Clinical evaluation of additional proteasome inhibitors of the next generation with greater efficacy is also needed. Three such proteasome inhibitors (carfilzomib, salinosporamide A and threonine boronic acid-derived proteasome inhibitor CEP-18770) have been recently tested in preclinical models of MM. Carfilzomib (PR-171; Proteolix), an epoxyketone related to epoxomicin inhibits the chymotrypsin-like proteasome activity as bortezomib does. However, carfilzomib is an irreversible inhibitor of all three proteasome proteolytic sites. Salinosporamide A (NPI-0052), a compound related to lactacystin binds irreversibly to the 20S proteasome and acts predominantly through caspase-8 activation. CEP-18770 is a reversible inhibitor of the chymotrypsin-like proteasome activity as bortezomib but it inhibits also the tryptic and peptidyl glutamyl activities of the proteasome.

Chapter 5 - Plasma cell dyscrasias (PCDs) include plasmacytomas and various forms of plasma cell myeloma (multiple myeloma-MM). Diagnosis of plasmacytoma requires demonstration of a monoclonal/aberrant plasma cell (PC) population in a tissue biopsy; whereas, diagnosis of a PCD involving the bone marrow (BM) (i.e., various forms of MM) requires quantitation of the PCs in the BM in addition to the demonstration of monoclonality/aberrancy. This chapter will describe the definitions of the various forms of PCD (including the International Staging System-ISS), the morphological variants and immunophenotypic features of neoplastic PCs, the diagnostic laboratory techniques useful in establishing a diagnosis (including immunophenotypic techniques), and the ancillary studies that may aid in diagnosis, prognostication, and therapeutic decision-making (i.e., immunophenotypic features, as well as cytogenetic and molecular findings).

Chapter 6 - Treatment of multiple myeloma, a B-cell cancer, is usually palliative. Bone disease affects 70% of multiple myeloma patients and causes complications such as pathologic fractures, severe bone pain, impaired mobility, spinal cord compression and hypercalcaemia, resulting in greater morbidity and poorer quality of life (QoL) for patients. Management of these complications can include treatment with bisphosphonates. The therapy choice for a multiple myeloma patient depends optimally on evidence that the selected treatment leads to better QoL and/or a lower risk of side effects. Therefore, a steady updating of the current knowledge of efficacy and safety of the therapy of choice is necessary. This chapter aims at a risk-benefit re-evaluation of bisphosphonates. This is achieved firstly by looking at new clinical studies examining the role of bisphosphonates on skeletal-related effect reduction and mortality, and secondly by analysing observational studies and case reports that constitute the only source of evidence for osteonecrosis of jaw (ONJ), a side effect that has been associated with intravenous bisphosphonates only in recent years, leading to a change in labelling.

Chapter 7 - Multiple myeloma (MM) is associated with many immune defects, that are responsible both for impaired anti-tumor responses, as well as frequent and recurrent infections. It was primary found that immune defects in MM patients included abnormalities in number and function of B, T and NK cells. More recent data revealed convincing evidences on an important role of dendritic cells (DC) and T regulatory cells in the impairment of the immune system.

B cell population in MM patients was found to be severely deficient. The suppression of $CD19^{+}$ B lymphocytes is reversible, correlates inversely with the disease stage, and specifically affects the early and late stages of normal B-cell differentiation. Low number of normal B cells results in reduced levels of polyclonal immunoglobulins (Ig). The inhibition of normal B cell proliferation and Ig secretion might be caused by altered cytokine activities, including decreased peripheral blood IL-4 level, or increased production of TGF-β by bone marrow stroma cells. DC are professional antigen-presenting cells which play a crucial role in initiation and potentiation of immune responses. Impaired DC function was described in a wide range of cancers. There is also a convincing evidence that defect in DC function may be responsible for the impairment of an immune system in MM. The reduced number of circulating myeloid (MDC) and plasmacytoid dendritic cells (PDC) characterized by low HLA-DR, CD40, as well as CD80 expression was found in patients with MM. Although MM is a B-cell malignancy, there are many abnormalities concerning T-cell compartment, such as impaired Th1/Th2 ratio as well as changes in regulatory T cells frequencies. In this chapter the authors summarized the current knowledge on the immune defects in MM.

Chapter 8 - *Objective:* Spinal myeloma is a disease requiring a multidisciplinary approach involving orthopaedic and oncology surgeons. Myeloma of the spine seriously affects spinal stability and can lead to compression of neural structures. The evaluation of security, possibilities, indications and efficiency of surgical management in patients with spinal myeloma are the main aim of our contribution.

Diagnostics: Imaging methods are essential for exact diagnostics as well as laboratory examinations. The techniques largely used are X-ray examinations, CT scanning and CT-myelography, MRI (magnetic resonance imaging), 99mTc-MIBI scintigraphy and FDG-PET (fluorodeoxyglucose positron emission tomography). The authors have to distinguish between solitary and multiple myeloma using all these diagnostic methods.

Therapeutic scheme: Instability of the spine, caused by pathological vertebral fracture without compression of the nerve structures, can be treated conservatively using an external orthosis. Surgery is indicated in patients whose survival prognosis is more than 3-6 month in a situation of existing or imminent spinal collapse or nerve damage. The primary aim of surgery is to stop the progress, improve or, in ideal case, prevent damage to the nerves. The surgery renews spinal stability and reduces or eliminates pain symptoms. The authors distinguish between posterior, anterior or combined surgical procedures.

Methods: The authors surgically managed 108 patients with spinal myeloma in the 1987-2008 period. Their average age was 58 years (range 28-78). There were 18 cervical, 59 thoracic and 31 lumbar spinal areas treated. The authors used the posterior approach in 47, anterior approach in 23, and combined surgery in 38 spines. The results, i.e. changes in neurological findings, were evaluated according to the Frankel grading system.

Results: In our group of surgically managed patients with spinal myeloma, 37 patients (38%) had improved neurological findings, 57 (58%) showed the same deficit, and only four patients (4%) had postoperative neurological deterioration.

Conclusions: Early diagnosis and urgent surgical decompression involving eventual stabilization of the spine can prevent irreversible damage to the nervous system due to pressure of the myeloma on the spine. Surgical treatment leads to complete consolidation in patients with solitary myeloma, and serves as a palliative treatment in patients with multiple myeloma.

Chapter 9 - Autologous peripheral blood stem cells (PBSCs) provide a rapid and effective hematopoietic recovery after the administration of chemotherapy alone or in combination with radiotherapy in patients with hematological malignancies, and guarantee a shorter time to engraftment and the lack of a need for surgical procedure necessary for bone marrow harvesting. For these reasons PBSCs have become the preferred source of stem cells for autologous transplantation in haematological and solid tumors. Multipotential and lineage-committed progenitor hemopoietic cells express the CD34 antigen, that represents the marker through which PBSCs are selected and collected. CD34+ PBSCs can be mobilized by the administration of G-CSF or GM-CSF alone or preceded by chemotherapy. The harvest of stem cells after mobilization can differ enormously inter-individually and for this reason several studies have been performed to identify those factors that can affect the yield of progenitors. Mobilized autologous peripheral blood stem cells have been increasingly used in the last decade within high-dose programs of therapy and represent by now the standard for many lymphoproliferative disease and in particular for multiple myeloma.

This comprehensive review tries to revisit the complex issue of the autologous peripheral blood stem cell transplantation in multiple myeloma patients focusing on all related aspect: biology of CD34+ stem cells, prognostic factor for mobilization, mobilizing regimens, high-dose approach of newly diagnosed patients, future perspective.

Chapter 10 - Multiple myeloma (MM) is an incurable plasma cell malignancy. Despite the use of conventional therapy or high dose chemotherapy with autologous stem cell support (ASCT) patients continue to relapse at constant rate. A small minority of patients are cured by allogeneic transplantation. Up to now, ASCT has been the treatment of choice for eligible myeloma patients aged below 65 years of age. Melphalan at a dose of 200 mg/m^2 is considered the standard conditioning regimen for ASCT in MM. Early ASCT seems to be beneficial. A planned double ASCT gives better results than a single ASCT, especially in cases who have not achieved a complete response (CR) after the first ASCT. ASCT is also a suitable procedure for myeloma patients with renal failure.

Allogeneic bone marrow transplantation is too risky to be considered for most patients but the possibility of a potentially curable graft-versus-myeloma (GVM) effect, which has been demonstrated in MM, gives this procedure the best chance for long-term disease control and may be considered as a possible treatment option for patients aged less than 50 years with an HLA-identical sibling. Registry data show that in patients who have undergone allogeneic matched sibling-donor transplantation, the long-term survival is around 25%. However, the median survival is comparable with patients who receive ASCT, mainly due to the high TRM rate of between 20%-40%, which seems to be higher in male patients. Allogeneic transplantations with matched unrelated donors have an even higher TRM and may be considered only in exceptional cases. Chronic graft-versus-host disease (GVHD) correlates with CR in allotransplant patients and provides evidence of an allogeneic GVM effect. In order to harness the GVM effect, current research is focused on allogeneic transplantation from HLA identical sibling after conditioning with a non-myeloablative or reduced intensity conditioning (RIC) regimens followed by DLI to eradicate residual tumour. In a significant proportion of patients disease response is preceded by GVHD, suggesting a clear relationship between GVHD and GVM.

However, many questions regarding the management of myeloma patients remain unanswered. How safe is ASCT in elderly patients? Is there a role for non-myeloablative allogeneic transplantation in MM and in which subgroup of patients? What is the role of novel agents, such as thalidomide, its analogues, and bortezomib, in maintenance therapy post ASCT or allogeneic SCT? This chapter will summarize all available data for the role of SCT in MM.

In: Multiple Myeloma: Symptoms, Diagnosis and Treatment ISBN 978-1-60876-108-1
Editors: M. Georgiev and Ev. Bachev

Chapter 1

Measurement of Proliferative and Apoptotic Indices in Myeloma Plasmocytes

J. Minarik and V. Scudla
Department of Internal Medicine III,
University Hospital Olomouc,
Czech Republic

Abstract

Multiple myeloma is a disease with a very heterogenous prognosis. Recent introduction of novel drugs with targeted mechanism of action has drawn the attention to those prognostic factors that have a close relation to internal properties of myeloma plasmocytes and reflect the behavior of the malignant clone.

Presented chapter summarizes the recent knowledge and clinical application of two biological parameters, proliferation and apoptosis of myeloma plasmocytes, which are regarded as the major factors of the tumor growth, accumulation and disease progression.

Our study presents a group of more than 300 patients with multiple myeloma (MM) and monoclonal gammopathy of undetermined significance (MGUS) in which the proliferative and apoptotic indices were measured at the time of diagnosis and in different phases of the disease course. The aim was to assess the prognostic significance of both of the parameters in patients treated not only with conventional chemotherapy, but also with high-dosed therapy with the support of autologous stem cell transplantation (HD-ASCT), and in patients treated with novel agents with biological mechanism of action (thalidomide, bortezomib). We also focused on longitudinal monitoring of proliferation and apoptosis in patients with MM with regard to the disease activity and the effect of chemotherapy. Finally we compared the behavior of both the indices in patients with long lasting stable MGUS and in a cohort of patients with the transformation of MGUS into overt symptomatic form of MM.

The results of our study revealed that the assessment of proliferative and apoptotic indices of myeloma plasmocytes has a prognostic significance in patients treated with conventional chemotherapy. HD-ASCT and the use of novel biological drugs overcome the adverse prognostic effects of unfavorable constellation of both of the indices, still maintaining certain differences in overall survival (OS) between groups of patients with different apoptosis. Both indices areuseful for the evaluation of malignant transformation of MGUS into MM, detection of progression/relapse of MM and monitoring of the persistence of stable/plateau phase of the disease.

Introduction

Multiple myeloma (MM) is a clonal disease characterized by neoplastic transformation, proliferation and accumulation of plasma cells in the bone marrow [1]. Under physiological conditions the amount of plasma cells are regulated by the delicate balance between processes that support the growth and regeneration of the tissue, and by the processes that cause natural selection and degradation of damaged cells. In the case of malignant transformation there is a disruption of this balance, and the dysregulation of proliferative and/or apoptotic features of the malignant clone determines the degree of the tumor activity as well as its expansion and the tissue damage.

Research dealing with internal processes of myeloma plasmocytes and response to therapy has recently become quite attractive, especially with regard to novel therapeutic approaches that considerably affect different pathways of cellular proliferation and apoptosis [2, 3] and thus are regarded as "targeted biological based treatment".

Biological Prognostic Factors

MM is a disease with a very heterogenous prognosis. With a proper stratification according to prognostic factors it is possible to actively search for patients with accumulation of adverse factors, and to choose an optimal individual therapeutic approach, either using a more intensive induction treatment and/or with the support of maintenance therapy. Essentially it is possible to divide the prognostic factors into three different categories: factors related to the patient, characteristics of the malignant clone, and the mutual interactions between the host and the tumor clone [4].

Substantial attention is drawn to the internal, biological properties of MM cells, their signaling, genetic aberrations, gene profiling etc. One of the first independent prognostic factors associated with adverse prognosis was the plasmoblastic morphology of plasma cells [5]. Immunohistochemical analysis of the produced immunoglobulin chain demonstrated the adverse effect of IgA type [6]. The progress in immunophenotyping revealed the relationship of immature myeloma cell population (expression of immature cell signs – CD20, sIg) with poor prognosis [4]. Down-regulation of adhesive molecules CD56 and CD11a, enabling growth of MM cells in bone marrow, together with high expression of CD44 are associated with extramedullary spreading of plasma cells. Expression of CD28 is linked to the increased activity of the disease and is often found in proliferating plasmocytes [7].

Cytogenetic analyses that demonstrated significance in acute leukemias [8] are recently being recognized as one of the most important prognosticators also in MM. Nearly all patients with MM have an abnormal finding of chromosomal aberrations in the form of deletions, aneuploidies or translocations [9]. Some of the primary cytogenetic changes are equally found in MGUS, MM and in plasma cell leukemia, most of the others (especially secondary changes) are specifically being found only in one of the forms, predominantly in active symptomatic MM. The most focused cytogenetic changes from the point of prognostic stratification are defects of chromosome 13 in the form of partial or complete deletions, abnormalities and deletions of chromosome 1 and 22, and some specific translocations such as t(4;14)(p16;q32), t(14;16)(q32;q23), presence of complex changes and hypodiploidy [9-12].

Dysregulation between oncogenes and tumor suppressor genes contributes to pathogenesis of MM. An association with progression or relapse was found in the case of e.g. mutation of p53, increased expression of c-myc, deletion of Rb gene, k-*ras* mutation or p16 methylation [4, 7, 13]. Several studies demonstrated a prognostic significance of increased microvascular density and some angiogenic cytokines especially in patients treated with conventional chemotherapy [14].

Recent studies assessing the prognosis of MM focus also on two parameters that determine the behavior of the tumor clone itself, proliferative and apoptotic index. Unlike other prognostic factors that usually assess the impact of the tumor on the organism, proliferative and apoptotic potential of myeloma plasmocytes are a specific measure of the tumor aggressiveness [4, 15-22]. Both proliferation and apoptosis are not single factors but reflect the interaction between several regulatory molecules and signaling pathways, and their imbalance contributes to the disruption of tissue homeostasis, activity of the disease, as well as the extent of tumor expansion.

Proliferation and Proliferative Index

Introduction

If we talk about the growth of malignant population, we mean the physiological, specifically the pathophysiological processes that cause its growth. It is the “escape” from natural regulatory mechanisms and the introduction of the tumor´s own pathogenetic pathway. Proliferation means the ability of cells to enter a new cell cycle and to undergo amplification of cell content with subsequent division of the cell. Proliferative potential or proliferative index is the measure of the rate of this ability.

Cell cycle impairment belongs among primary features of MM pathogenesis leading to the tumor expansion [23]. Defect in the expression of cell cycle inhibitors leads to the activation and over-expression of genes responsible for cell cycle acceleration, especially in MM precursor cells. These cells subsequently avoid the physiological selection caused by regulatory mechanisms of the organism and together with genetic modifications and other intracellular changes undergo differentiation into proliferating plasmoblasts and finally into differentiated myeloma cells.

Cell Cycle Regulation

The functionality of cell cycle in healthy as well as malignant cells is generally mediated by a series of enzymatic and non-enzymatic factors that are able to accelerate or decelerate the cell cycle or alternatively modify its course. These factors may be of both the intracellular and extracellular origin, i.e. intracellular signaling and external receptor mediated events. The major regulators affect the checkpoint at the end of G1 phase, which decides about the cell arrest or the entrance of the cycle. Their influence may be either stimulating or inhibitory. Among the characteristic stimulating molecules are two cyclin-dependent kinases (CDK4 and CDK6) together with three D-cyclins – cyclin D1, cyclin D2 and cyclin D3 (in multiple myeloma there is a typically increased expression of cyclin D1 and D3), (figure 1) [23]. Their activation leads to phosphorylation of "retinoblastoma" protein pRb (p105) followed by the release of transcription factors that lead to the entrance of cells into S-phase of the cell cycle [23]. Other stimulating factors are e.g. oncogene *ras* mutation, loss of p53 or the increased expression of c-myc, which are, however, relatively rare in newly diagnosed myeloma but are frequently found in progressive disease [4, 7].

In contrast, the catalytic activity of cyclin dependent kinases CDK4 and CDK6 is negatively regulated by the inhibitory proteins of the INK4 family ($p16^{INK4a}$, $p15^{INK4b}$, $p18^{INK4c}$ and $p19^{INK4d}$) [23]. INK4 proteins form stable complexes with CDK4 and CDK6 thus disabling their action during Rb gene phosphorylation. In MM the most important inhibitory proteins of the cell cycle are p16 and p15 [23].

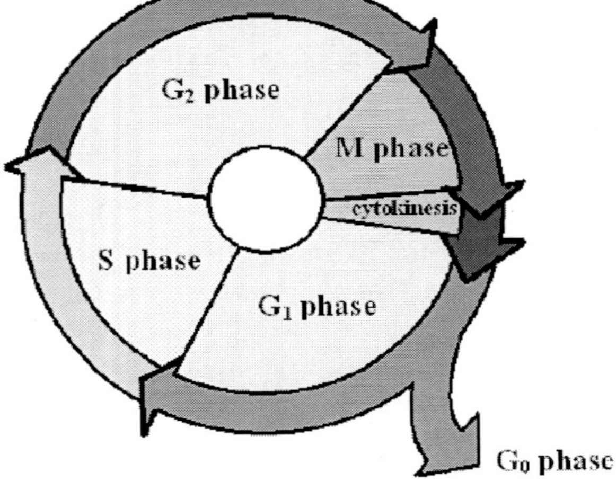

Figure 1. Cell cycle model and its regulation in multiple myeloma.

Presented simple model shows individual phases of cell cycle in eukaryotic as well as tumor cells. The time for one cycle duration is also called the „generation time". Most of the regulation takes part at the major checkpoint at the end of G1 phase, that decides about the cell arrest (G_0 phase) or the entrance of the cycle. Typical stimulating factors are cyclin dependent kinases (CDK4 and CDK6) and cyclins D1-D3. Negative regulation is mediated by inhibitory proteins of INK4 family that form stable complexes with CDK4 and CDK6.

Deletion of the genes for p16 and p15 is only rarely found; on the other hand, they usually have higher percentage of methylation that inhibits their transcription and leads to their lower activity and subsequently to disease progression [23, 24].

Growth Factors

In addition to the molecules directly affecting the cell cycle there is a variety of other factors that influence cell growth and as such are called "growth factors". Recent therapeutic approaches attempt to target these molecules, specifically the cytokines and their signaling pathways that belong to the most significant mechanisms of growth, drug resistance and prolonged survival of myeloma plasmocytes [7].

The major growth factor of myeloma cells is interleukin-6 (IL-6), formerly called the B-cell growth factor [7]. IL-6 is one of the strongest factors of proliferation and cell death protection. It is produced by stromal cells of the bone marrow microenvironment – the fibroblasts, osteoblasts, osteoclasts, monocytes and macrophages. Lesser amount of IL-6 is produced also by myeloma cells themselves (autocrine production). MM cells express on their surface IL-6 receptor which enables the IL-6 stimulation. The signal from IL-6 is transferred into the cell by a transduction protein gp130 which is then able to activate two pathways – the JAK2-STAT pathway (Janus kinase 2 – signal transducer and activator of transcription) and Ras-MAPK pathway (mitogen activated protein kinase). The JAK2-STAT pathway activates a series of anti-apoptotic proteins and the Ras-MAPK pathway leads to an increase in the production of transcription factors, such as ERK-1, AP-1, NF-IL-6 that cause an increase in proliferation [7, 25-31]. Although IL-6 is the most potent growth factor of myeloma plasmocytes, several studies indicate that it is not the only factor responsible for growth of tumor cells as many cell lines appear to be IL-6 independent, and some approaches (such as introduction of mutant *ras*) can even induce IL-6 independence [32, 33].

Another well known growth factor responsible for MM proliferation and growth regulation is IL-1β [7, 26]. The excess expression of IL-1β can contribute to the transformation of MGUS into MM. IL-1β also supports the production of IL-6, changes the expression of cytoadhesive molecules, and has a role in the activation of osteoclasts [26]. Similar properties have been found also in vascular endothelial growth factor (VEGF). It is a protein secreted by MM cells as well as by the bone marrow stromal cells, and in the contact with cellular stroma it induces the formation and excretion of IL-6 [26]. It also leads to an increased angiogenesis and induces the migration of myeloma cells.

Insulin-like growth factor 1 and 2 (IGF1 and IGF2) are direct stimulators of cell cycle [7]. Their signaling pathway uses PI3K (phosphatidylinositol-3′-kinase) and MAPK. In addition to their direct stimulation they increase the sensitivity of MM cells to IL-6 and induce drug resistance [7]. Interleukin-15 (IL-15) induces proliferation and prolongs the survival of human B and T lymphocytes, NK cells and neutrophils [26]. Plasma cells constitutively express on their surface IL-15 receptor (IL-15R) and similarly as in the case of IL-6 are able to produce this cytokine with autocrine secretion. Another potential growth factor is interleukin-10 (IL-10), supporting the growth of myeloma cells and increasing their proliferation activity [26]. Its specific effect is still not known, nevertheless, it is assumed to have an impact on the expression of some cytokines and regulation of their receptors. Finally there are many other stimulating growth factors (usually not as specific and potent in MM) such as granulocyte-macrophage colony stimulating factor (GM-CSF), stem-cell factor (SCF), IL-3, tumor-necrosis factor α (TNF-α), hepatocyte growth factor (HGF) [7, 26]. It has been shown that also some proteins that decelerate growth of plasma cells may have an important regulatory role in MM. An inhibitory effect has been demonstrated for example in the case of interferon gamma (IFN-γ) or Fas antigen (CD95) [34].

Proliferation of Plasma Cells in Multiple Myeloma

In MM the generation time, or the "doubling time" of myeloma cells is relatively long – 5 to 15 months [7]. The reason why the tumor mass grows faster than normal plasma cell population is therefore not in the speed of cell cycle itself but in the percentage and total amount of cells that enter the cell cycle. The total myeloma mass can be divided into three mutually interconnected compartments [35-37]. It is the small compartment of stem cells that is formed by pluripotent cells supplying the other compartments. Then it is the expansion compartment, or the "growth fraction" in which the cells repeatedly enter the cell cycle, divide and form the definite amount of cells which subsequently undergo differentiation. Finally the third, differentiation compartment is the largest, and contains cells with fading proliferation and beginning maturation. At the same time there appears the process of cell apoptosis and necrosis. Total mass of bone marrow myeloma cells is therefore comprised of a small pool of fast proliferating cells and a number of non-proliferating differentiated elements that are slowly being degraded by programmed cell death and secondary necrosis.

Generally, the proliferating cells are described as cells that synthesize DNA. Even though they usually form only a small percentage of the whole tumor mass (about 1-3% of all MM cells), they are still the substantial marker for the clone expansion, aggressiveness and drug resistance. This small percentage in proliferating pool exceeds several times the proliferating capacity of normal bone marrow elements. Even a small change has an immense influence on the proliferating activity of the whole tumor population. Myeloma cells that afterwards undergo maturation have a decreased capability of apoptosis and accumulate in the bone marrow microenvironment. This leads to the increase of the total myeloma mass and causes the manifestation of clinical symptoms of the disease [1, 28, 29].

Apoptosis and Apoptotic Index

Introduction

Although MM was formerly regarded as a disease with increased proliferative activity, a closer insight into the biological properties of myeloma cells revealed that only a small percentage of the cells are actively proliferating, whereas the majority of the cells do not enter the cell cycle. The actual cause of accumulation and tumor expansion is the loss of apoptotic controls [20, 22]. The final apoptotic process is, however, a consequence of the disruption of various different molecular pathways, including the transformation of oncogenes as well as the interaction between the cell and its microenvironment. Monitoring of apoptosis is among the most intensively investigated cellular processes. The percentage of plasma cells undergoing apoptosis is generally known as the apoptotic index.

Apoptosis plays several roles in the pathogenesis of MM. Quite obvious is the participation in prolonged survival and accumulation of differentiated myeloma plasmocytes. Nevertheless, the loss of apoptotic control very significantly contributes to the growth of neoplastic tissue itself even during the process of transformation of "premalignant" into tumor cell [40]. Differentiation of the plasma cells is a multistep process in which each of the individual steps is influenced by the cell cycle, apoptosis and cell migration [23]. Most of the normal plasma cells are eliminated relatively quickly by apoptosis. Even the neoplastically transformed cells undergo apoptosis and have therefore very little or no chance to express their malignant potential. Apoptosis thus represents the critical determinant of the tissue homeostasis of plasma cells. Only in the case of the disruption of apoptosis are the neoplastic cells able to live long enough to divide and set up the pathogenetic pathway leading to the development of MM. The upfront feature of overt MM – the accumulation of myeloma cells – is represented predominantly by the defect in apoptosis. Block of apoptosis stabilizes cells that may overexpress cell cycle activation that would normally lead to genetic instability. Cumulative genetic events can take place leading to the gross abnormalities often observed in myeloma plasmocytes. Targeted therapy may stop or slow the growth of the tumor population but if it does not activate the apoptotic pathway of myeloma plasmocytes, the surviving cells may develop resistance and lead to a fast progression of refractory MM. Disruption of apoptotic mechanisms of plasma cells is therefore regarded as one of the major factors in pathogenesis and chemoresistance in MM [41].

Major Apoptotic Mechanisms in MM

Apoptosis of myeloma cells is controlled by complex mechanisms that maintain the equilibrium between cellular survival factors and death specific factors. The survival factors (e.g. Bcl-2, NF-κB) lead to long survival of the cells by the blockade of programmed cell death. Death specific factors trigger a cascade of signals leading to the apoptosis of myeloma cells. The tumorigenesis and malignant phenotype is caused by both the loss of proapoptotic signals and the activation of antiapoptotic mechanisms [42-44].

The changes in MM apoptotic mechanisms are often very variable and depend not only on genetic aberrations but also on the interaction between myeloma plasmocytes and the bone marrow microenvironment [7]. In early stages of the disease, the growth of the cells depends on the supporting role of bone marrow, and the stroma itself produces some anti-apoptotic factors. In advanced stages the plasmocytes are often able to regulate the formation of anti-apoptotic mechanisms themselves. Due to the uniqueness of every individual are also the mechanisms of apoptosis and especially of its disruption various. In MM there are several combinations of anti-apoptotic mechanisms of intracellular as well as extracellular origin, and their individual contribution may be different in individual stages of the disease – in early or late phase, in smoldering or aggressive MM [7]. Recently some processes have been described that are common to most myeloma populations.

Fas Induced Apoptosis

One of the major apoptotic mechanisms in plasma cells is the activation of the extrinsic apoptotic pathway through the Fas receptor. Fas receptor or CD95 (Fas/Apo1) is a "death receptor" which belongs to the TNFR family (tumor necrosis factor receptor) [45]. After binding to a specific external cytokine stimulus it changes the conformation of C-terminuses of the receptor molecule – the "death domain" at the inner part of cell membrane and together with adapter molecules causes oligomerisation with cytoplasmatic proteins and forms macromolecular complex DISC (death-inducing signalling complex), which activates caspase 8 and starts the proximal (or initiator, apical) caspase pathway (figure 2) [46]. In the case of Fas induced apoptosis the specific cytokine binding to the receptor is Fas-ligand (FasL), which is a product of T-lymphycytes. The specific adapter molecule bound to death domain of activated Fas receptor is FADD (Fas associated death domain). The whole DISC complex consists of following molecules:

1. Fas ligand activating the Fas death receptor
2. The molecule of Fas death receptor itself with activated death domain
3. Cytoplasm adapter protein FADD
4. Procaspase 8
5. Some other cytoplasm signaling proteins (such as caspase 10, c-FLIP, RIP, Dap3)

Activated caspase 8, the key molecule of the extrinsic apoptotic pathway, subsequently activates effector proteases (caspase 3, 6 and 7) responsible for the effector (executioner) phase of apoptosis [23].

In myeloma cells Fas expression on the surface of cell membrane is usually reduced [23, 45-47]. The reasons for the disruption of apoptosis in MM are, however, not mainly due to quantitative decrease of Fas expression but predominantly due to the alteration of its function. Fas receptor is commonly found on the surface of MM cells, but it is usually altered and less sensitive to extrinsic stimuli than in normal cells [45]. The reasons for diminished sensitivity are the disequilibrium between pro and anti-apoptotic signals both extra and intracellular that influence the function of Fas receptor, such as the secretion of anti-apoptotic factors by the bone marrow microenvironment, adhesion of MM cells to fibronectin, increased expression of bcl-2 and others [45].

Another potential resistance mechanism is the constitutive expression of FasL on myeloma cells. FasL of myeloma plasmocytes binds to the Fas receptor of T-cells, and destroys the T-lymphocytes by their own weaponry, thus allowing the myeloma cells to escape from their immunological control [23].

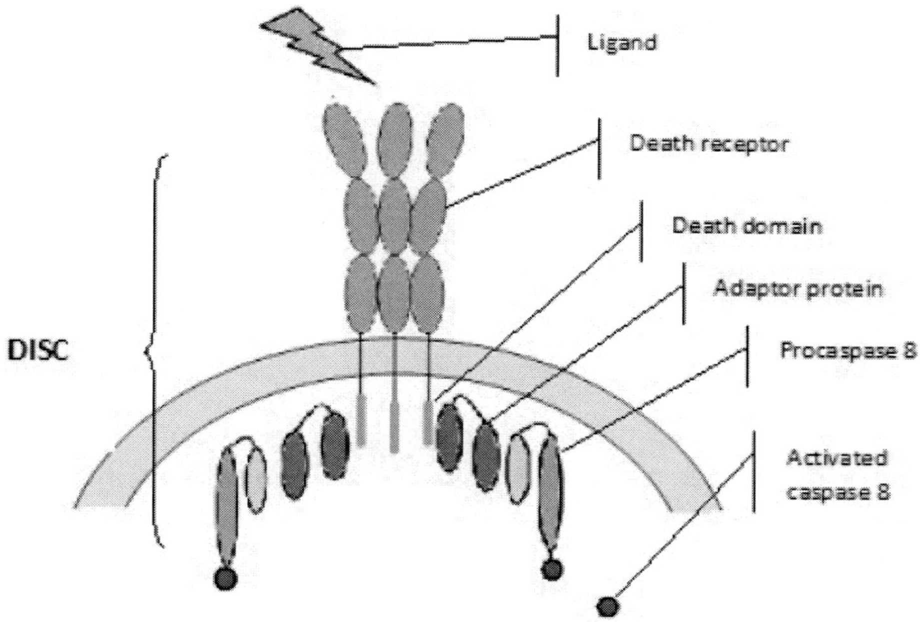

Figure 2. Extrinsic apoptotic pathway and formation of DISC

Binding of specific ligand to „death receptor“ (e.g. Fas, TRAIL) changes the conformation of death domain at the inner part of cell membrane and causes oligomerisation with adaptor protein (FADD, respectivelly TRADD), procaspase 8 and some other signalling proteins. This whole complex DISC (death-inducing signalling complex) activates caspase 8 and starts proximal apoptotic pathway.

CD40 Regulated Apoptosis

One of the known apoptotic regulatory mechanisms in MM is mediated by the surface receptor CD40 [23]. It is another TNFR family receptor and it is activated by ligand CD40L on the surface of T-lymphocytes. Activation of CD40 leads to a series of biological effects. It induces the secretion of IL-6, one of the most powerful growth factor that increases proliferation of plasma cells, expression of adhesion molecules enabling the migration and binding to the bone marrow, induction of VEGF leading to increased angiogenesis, and the overexpression of some other surface molecules including Fas [23].

Although the CD40 molecule may induce apoptosis by increased expression of Fas receptors, its effect in MM is predominantly antiapoptotic [49]. The known mechanisms of apoptosis inhibition and cell cycle promotion by CD40 molecule are the activation of protein kinase Akt by the “secondary messenger” PIP3 (phosphatidyl inositol triphosphate) [23]. Akt proteinkinase inhibits apoptosis by the inhibition of the intrinsic pathway (by stabilization of mitochondrial membrane) and by the activation of NF-κB and inhibition of caspase 9. Cell cycle is induced by the activation of the proteinkinase MAPK, leading to an increased production of transcription factors [23, 48, 49].

TRAIL Induced Apoptosis

TRAIL (TNF-related apoptosis-inducing ligand) is a signaling molecule for DR-4 and DR-5, other receptors of the TNF family. The mechanism of the triggering of an apoptotic cascade is similar as in Fas induced apoptosis [45]. Binding of the ligand activates the death receptor and subsequent start of the extrinsic apoptotic pathway. TRAIL is preferentially bound to MM death receptors and causes their apoptosis [50]. Increased apoptosis of MM plasmocytes is associated with their ability to produce and express their receptor. Sensitivity of plasma cells to TRAIL induced apoptosis correlates with decreased expression of Fas and CD40 and the inactivation of NF-κB [23]. Some of the drugs used for MM treatment act through the activation of TRAIL, for example interferon alpha and beta or arsenic trioxide. [50, 51].

The anti-myeloma effect of TRAIL is in a large part inhibited by the action of osteoprotegerin (OPG), released by osteoblasts [23, 52]. The feedback activation of OPG ligand (OPGL) induces an increased osteoclast differentiation. The TRAIL-OPG interaction leads to a defect in apoptosis as well as to a disruption in the bone marrow microenvironment regulation. In patients with aggressive clone TRAIL is excessively expressed on the cell membrane together with FasL. It has been shown that FasL+/TRAIL+ plasma cells negatively regulate the maturation of erythroblasts and can be one of the key mechanisms of anemia in MM [53]. Recent therapeutic approaches are therefore aimed to development of specific agonists of DR-4 and DR-5 receptors, which would not interfere with OPG but would more effectively activate the apoptotic cascade [54].

Inhibition of Apoptosis by Insulin-Like Growth Factor-1 Receptor

Increased expression of insulin-like growth factor-1 receptor (IGF-1R) has been a frequent finding in MM plasmocytes [55-57]. IGF-1R regulates the transcription and synthesis of proteins, proliferation, migration and the inhibition of apoptosis. Its major ligand is IGF-1 although it might be activated by insulin itself or by IGF-2, usually with a lesser affinity [57]. Binding of the ligand causes dimerisation of IGF-1R followed by the activation of two signaling pathways – MAPK (mitogen activated proteinkinase), leading to the increase of proliferation impulses, or PIP3 (phosphatidyl inositol triphosphate) [55]. The pathway of second messenger PIP3 leads via PDK1 (3-phosphoinositid dependent protein kinase 1) to the activation of Akt protein kinase (also called the protein kinase B) [58]. Akt proteinase blocks apoptosis by several mechanisms. It causes the inhibition of cytochrome-c release from mitochondria by the phosphorylation of proapoptotic protein Bad – the phosphorylation blocks the function of Bad which is responsible for mitochondrial membrane destabilisation. Akt proteinase activates NF-κB by the phosphorylation of IKK (IκB kinase), unbinds NF-κB from its inactive complex with IκB, and directly phosphorylates caspase 9 thus blocking its activation [58]. Moreover, it increases the production of some intracellular antiapoptotic proteins, such as FLIP, survivin, cIAP-2 and XIAP. In MM most of the signaling activates the PIP3 second messenger pathway and not the MAPK, leading to a more intensive antiapoptotic activity [58-60].

Regulation of Apoptosis by Nuclear Factor Kappa B

One of the most intriguing regulatory systems, that has received recent attention, is the ubiquitin-proteasome system. The proteasome is a complex of proteins with protease activity and belongs, together with lysosomes, among the major proteolytic mechanisms of the cell. The proteasome is able to distinguish protein molecules determined for degradation, which are marked by ubiquitinylation – the binding of at least 4 molecules of ubiquitine [61]. With the use of proteasomes the cell regulates protein concentration by degrading excessive and damaged or unfolded proteins. With the exception of molecules intended for degradation, the proteasome specifically recognizes the transcription factor NF-κB (nuclear factor kappa B) and releases it from the inactive complex with its inhibitor I-κB. NF-κB belongs to a family of homo and heterodimer transcription factors that specifically bind to a sequence κB. The inactive complex NF-κB-IκB is commonly found in cytoplasm and is activated by extracellular stimuli (e.g. inflammatory cytokines TNF-α or IL-1). NF-κB is then translocated to the nucleus where it regulates the transcription of genes for several anti-apoptotic proteins, cytokines (IL-6, angiogenic factors), proliferation regulating proteins, and adhesive molecules [62]. NF-κB supports proliferation and blocks apoptosis (especially by the inhibition of caspase 8), and as such can widely facilitate tumor growth and setting up metastases. Inhibition of NF-κB, on the other hand, inhibits proliferation and enables the apoptotic pathway [61, 62].

In MM an increased activation of NF-κB has been found. The former explanation was due to the influence of extracellular stimulating factors such as IL-6. Recently some genetic aberrations have been found that lead to an excessive activity of this factor [63, 64]. One of them is the deletion or mutation of TRAF3, the tumor suppressor gene associated with the inhibition of NF-κB inducing kinase (NIK). If TRAF3 gene is altered, quite a frequent variant found in MM, NIK alters its function and leads to the activation of NF-κB [63]. Some other regulatory gene aberrations that lead to an increased activation of NF-κB are, for example, biallelic loss of CYLD gene and the deletion of BIRC2/BIRC3 genes that code for cIAP1 and cIAP2 [63].

The proliferating and anti-apoptotic activity of NF-κB itself is caused by its translocation to the nucleus and its initiation of transcription pathways. NF-κB moreover regulates the formation of a series of adhesive molecules responsible for the interaction of myeloma cells with the bone marrow microenvironment including intracellular adhesion molecule-1 (ICAM-1), vascular cellular adhesion molecule-1 (VCAM-1), fibronectin, laminin. In this way NF-κB also affects the growth of the tumor and the initiation of new metastases. It also regulates the formation and function of surface proteases (such as matrix metalloproteinases), which are responsible for local invasivity of the tumor [61].

Bcl-2 Family

Most conventional chemotherapeutics used in MM treatment (such as anthracyclines) cause the activation of apoptosis primarily by a mechanism which releases cytochrome-c from the mitochondria. Overexpression of some anti-apoptotic factors that inhibit cytochrome-c release is, therefore, often accompanied by resistance of MM to chemotherapy. Attention has been largely drawn to the Bcl-2 gene family.

Increased levels of Bcl-2 protein are present in majority of MM patients. The gene product of Bcl-2 is a prototype of anti-apoptotic factor that blocks both the extrinsic and especially the intrinsic apoptotic pathway. Excessive production of Bcl-2 likely causes a failure of apoptotic mechanisms and contributes to the lifespan of myeloma cells, increasing the tumor mass even without increased proliferative activity [5].

Another member of the Bcl-2 family, Bcl-xL is often found in relapsing patients and is connected with resistance to chemotherapy. Overexpression of Bcl-xL is linked to IL-6 signaling, and it has been demonstrated that essentially all human primary myelomas express Bcl-xL constitutively [33]. MM patients have also often increased levels of Mcl-1 (myeloid cell factor-1). Suppression of Mcl-1 activity induces apoptosis, whereas high levels lead to an even stronger resistance to cellular death. Down-regulation of Mcl-1 is one known mechanisms of proapoptotic activity of melphalan on sensitive cells [65]. It is quite interesting that increased expression of Bcl-2, Bcl-xL and Mcl-1 is not subject to a frequent genetic aberration like in follicular lymphoma [66]. It is more likely that their regulation is largely under the influence of the bone marrow microenvironment, especially the growth factor IL-6 [67-70].

Interleukin-6

Interleukin-6 (IL-6) is the most important growth factor in MM. Its effects contribute also to the regulation (blockade) of apoptosis. By the activation of STAT3 (signal transducer and activator of transcription 3), it induces the expression of antiapoptotic proteins, especially Bcl-xL and Mcl-1, which are potent antiapoptotic factors belonging to the Bcl-2 family [23, 41, 71]. Although microarray analyses have revealed that the vast majority of IL-6 target genes are controlled through STAT3, different expression of known apoptotic regulators (such as the members of Bcl-2 family) does not sufficiently account for the observed STAT3-mediated survival effect [31]. Some recent studies revealed that microRNAs (especially miR-21) mediating promoter activity is likely the mechanism through which STAT3 may suppress apoptosis of neoplastic cells [31, 72]. IL-6 can block apoptosis using the Akt protein kinase (via the second messenger PIP3), that can effectively lead to the inhibition of apoptosis by the activation of NF-κB and other factors. Reversely, the IL-6 receptor (IL-6R) antagonists that block the stimulation of IL-6 play the role of proapoptotic factors [71].

Role of p53 Mutation, P-Glycoprotein and Other Molecules

Abnormalities of the p53 gene are quite rare in MM, although they are frequently found in relapsing patients, and particularly in plasmocellular leukemia. Disruption of the normal p53 signalling leads to a blockade of apoptosis [23].

P53 protein is regarded as the major receptor of the intrinsic apoptotic pathway. In healthy tissue p53 is activated by irreversible damage to nuclear DNA. In the case of a minor damage, it can catalyse renaturation of DNA, its synthesis and reparation [39]. But, if the changes to the genome exceed its reparation capacity, p53 expression is largely increased leading to extranuclear effects, in the form of a transcription factor [39]. In the cytoplasm, p53 induces the formation of p21 protein (cyclin dependent kinase inhibitor) and PIGs (p53-induced genes), whose products subsequently damage mitochondria by free radicals – ROS (reactive oxygen species). Mitochondria, which are responsible for energetic metabolism of the cell, lose their membrane potential leading to increased mitochondrial membrane permeability with the release of cytochrome c and other proapoptotic molecules (apoptosis inducing factor – AIF, Smac/Diablo protein, other ROSs and calcium ions) with the formation of the apoptosome (figure 3) [73]. Abnormities of p53 cause a defect in function, and cells with damaged or neoplastically changed genomes are able to prolong their survival. P53 is, moreover, responsible for the induction of death receptor translocation onto the cell membrane. This activity is independent from transcription activity, and in the case of p53 disruption it may cause a defect in the extrinsic apoptotic pathway as well [23, 39, 45].

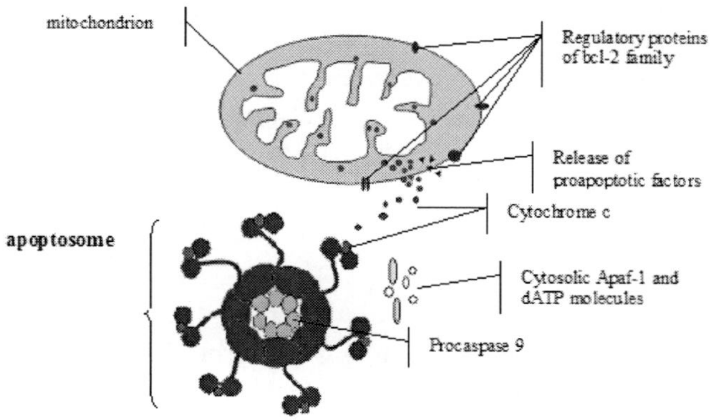

Figure 3. Intrinsic apoptotic pathway and formation of the apoptosome

The intrinsic apoptotic pathway is started by the damage of mitochondrial membrane with subsequent loss of membrane potential and increase of membrane permeability. Members of bcl-2 family have essential regulatory influence on both proapoptotic (Bax, Bad, Bid, Bak, Bok, Diva, Bcl-X_S, Bik, Bim, Hrk, Nix, PUMA, NOXA) and antiapoptotic functions (Bcl-2, Bcl-w, Bcl-X_L, Mcl-1, Nr13, A1/Bfl-1). Increased permeability of mitochondrial membrane enables the release of proapoptotic molecules, especially cytochrome c and some other factors, such as AIF (apoptosis inducing factor), Smac/Diablo protein, free oxygen radicals and calcium ions. Subsequently, by the cooperation of cytochrome c, cytosolic Apaf-1 (apoptotic protease activating factor-1) and dATP (deoxyribonukleotidtrifosfát) is formed the macromolecular complex apoptosome, which is responsible for the activation of procaspase 9 into caspase 9, the initiation molecule of the intrinsic apoptotic pathway.

One of the most important mechanisms of multidrug resistence (MDR) in MM is mediated by the gene for P-glycoprotein (P-gp), which codes a transmembrane protein [23]. Altered P-gp is able to block several heterocyclic compounds including anthracyclines, vinca alkaloids and others. The MRP (multidrug resistance-associated protein) family has similar effects – their overexpression blocks the activity of several cytotoxic drugs. P-gp, MRP and some others are also known as "classical inhibitors of apoptosis".

Proteins called IAPs (inhibitor of apoptosis proteins) can block apoptosis that has already started. The IAPs family consists of several proteins (e.g. c-IAP1, c-IAP2, XIAP, survivin, apollon) that have a common BIR (baculoviral IAP repeat) domain that is able to bind caspases. Their wide range of action is based on their ability to directly bind to activated caspases (especially caspase 3, 7 and 9) and block their activity [74-77]. IAP members can be activated by NF-κB. Altered expression of IAPs may thus affect the sensitivity of MM to some anti-myeloma drugs, especially those which interfere with NF-κB.

Detection Methods Assessment of Proliferative Potential of Myeloma Plasmocytes

In the past, several methods have been established for the assessment of myeloma cell kinetics. Measurement of proliferative potential of myeloma plasmocytes has been an acknowledged method since 1980´s, although the first attempts at the evaluation of the cellular replication ability were conducted even two decades earlier – the so called "mitotic index" [78-83]. Proliferation has been evaluated using different systems that mostly reflect the percentage of cells in a specific phase (usually S-phase) of the cell cycle.

Autoradiography

Based on this characteristic method of detection, the measurement of proliferative potential has been known as the"labeling index". The replicating DNA of proliferating cells was marked or "labeled" by a specific reagent which was then detected and quantified [16, 18, 84]. The very first attempts utilized autoradiography with an incorporated radioactive element, mostly tritiated hydrogen in the thymidine molecule - [^{3}H]TdR LI (tritiated thymidine labeling index, H-3 thymidine labeling index) [18, 84, 85]. Experimentally other elements were also used, such as radioactive carbon [^{14}C]. The technique of [^{3}H] thymidine incorporation required, however, specialized laboratories for dealing with radioactivity. Moreover, the assessment was time consuming including several days for material preparation. Therefore, it did not find a wider use in clinical practice.

Bromdeoxyuridine and Flow Cytometry

Newer methods of detection tried to avoid radioactive materials. One of the most important steps was the introduction of 5-bromo-2-deoxyuridine (BrdUrd LI - bromdeoxyuridine labeling index) with immunofluorescent or FACS (fluorescence-activated cell sorting) detection of specific monoclonal antibody against bromdeoxyuridine [85-89]. The method was faster than autoradiography (approximately 7 hours) with similar results, and in particular much easier. It had a great advantage in preservation of cellular morphology and immunological features as it did not necessarily denature the DNA like autoradiography [88]. However, in the case of a smaller number of plasma cells in a sample it had only a limited sensitivity. Therefore several departments tried to use flow cytometry which had already proved its relevance in cell cycle evaluation in other hematological malignancies like acute and chronic leukemias and some non-hodgkin lymphomas [90-93].

The first studies, however, did not confirm the prognostic relevance of the evaluation of the plasma cells S-phase using flow-cytometry [94]. Unlike the other hematological malignancies, in MM the bone marrow (BM) is usually not completely embedded by pathological elements but instead consists of a mixture of normal and tumor cells in a different ratio. In leukemias or lymphomas the BM is mostly packed with the tumor, whereas MM cells can be present in focuses and in different distributions in histological samples. The previous methods did not meet such issue as they were evaluated by experienced technicians who unambiguously recognized plasma cells from the other population. The newer techniques based on cell sorting, therefore, had to be designed in two steps (double staining). The first step identified the plasma cells, usually using specific characteristics, such as cIg [94] or surface markers CD38 [95] or CD138 [96]. The next step included labeling of cellular DNA with bromdeoxyuridine, propidium iodide or other stains [97].

Propidium-Iodide Staining

Together with flow-cytometry evaluation of proliferative potential, newer staining methods emerged that were capable of better cell cycle evaluation. One of the most used has been propidium iodide, which is a fluorescent intercalating agent that binds between the bases of double-stranded DNA (intercalates) and enhances its fluorescence 20-30 times with excitation maximum shift of 30-40 nm [97]. Because of these effects it is easily detectable by accessible methods, such as fluorescent microscopy or flow cytometry. Using an appropriate software, and with the help of mathematically defined DNA histogram, it is possible to display the percentage of cells in G1, S and G2/M phase. Detection of S-phase is similar as in the case of BrdUrd, with a double staining technique. Myeloma elements are identified using a monoclonal antibody (specific monoclonal antibody anti CD138) and S phase detected by propidium iodide stain [97]. The results are similar and significant as in the [^{3}H]TdR LI and BrdUrd technique, still with an easier method and a faster and more precise evaluation [98].

Other Detection Techniques

Recently several different methods of detection have been established, that have a relation to growth characteristics of the tumor population. Some of the well-known methods are: the "triple staining" which differentiates also immature primitive plasma cells [99, 100], detection of nuclear antigen Ki-67 [101-103], cyclin D1 detection [23], immunohistochemical analysis of PCNA (proliferating cell nuclear antigen) [104, 105], detection of AgNORs (argyrophillic proteins associated with the nucleolar organizer regions) in histological samples [106], monitoring of serum thymidine kinase [107], and some others [39, 108-110]. The advantage of micromolecular techniques reposes upon the precise detection of intracellular processes, histological analyses are able to reflect the distribution of proliferating cells and BM elements, and are capable even for older fixed samples. Indirect measurement of serum levels of thymidinekinase is fast and non-invasive. It is always necessary to decide about the specific utilization of each method as they detect slightly different aspects of proliferation and do not always correlate with each other.

Expression of Ki-67

One of the newest detection methods in the evaluation of MM proliferation is the assessment of Ki-67. Ki-67 is a nuclear antigen present in all cells that are in an active cell cycle, in G1, S, G2 and M – phase, with gradual increase from G1 phase (in which it has lowest levels) to G2 and M phase with highest levels of the antigen [102]. Unlike most techniques that assess only the S-phase of cell cycle with relatively low representation of proliferating cells (median from 0.1 – 3.0%), Ki-67 reflects the percentage of all cells except of G_0 and initial G_1 phase with 5-10 fold higher values of the index (median 1 – 5%) [102]. A regression between Ki-67 and bromdeoxyuridine proliferative index was found enabling "conversion" of the values from one index to another [103]. The real significance of this parameter is, however, a bit attenuated by the fact that it does not directly measure the proliferative but rather "cycling" potential of plasma cells.

Detection of Proliferation Using Nuclear Antigen PCNA

PCNA (proliferating cell nuclear antigen – co-factor of deltaDNA dependent polymerase) is a 36kDa nuclear protein with varied percentual representation during proliferation. It is necessary for DNA replication and participates in DNA repair and RNA transcription [104]. The concentration of PCNA increases from G1 phase with a peak in S-phase followed by a decrease in G2/M phase [105]. It can be assessed using conventional immunohistochemical techniques with a specific anti-PCNA monoclonal antibody. The results are similar to the Ki-67 technique, up to now more within experimental assessments, without a wider clinical utilization. Some correlation was found between PCNA values and cell morphology with a higher percentage of proliferating cells in immature cells and the highest (nearly 100%) levels in plasmoblastic MM and plasmocelular leukemia [104, 105].

PCNA is, however, not able to distinguish between proliferation in tumor and inflammatory cells, and its sensitivity is bound by the infiltration of bone marrow by tumor elements.

Cyclin D1

Normal hematopoetic cells, including normal lymphycytes and plasma cells, express predominantly cyclin D2 with a lower level of cyclin D3, but they usually do not express cyclin D1 [39]. MM on the other hand has an evident increase in D1 cyclin with a low D2 cyclin level. Cyclin D1 plays a crucial role in the control of the cell cycle from G1 to S phase. Its overexpression leads to an increased proliferation rate. Detection of D1 cyclin is a promising method, evaluating proliferative potential in adherence to a specific genetic aberration - t(11,14) [39]. Interestingly, increased cyclin D1 expression itself has not been associated with a marked increase in plasmocyte proliferation. D cyclins are highly active functionally, which was confirmed by the ability of cyclin D3 to compensate for the cyclin D2 activity loss in active lymphocytes [39]. Therefore, it is possible that increased expression of cyclin D1, without adequate increase of cyclin dependent kinases CDK4 and CDK6, is not sufficient for the increase of myeloma cell proliferation [23].

Serum Thymidinekinase

The cell cycle is largely influenced by enzymatic factors that are necessary for correct regulation of other intracellular processes. Some of the factors that take part in these processes encompass the whole cell cycle, where others are specific for only some parts of it. Synthesis of DNA in S-phase is strictly connected to enzymes such as thymidinekinase, DNA-polymerase, dihydropholatereductase or ribonucleotide-reductase [107]. Evaluation of serum levels of thymidinekinase (TK) has therefore become another possibility of indirect assessment of proliferative potential. TK is an enzyme catalysing phosphorylation of thymine to deoxythymidinemonophosphate. Higher level of TK means a more active cell population with a worse prognosis. On the other hand the assessment of TK correlates very poorly with other prognostic factors. The reason for this very low specificity of the assessment is because TK is not strictly tumor-bound, and it is often increased in other neoplastic and benign diseases (herpes simplex infection, CMV, EBV, viral hepatitis, impairment of B12 and folic acid metabolism) and even in some physiological states accompanied by increased tissue proliferation (although the values scarcely exceed normal laboratory range). Moreover, increased TK levels are found only in a third of patients with increased proliferating potential [107].

Proliferative Potential Assessment Using AgNORs

The reason for the introduction of AgNORs (argyrophillic proteins associated with the nucleolar organizer regions) was because the common measurement of proliferative potential could not be applied on routinely fixed BM biopsies samples [106]. After staining with silver nitrate and incubation with methyl green, even older samples can be used for proliferation detection using this technique. Argyrophillic proteins associated with the nucleolar organizer regions are regarded as parameters of DNA transcriptional activity or the DNA transcriptional potential. They correlate with cell proliferating and duplicating activity, and they have a relation to the prognosis of MM [106]. The disadvantage is in the manual evaluation based on subjective examination by experienced technicians, and also in the quality of histological samples in which a low percentage of tumor cells diminishes both sensitivity and specificity of the method. On the other hand, even "very old" histological samples are capable of AgNORs assessment enabling thus the evaluation of patients who were previously not examined.

Interleukin-6

Interleukin-6 (IL-6) has already been reported as the most important growth factor of MM plasmocytes. Measurement of its serum levels can also indirectly indicate the proliferative activity of myeloma plasmocytes. IL-6 is a pleiotropic, multifunctional cytokine playing roles in different physiological processes such as bone metabolism, acute phase reactions, hematopoesis and B-cell differentiation [7, 26]. In contrast, it has been shown to be a potent mitogen and survival factor for myeloma cells and cell lines, and it plays a crucial role in MM pathogenesis [111]. It is strongly expressed by the bone marrow microenvironment, and its high levels in serum indicate poor prognosis. Clinical studies have confirmed the relation between IL-6 and clinical activity of the disease [26, 29, 30, 112]. Because of its wide expression within pathophysiological as well as nespecific, infectious or inflammatory processes, IL-6 is at present regarded as a relatively low sensitive factor for the differentiation of prognostic groups. As a parameter with a relationship to stroma, the levels of IL-6 are non-specific and reflect the activity of bone marrow rather than MM itself. Moreover, certain interpretation issues come up due to significant differences in IL-6 measurements using different techniques. Very sensitive methods such as the bioassay confirmed the relation between IL-6 and the prognosis of MM, whereas less sensitive techniques (e.g. RIA and EIA) did not confirm this relationship [27, 29, 30].

Soluble IL-6 Receptor and Other Cytokines

Interleukin-6 is bound to a specific membrane receptor (IL-6R) and this complex (IL-6/IL-6R) induces the dimerisation of the membrane transduction glycoprotein gp130 [113]. Intracellular signaling pathway initiated by gp130 activates Janus tyrosine kinases (JAK) JAK1, JAK2 and Tyk2. These tyrosine kinases subsequently initiate several signaling cascades that lead to the activation of STAT (signal transducer and activator) which blocks apoptosis, and MAPK (Ras/mitogen-activated protein kinase) that induces proliferation [113]. *In vitro*, sIL-6R potentiates the growth effect of IL-6 on myeloma cells. First, it links to IL-6, and then forms a complex with the gp130 molecule on the surface of myeloma cells.

It activates the tyrosine kinase that initiates proliferation of plasma cells. Measurement of sIL-6R demonstrated a relationship to MM prognosis which is more significant than in the case of IL-6 [29, 30]. However, it has only a limited specificity and is widely influenced by the activity of other cytokines.

Other IL-6 related cytokines that may have an impact on MM pathogenesis include: interleukin-11 (IL-11), leukemia inhibitory factor (LIF), IL-2 as a potential factor stabilizing proliferation, oncostatin M (OSM) and ciliary neurotrophic factor (CNTF) [114, 115]. There exist other cytokines that have a certain impact on the induction of proliferation and blockade of apoptosis in MM plasmocytes and that act outside the glycoprotein gp130 pathway, such as IL-10, IL-15, insulin-like growth factor-1 and others. Their assessment has not, however, become a routine part of MM diagnostics [39].

Detection of Apoptosis of Myeloma Plasmocytes

Assessment of apoptosis in myeloma plasmocytes is relatively difficult. Several factors may influence intracellular processes and especially the loss of contact with the natural microenvironment can lead to the initiation of the apoptotic and necrotic cascade. Therefore it is vital to evaluate apoptosis soon after the material is withdrawn or to use an adequate preserving agent to block the initiation of the apoptotic cascade by contact with the outer environment [116]. Moreover, it is necessary to clearly distinguish living cells from apoptotic and primarily necrotic cells.

Microscopy

One easy method is the microscopic evaluation of characteristic morphologic features of apoptosis using light or electron microscopy [116]. After staining of the samples (eg. using May- Grünenwald-Giemsa stain, MGG) the cells are separated into groups of vital, apoptotic or necrotic cells. Apoptotic cells have a characteristic morphology – condensation of chromatin and cytoplasm (apoptotic cells), cytoplasmatic fragments with and/or without the presence of condensed chromatin (apoptotic bodies), and intra or extracellular fragments of chromatin (micronuclei). A limitation is the total number of evaluated cells (usually only 200-500) and the requirement of an experienced morphologist. Electron microscopy of DNA fragmentation is, however, regarded as one of the most reliable methods.

Gel Electrophoresis

Very fast and relatively inexpensive is the assessment of DNA fragments using gel electrophoresis [116]. Formation of oligonucleosomal "ladder fragments" by specific endonucleases is a characteristic feature of apoptotic cells. These oligonucleosomal fragments of 180-200 pairs of bases (180-200 pb) can be detected using conventional gel electrophoresis. The technique is easy and fast. Nevertheless, it loses its specificity in the presence of necrotic cells. In addition, recent findings revealed that the formation of low-molecular ladder fragments as a late sign of apoptosis is forerun by the cleavage of DNA into bigger fragments (about 300 pb – 50 kpb), and in some cell types the cleavage stops at this moment and does not continue [116]. These fragments are not detectable using conventional techniques, but only by pulse electrophoresis with a periodically changing electrical field.

DNA Staining

The most used methods for the detection of apoptosis are based on DNA staining [117, 118]. Even a small percentage of apoptotic cells can be detected by special staining of nucleic acids or DNA breaks.

Among the techniques which stain nuclear DNA belongs 7AAD (7-amino actinomycine-D). 7AAD is a fluorescent agent which detects cytosine and guanine bases. Using FACS (fluorescence-activated cell sorting), it is possible to sort out cells with different intensities of fluorescence. Vital cells are usually negative for the stain (no stain – 7AAD did not penetrate nuclear membrane to DNA), apoptotic cells have a dim stain (certain increase of membrane permeability, yet with maintained integrity causes limited penetration of 7AAD), and late apoptotic/necrotic cells are usually with clear fluorescence (loss of membrane integrity) [119].

Immunohistochemical methods are often used for the detection of DNA-breaks including: TUNEL, ISNTA and ISEL [117]. Before the apoptotic cell forms definite fragments of DNA, minor morphological changes of DNA can be observed in the form of DNA breaks. TUNEL (terminal deoxynucleotidyl transferase [TdT]-mediated desoxyuridinetriphosphate [dUTP] - biotin nick end-labeling), is based on the detection of structural alterations of DNA (DNA breaks) in histological tissue samples using biotin-dUTP. This technique stains the cells in the beginning and in the middle part of apoptosis, and it detects the necrotic or damaged cells as well. DNA breaks, however, occur also in cells undergoing DNA reparation, during electrocoagulation, autolysis, and even during fixation and paraffin embedding, which might artificially increase the values of the apoptotic index. The avantage of TUNEL is in long-term preservation and the possibility to compare individual samples. On the other hand, fragility of cells during fixation, low sensitivity and time consumption during the assessment make this method inconvenient for fast and routine assessment in clinical practice. Detection of apoptosis using ISNTA (in situ nick translation assay) is similar to the previous TUNEL method except for the detection of late phase apoptosis [117]. DNA-polymerase synthesizes DNA where breaks occur. These newly synthesized segments are stained by biotynylated dUTP. The more breaks in the DNA (the more is the nucleus damaged and the cell in later phase of apoptosis), the more intensively the cell will stain with dUTP. ISEL (in situ end-labeling) also uses the detection of DNA breaks. At first, biotynylated nucleotides are incorporated into the breaks with subsequent specific staining (DAB) and final apoptotic evaluation.

Protease Activity Detection and Mitochondrial Stains

Very sensitive methods assessing apoptosis are based on the detection of caspases, either by the evaluation of amino acid sequences specific for individual caspases or, more recently, directly by specific monoclonal antibody or non-fluorescent substrates which are downgraded by the caspase to fluorescent products [74-77]. Evaluation of specific caspases helps to predict which of the apoptotic pathways was initiated and how the process of apoptosis is being regulated in different conditions.

Typical feature of the internal apoptotic pathway is the disruption of the mitochondrial membrane by the formation of pores and by the change in redox potential, followed by the leak of cytochrome-c into the cytoplasm. These processes can be used for apoptotic detection – either by stains that normally do not penetrate the impermeable mitochondrial membrane (only after its disruption), or by specific detection of molecules expressed on the mitochondrial surface only during apoptosis (e.g. Apo2,7 specifically detects 38kd mitochondrial membrane antigen 7A6) [116]. Other possibilities include the detection of a change in the mitochondrial membrane potential - „potential-dependent spectral shift“, or directly assessing the leak of cytochrome-c.

Experimentaly it is possible to measure apoptosis using increased production of ROS, a change in ion concentrations (apoptosis causes change in pH, Na^+, K^+ and Ca^{2+} concentration), ATP/ADP ratio, the analysis of forward and side scatter in flow cytometer and some others.

Annexin-V Evaluation

In our department we have confirmed the significance of apoptotic detection using Annexin-V and flow cytometry [120, 121]. Annexin-V is a calcium dependent protein that preferentially binds to negatively charged phospholipids such as phosphatidylserine. Phosphadidylserine in vital cells is found only on the intracellular side of the cell membrane. In the case of apoptosis, it is exposed at the cell surface and may be bound to annexin-V, which can be visualized by several fluorescence stains (FITC fluorescein isothiocyanate, Alexa488, Cy3 or PE phycoerythrin) [120].

For distinguishing between apoptotic and necrotic cells it is possible to use propidium iodide which stains intracellular DNA in late phases of apoptosis when the cell membrane is disrupted and fully permeable to its molecule [122].

The advantage of this method is in fast, accessible and an inexpensive evaluation of apoptosis both of extrinsic or intrinsic origin, without a need for specialized assessment of different cytokines or other molecules, and it provides an easy distinction of apoptotic and necrotic cells. On the other hand, even this technique requires standardized extraction of the sample with early assessment, as many environmental factors may affect the final result.

Measurement of Proliferative and Apoptotic Indices and Their Clinical Application

The possibility of measuring and quantifying the growth potential of myeloma cells meant a significant advance in the knowledge of myeloma population kinetics, and contributed to a better understanding of biological properties of myeloma plasmocytes. The pivotal parameter of tumor dynamics is the speed of its replication represented by the proliferative index. The first experience with the proliferative index has soon placed the parameter among significant factors in MM, not only in experimental medicine but also in clinical practice. The aim of surveys in MM was predominantly to assess two dominant aspects, the relationship of the proliferative index to MM prognosis [15, 16, 123], and the comparison of PI in overt MM and in MGUS [18, 85, 124].

Although myeloma is regarded as a predominantly accumulative disease, only a very few clinically oriented studies reported on apoptosis in MM. The reason is likely due to its fragility and possible influence of several internal as well as external effects. Although there are several laboratory methods enabling the analysis of cell death, up to now there has not been a generally accepted and easily accessible method for routine assessment of apoptosis in myeloma plasmocytes [20, 21, 121], and most of the published studies dealing with MM apoptosis are based on *in vitro* observations or animal models.

Prognostic Significance of Proliferative and Apoptotic Index

Clinically oriented studies demonstrated a strong predictive significance of PI measurement, where high (or better higher) values of the proliferative index at the time of MM diagnosis together with vast tumor mass sorted out a group with a very poor prognosis and short median of survival [125]. Several studies have shown that the evaluation of proliferative potential of myeloma cells is a strong and independent prognostic factor of overall survival [15-22]. Unlike other parameters that usually reflect the impact of tumor expansion on the organism, the proliferative index is a specific measure of the tumor´s aggressiveness [21]. Concordant results of these studies and multivariation analyses helped to develop newer and easier methods of PI detection, and lead to a more intensive view of molecular biology within myeloma populations. Comparison to plasma cell morphology (as one of the pivotal prognostic factors in the past) found significantly lower values of PI in differentiated, "mature" cells than in "intermediate" or undifferentiated, "immature" cells [126]. Correlation with the maturation of plasma cells was then confirmed by Joshua et al, who found significantly higher values of PI in primitive plasmoblastic cells characterized by immunophenotyping with the presence of markers CD38, CD45, VLA5 and CD56, than in the whole MM population [99]. Analyses have repeatedly confirmed the independence of PI from β2M [15, 16, 86, 126]. Both the factors, although being very potent prognosticators, reflect totally different features of myeloma population. Proliferative index expresses the kinetic aggressiveness of tumor cells whereas β2M is a static indicator of tumor mass and renal functions.

Most of the studies, however, analyzed patients treated only with conventional chemotherapy. With the introduction of high dose chemotherapy with support of autologous stem cell transplantation (HD-ASCT), and particularly the novel agents with biological mechanism of action (such as thalidomide, bortezomib), many "classical" prognostic factors lost their significance. The results from our study hold on to the previous findings and present up-to-date evaluation of proliferation and apoptosis in the era of new biological based treatment. In a cohort of more than 200 patients incapable for HD-ASCT we have found that the prognostic significance of PI loses its predictive potential with time. The curves of overall survival had a different course in the first 35 months, however, after 40 months they merged, and the prognosis was the same in patients with high or low values of PI (figure 4). The reason for the loss of prognostic significance was traced in the inclusion of patients treated in their second or third relapse/progression also with novel drugs, thalidomide and/or bortezomib.

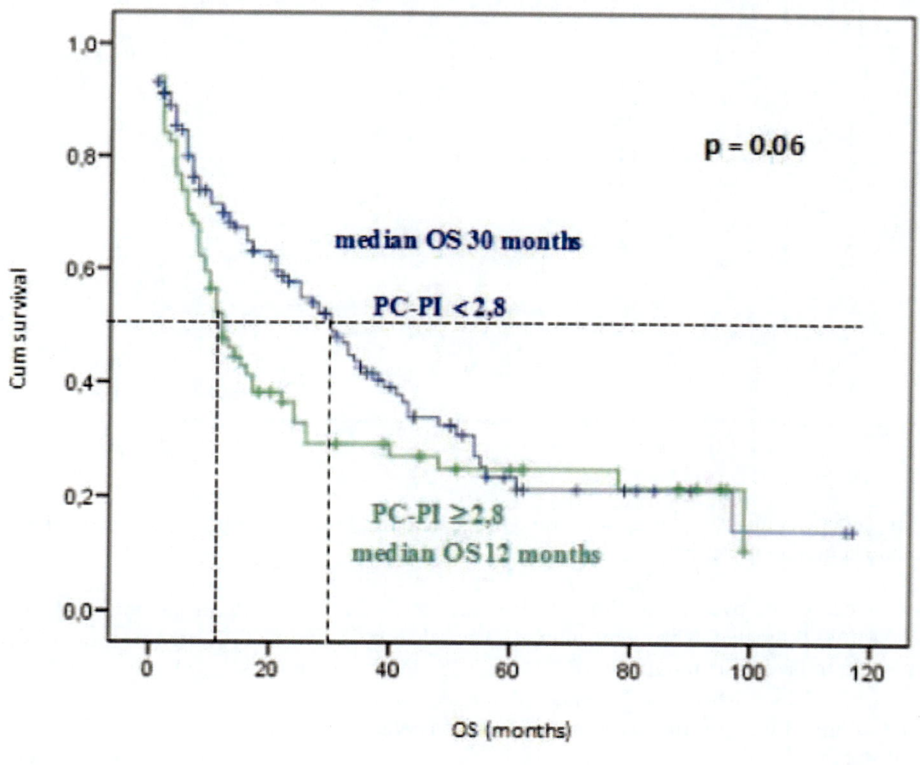

Figure 4. Overall survival in multiple myeloma patients according to proliferative index

Kaplan-Meier curves show a difference in the overall survival in multiple myeloma (MM) patients treated with conventional and biological therapy (n=217). Patients with high PC-PI ≥ 2.8% have worse prognosis (M = 12 months) than patients with low value of PC-PI < 2.8% (M = 30 months), with borderline significance (log rank test p = 0,06). Merging of both curves after 40 months is very likely due to the effect of new drugs with biological effect (thalidomide and bortezomib).

PC-PI = propidium iodide (proliferative) index of plasma cells.

OS = overall survival.

After separating the whole cohort according to their treatment, there was still a significant difference in OS in patients treated with conventional chemotherapy only (figure 5) whereas in the group treated also with thalidomide and/or bortezomib there was no difference and the curves had a similar course, moreover, with better OS (figure 6).

Similar results were observed in patients treated with HD-ASCT. Rare observation from previous studies have already assessed proliferative index in patients treated by HD-ASCT. In the study of Boccadoro et al, patients with unfavorable prognosis (high values of PI) profited from HD-ASCT, whereas in patients with low PI, there was no significant difference according to the therapeutical approach [127]. Moreover, HD-ASCT suppressed the prognostic potential of PI in patients treated by HD-ASCT.

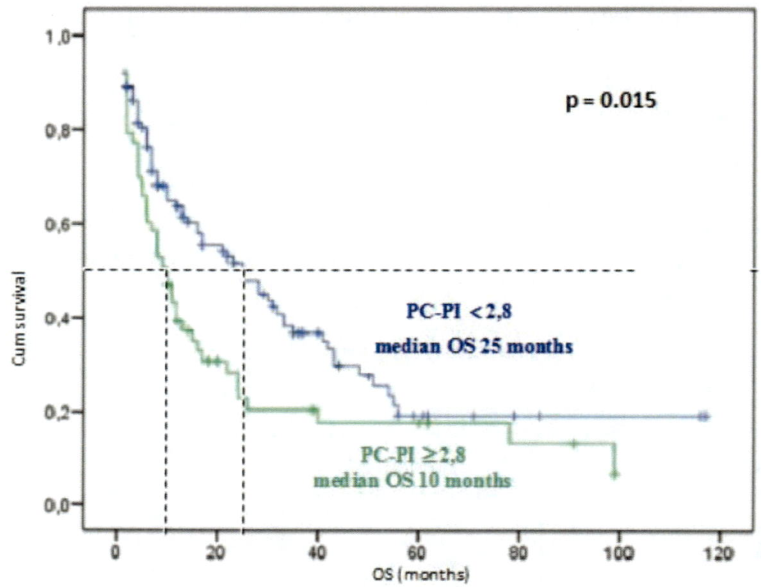

Figure 5. Prognostic significance of proliferative index in multiple myeloma patients treated with conventional chemotherapy only

Kaplan-Meier curves of overall survival present, that the value of PC-PI in patients with multiple myeloma (MM) treated with conventional chemotherapy only (n=167) significantly separate a group with unfavorable prognosis (PC-PI ≥ 2,8%, M = 10 months), and a group with better prognosis (PC-PI < 2,8% M = 25 months) , log rank test p = 0,015.

PC-PI = propidium iodide (proliferative) index of plasma cells.

OS = overall survival.

In the study of Gertz there was no significant difference between the time to progression (TTP) in transplanted patients divided according to low or high levels of PI [128]. In his study, however, the PI was assessed in the persisting circulating cells in the graft, i.e. in already treated patients. Rajkumar and Winkler on the other hand found maintained significance of PI in patients treated by HD-ASCT, unlike other prognostic factors such as the cytogenetic profile and β_2M levels [129, 130].

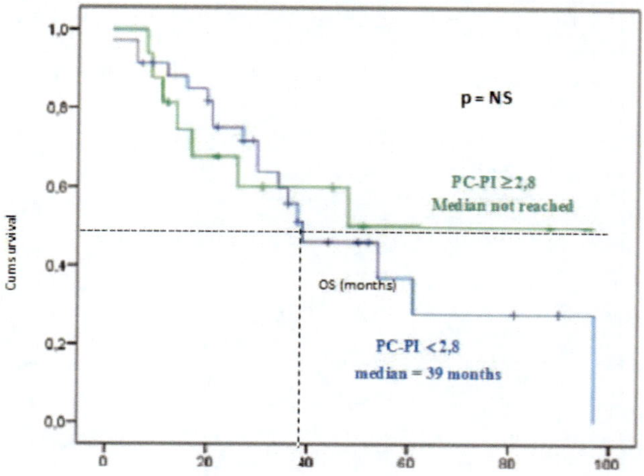

Figure 6. Prognostic significance of proliferative index in multiple myeloma patients treated with biological therapy

In multiple myeloma patients (n=50) treated within the course of the disease with novel biological therapies (thalidomide, bortezomib), there is no significant difference in the Kaplan-Meier overall survival curves, log rank test p = 0,677, suggesting that novel drugs overcome the prognostic significance of PC-PI. The overall survival is prolonged in both groups, median > 39 months.

PC-PI = propidium iodide (proliferative) index of plasma cells.

NS = statistically non-significant value.

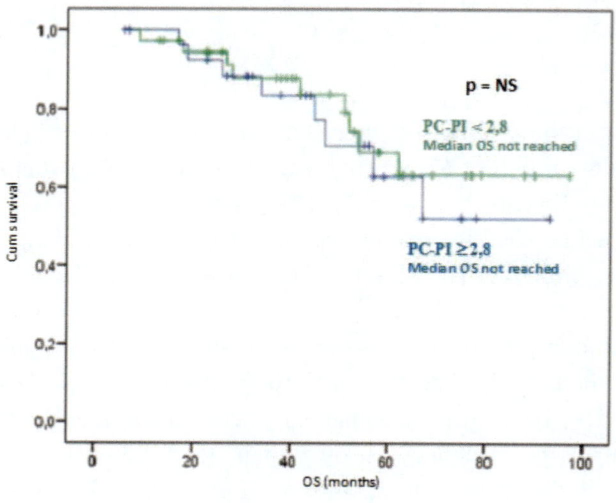

Figure 7. Prognostic significance of proliferative index in multiple myeloma patients treated with high-dosed chemotherapy with support of autologous stem cell transplantation

In the group of patients with multiple myeloma (MM) treated using high-dosed chemotherapy with support of autologous stem cell transplantation (n=67) there was no significant difference in the curves of overall survival (OS) according to Kaplan-Meier. Both the groups of patients with high proliferative index PC-PI ≥ 2.8% (n = 42) and patients low proliferative index PC-PI < 2,8% (n = 25) have similar prognosis with median OS > 80 months, log rank test p = 0.388.

PC-PI = propidium iodide (proliferative) index of plasma cells. NS = statistically non-significant value.

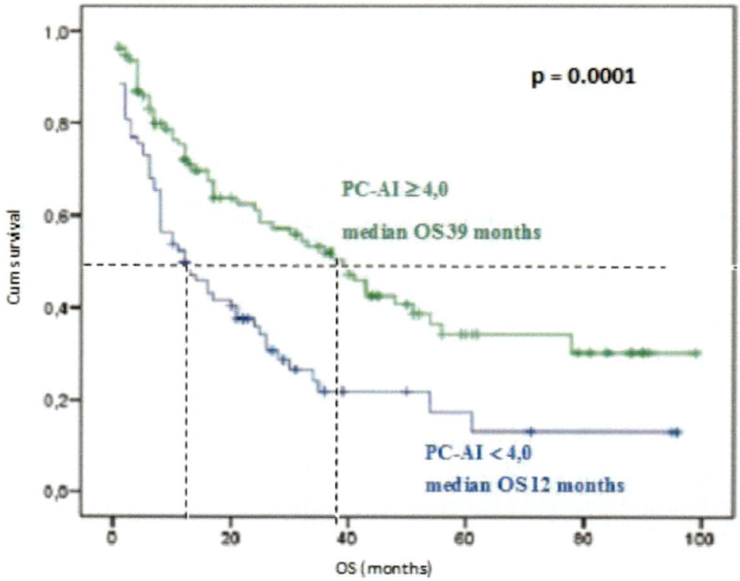

Figure 8. Overall survival in multiple myeloma patients according to apoptotic index

Patients with newly diagnosed multiple myeloma (n=189) treated by conventional chemotherapy and/or with the use of novel biological drugs (thalidomide, bortezomib) can be divided according to the levels of PC-AI into a group with unfavorable prognosis with PC-AI < 4.0% (M = 12 months) and a group with better prognosis, PC-AI ≥ 4.0% (M = 39 months), as shown on the Kaplan-Meier curves of overall survival (log rank test p = 0.0001).
PC-AI = annexin-V (apoptotic) index of plasma cells.
OS = overall survival.

Our results support the findings of Boccadoro and Gertz with PI being overcome by the HD-ASCT therapy. In a group of 67 patients undergoing HD-ASCT there was no significant difference in OS according to PI (figure 7). Due to a prolonged survival over 80 months, none of the groups had reached the median yet, but the curve course together with statistical estimation imply the strong effect of HD-ASCT even on proliferation characteristics of myeloma cells.

With the use of our previous experience with the propidium-iodide index, we have adopted a similar method for the detection of apoptosis, using annexin-V and flow cytometry [22, 120-122]. Analysis of a cohort of 190 patients inconvenient for HD-ASCT confirmed the presumption that myeloma plasmocytes owe their long survival, except of cell cycle dysregulation, also to the defect of apoptosis. High levels of apoptotic index clearly distinguished patients with favorable prognosis from patients with low apoptotic index and poor prognosis (figure 8). Low apoptotic levels thus suggest the accumulation of highly anaplastic population of tumor cells with resistance to conventional chemotherapy. The difference in OS was observed not only in the whole group but also in patients treated with conventional chemotherapy only (figure 9), and in patients treated with novel biological drugs, thalidomide and bortezomib (figure 10). In the group of 67 patients undergoing HD-ASCT there was a certain trend prognostically favoring patients with higher apoptotic levels.

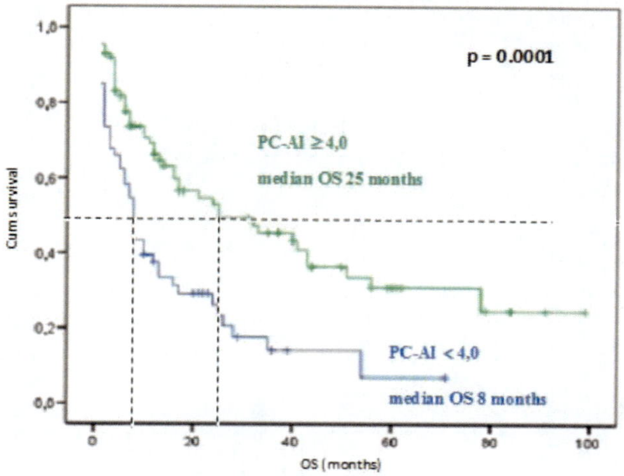

Figure 9. Prognostic significance of apoptotic index in multiple myeloma patients treated with conventional chemotherapy only

The values of PC-AI in multiple myeloma patients treated only with conventional chemotherapy (n=139) significantly separate a group of patients with unfavorable prognosis with low PC-AI < 4.5% (M = 8 months), and a group of patients with better prognosis, PC-AI ≥ 4.5% (M = 25 months). The graph shows the Kaplan-Meier analysis of overall survival, log rank p = 0.02.

PC-AI = annexin-V (apoptotic) index of plasma cells.

OS = overall survival.

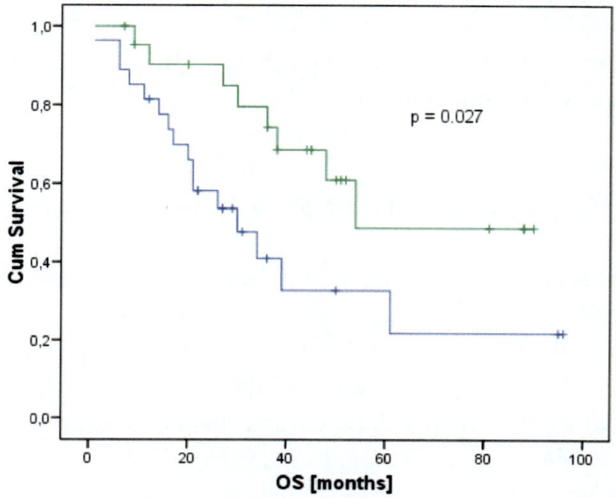

Figure 10. Prognostic significance of apoptotic index in multiple myeloma patients treated with biological drugs

Apoptotic index in multiple myeloma patients (n=50) treated in the course of the disease with novel biological drugs (thalidomide and bortezomib) divides the whole cohort into a group of poor prognosis with PC-AI < 4.5% (M = 30 months), and a group with good prognosis, PC-AI ≥ 4.5% (M = 54 months), as shown on Kaplan-Meier curves of overall survival, log rank test p = 0.027.

PC-AI = annexin-V (apoptotic) index of plasma cells.

OS = overall survival.

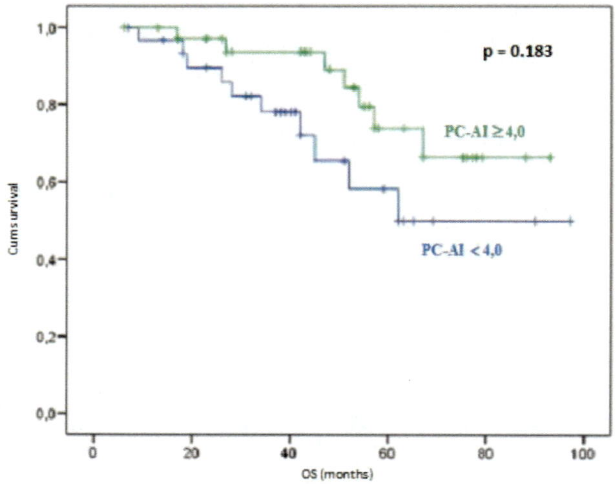

Figure 11. Prognostic significance of apoptotic index in multiple myeloma patients treated by high-dosed chemotherapy with support of autologous stem cell transplantation

Kaplan-Meier curves according to the values of PC-AI in a group of patients with multiple myeloma (n = 67) treated by high-dosed chemotherapy with support of autologous stem cell transplantation (HD-ASCT). Presented results show a trend favoring patients with high apoptosis PC-AI ≥ 4.0% (n = 39) in contrast to patients with low apoptosis PC-AI < 4.0% (n = 28). Due to a prolonged survival with OS > 80 months (not reaching median OS in any of the groups), the result is preliminary and not statistically significant, p = 0.183. PC-AI = annexin-V (apoptotic) index of plasma cells. OS = overall survival.

In just a short interval of observation, not reaching the medians of OS (over 80 months), the result was not statistically significant (figure 11).

Longitudinal Measurement of Proliferation and Apoptosis

Unlike most prognostic factors that are used in MM at the time of diagnosis, proliferative and apoptotic indices are regarded as kinetic parameters that may vary during the course of the disease. Because of their kinetic potential they are able to reflect changes in myeloma clone and to estimate the actual aggressiveness of the tumor. Previous studies have already confirmed the difference between proliferation and apoptosis in patients with active and stable/remission phase MM [18, 20, 85, 121, 131]. High values of PI together with low apoptotic index are very coherent indicators of the disease activity and the loss of stable/plateau phase [15, 16, 22, 84, 99, 123, 132]. Respectively, low proliferation and high apoptosis of myeloma cells indirectly indicate stability of the disease. Rajkumar describes higher proliferation together with increased angiogenesis and the amount of circulating plasma cells as factors increasing the progression risk in patients with asymptomatic myeloma [133]. The study of Steensma et al. revealed that measurement of PI in stable MM can sort out a group of patients with increased values of PI who have a shorter time to progression (about 8 months) in comparison with patients with low values of PI (stable phase was maintained for 39 months) [134].

Our study of 310 patients treated by conventional chemotherapy or HD-ASCT questioned the outcome of longitudinal measurement of both proliferation and apoptosis within the course of MM. We found that patients reaching at least partial remission had significantly decreased levels of PI together with increased apoptosis. Patients with resistant disease, on the other hand, maintained high proliferative index together with low apoptosis (figure 12). The results were the same with similar absolute values of both indices regardless of the treatment used (i.e. the conventional therapy or HD-ASCT) and even regardless of treatment line (i.e. patients after frontline therapy had similar results as patients after treatment of progressions/relapses, data not shown). The relationship is even clearer when evaluated according to the McNemara test of symmetry (figures 13-16).

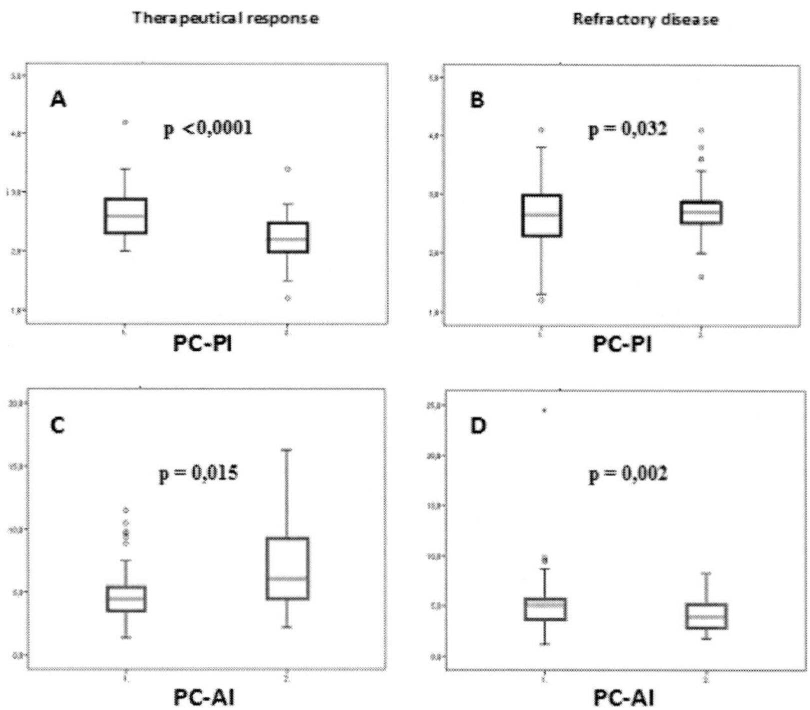

Figure 12. Comparison of proliferative and apoptotic indices in multiple myeloma patients with respect to treatment response

Patients with active multiple myeloma (at the time of diagnosis or progression/relapse) have different behavior of both proliferative and apoptotic indices with respect to the effect of therapy. In the group reaching therapeutical response (at least PR according to IMWG criteria) there is simultaneous decrease in proliferation (A, median PC-PI 2.6 vs 2.2) together with an increase of apoptosis (C, median PC-AI 4.5 vs 6.05). Non-responders (patients not reaching PR according to IMWG criteria) maintained high levels of proliferation (B) even with a mild increase (median PC-PI 2.6 vs 2.7), together with stable or decreasing apoptosis (D, median PC-AI 5.05 vs 3.9).

PC-PI = propidium iodide (proliferative) index of plasma cells.

PC-AI = annexin-V (apoptotic) index of plasma cells.

PR = partial remission.

Patients who reached remission displayed a significant shift of PC-PI from a higher into a lower category (figure 13) with no one having an increase of PC-PI into a higher category. In patients with refractory myeloma there was no significant change with a tendency toward increased values of PC-PI (figure 14). Apoptosis showed reversed relationships with a significant increase in higher categories in the case of the sensitive disease (figure 15) and a significant decrease in the case of refractory myeloma (figure 16).

Since MM is still an incurable disease, the aim of its treatment is to induce remission and to maintain it as long as possible. Many recent studies put stress on reaching complete remission (CR) [135-137], although the results of some authors did not unambiguously confirm the superiority of CR for overall survival [138-141]. Inconsistence in these results puts forward the issue of internal properties of residual myeloma population, especially its growth and survival characteristics that may cause early progression even in patients with CR. We have confirmed that patients with long lasting stable MM after the previous treatment maintain low values of PI and high level of apoptosis, whereas patients with subsequent progression owe its ascension to the increase of proliferation and decrease of residual myeloma cells apoptosis (figure 17).

The observation, however, does not have absolute validity and little or no change in either of the indices in progressing patients suggests a participation of other possible factors (such as presence of growth factors, bone marrow microenvironment changes etc.) in the set up of MM progression. Nevertheless, patients with high proliferation or low apoptosis in residual myeloma cells should be carefully observed as a potential risk group for early progression and should be considered as candidates for maintenance or consolidation therapy.

		PC-PI after treatment			
	p = 0,0002	≤2,3	2,4-2,8	>2,8	Total
PC-PI initial	≤2,3 % of total	10 26,3%	0 0%	0 0%	10 26,3%
	2,4-2,8 % of total	11 28,9%	7 18,4%	0 0%	18 47,4%
	>2,8 % of total	3 7,9%	6 15,8%	1 2,6%	10 26,3%
	Total	24 63,2%	13 34,2%	1 2,6%	38 100,0%

Figure 13. Behavior of proliferative index in multiple myeloma patients reaching remission after conventional chemotherapy

McNemara test of symmetry proves that patients with multiple myeloma (MM) who reach remission after conventional chemotherapy (n=38) display significant decrease of PC-PI from a higher into a lower category. In neither of the patients was detected a shift of PC-PI into a higher category.

PC-PI = propidium iodide (proliferative) index of plasma cells.

p = NS		PC-PI AFTER TREATMENT			TOTAL
		≤2,3	2,4-2,8	>2,8	
PC-PI INITIAL	≤2,3 % OF TOTAL	10 13,5%	8 10,8%	3 4,1%	21 28,4%
	2,4-2,8 % OF TOTAL	2 2,7%	19 25,7%	9 12,2%	30 40,5%
	>2,8 % OF TOTAL	0 0%	9 12,2%	14 18,9%	23 31,3%
	TOTAL	12 16,2%	36 48,6%	26 35,1%	74 100,0%

Figure 14. Behavior of proliferative index in multiple myeloma patients refractory to conventional chemotherapy

In patients with refractory myeloma (n=74) there is no significant change in PC-PI according to McNemara test of symmetry and most of the patients stay within the same discrimination category.
PC-PI = propidium iodide (proliferative) index of plasma cells.
NS = statistically non-significant value.

Proliferation and Apoptosis as Diagnostic Parameters

One of the most fundamental requirements in evaluating monoclonal gammopathies is the distinction between monoclonal gammopathy of undetermined significance (MGUS) and multiple myeloma, especially in its early stages. Recent diagnostic criteria (IMWG criteria) are based on arbitrarily determined parameters evaluating also the presence of tissue damage CRAB, in addition to plasma cell bone marrow infiltration and presence of M-protein in serum and/or urine [142].

p = 0,041		PC-AI AFTER TREATMENT			TOTAL
		≤3,5	3,5-5,0	>5	
PC-AI INITIAL	≤3,5 % OF TOTAL	1 2,7%	3 8,1%	4 10,8%	8 21,6%
	3,5-5,0 % OF TOTAL	0 0%	5 13,5%	11 29,7%	16 43,2%
	>5,0 % OF TOTAL	2 5,4%	3 8,1%	8 21,6%	13 35,1%
	TOTAL	3 8,1%	11 29,7%	23 62,2%	37 100,0%

Figure 15. Behavior of apoptotic index in multiple myeloma patients reaching remission after conventional chemotherapy

McNemara test of symmetry shows in majority of multiple myeloma patients, who reach remission after conventional chemotherapy (n=37), a significant shift from a category with lower PC-AI into a category with higher values of PC-AI. Only a minority of patients (5 individuals, 13.5%) displayed a decrease of the index.
PC-AI = annexin-V (apoptotic) index of plasma cells.

p = 0,038		PC-AI after treatment ≤3.5	PC-AI after treatment 3,5-5,0	PC-AI after treatment >5	Total
PC-AI initial	≤3,5	9	5	1	15
	% of total	12,2%	6,8%	1,4%	20,3%
	3,5-5,0	7	7	8	22
	% of total	9,5%	9,5%	10,8%	29,7 %
	>5,0	8	16	13	37
	% of total	10,8%	21,6%	17,6%	50%
	Total	24	28	22	74
		32,4%	37,8%	29,7%	100,0%

Figure 16. Behavior of apoptotic index in multiple myeloma patients refractory to conventional chemotherapy

Patients with multiple myeloma who are refractory to the treatment (n=74) have a significant shift of PC-AI from a higher into a lower category according to Mc Nemara test of symmetry.

PC-AI = annexin-V (apoptotic) index of plasma cells.

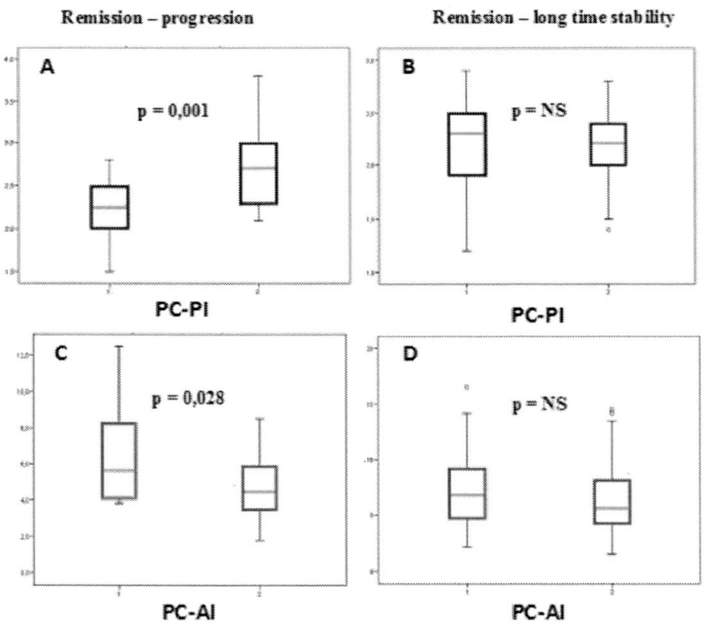

Figure 17. Behavior of proliferative and apoptotic index in remission of multiple myeloma

Proliferative and apoptotic index of myeloma plasmocytes show different behavior in a group of patients in remission of the disease (n = 72) with respect to the activity of MM. In the case of subsequent progression there is a significant increase in proliferation (A, median PC-PI 2.25 vs 2.7) together with decrease of apoptosis (B, median PC-AI 5.6 vs 4.45) whereas in long lasting stability of MM there was no change in both the proliferative index (B, median PC-PI 2.3 vs 2.2) and the apoptotic index (D, median PC-AI 6.75 vs 5.6).

PC-PI = propidium iodide (proliferative) index of plasma cells.

PC-AI = annexin-V (apoptotic) index of plasma cells.

NS = statistically non-significant value.

Similar principles were used for standard clinical staging according to Durie-Salmon, expressing the mathematical model of total tumor mass, and the up-to-date staging according to IPI (International Prognostic Index), evaluating the total tumor mass with the help of serum levels of β2-microglobulin and albumin [143].

More sophisticated knowledge of myeloma biology attenuated the prognostic significance of classical staging systems that revealed the character and load of tumor burden rather indirectly, according to the tissue damage (degree of anemia, hypercalcemia, bone involvement, renal impairment etc.). Newer staging systems have been therefore established that reflect the internal properties of tumor population.

For the dynamic description of malignant clone character, critical are the tumor mass and the speed of neoplastic growth. Based on these facts, an ECOG staging system was established that was based on a combination of BrdUrd proliferative index (parameter of the speed of tumor growth) and β2-microglobulin (parameter of tumor load) [15]. The staging system was simple, with significant distinction of three prognostic groups. Necessity of specialized laboratories and only a limited use of proliferative index in diagnostic centres caused this staging system to fall into oblivion. San Miguel et al have later proposed a new staging system based on the tumor load, activity of the disease and characteristics of the host. Tumor burden was represented by β2M, myeloma activity by the means of proliferative index (measured with the use of propidium iodide) and the host was defined by performance status. Individual prognostic groups had significantly different prognosis with median OS 9, 36 and 80 months [95]. Strong prognostic potential of this staging system was verified also by our department [21].

The early studies on myeloma biology put forward a question whether the kinetic properties of plasma cells (especially the proliferative index) could be the determinant clearly separating "benign" MGUS from MM, particularly in its early stage (smoldering myeloma, MM st. IA, asymptomatic myeloma) [18, 95, 99, 123]. Parameter reflecting proliferation was regarded as the most significant and independent factor of survival in patients with MM [144]. Active myeloma usually had significantly higher value of PI than MGUS and SMM with relatively low values of PI [5, 18, 20, 85, 124]. Its considered inclusion in diagnostic criteria was, however, limited by significant overlapping of the values in each of the disease, i.e. MM, SMM and MGUS. The reason is very likely in the growth characteristics of the tumor clone. Contemporary technical and laboratory methods are usually able to detect MM with a mass of $>10^{12}$ cells. According to Gompertzian function, the initial growth is extremely fast (exponential) with subsequent progressive reduction after reaching the steady state. In the measurement of PI after reaching steady state the values of PI are decreasing [7, 20, 84, 145, 146]. This phenomenon explains surprisingly low values of proliferation in some patients with a large tumor mass with unfavorable disease course, and also the lack of correlation between proliferative index and stage of the disease [37]. In the majority of patients the measurement is carried out in different stage of the exponential expansion of the tumor population. The same mechanism explains higher values of PI in relapse of MM when the beginning of relapse/progression is usually detected earlier, when the tumor mass is less than 10^{12} myeloma cells.

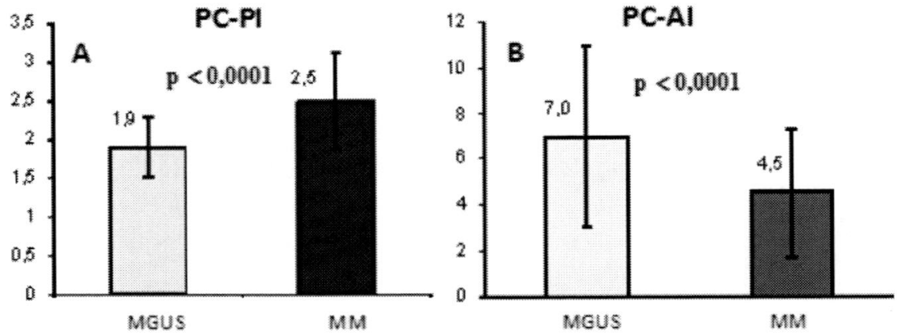

Figure 18. Comparison of proliferative and apoptotic indices in monoclonal gammopathy of undetermined significance and multiple myeloma

Within the comparison of MGUS (n = 78) and multiple myeloma (n = 303) we can see in MM significantly higher values of proliferative index (A) together with lower apoptotic index (B). Certain overlapping of borderline values, however, limits their diagnostic use.

PC-PI = propidium iodide (proliferative) index of plasma cells. PC-AI = annexin-V (apoptotic) index of plasma cells. MGUS = monoclonal gammopathy of undetermined significance.

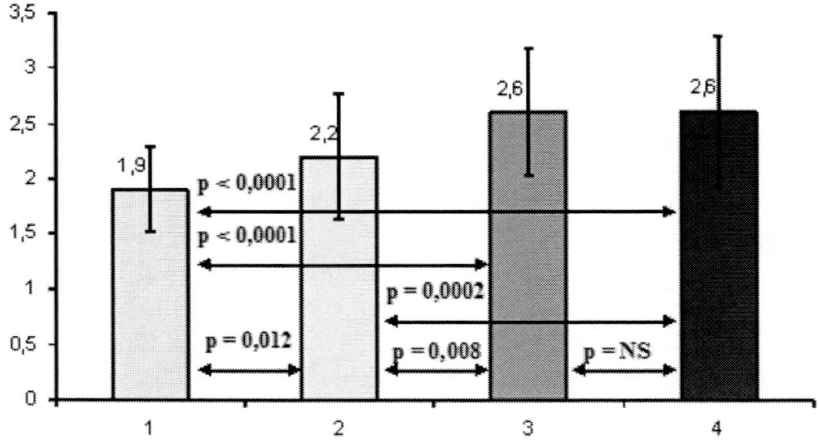

Figure 19. Comparison of proliferative index in monoclonal gammopathy of undetermined significance and individual stages of multiple myeloma according to Durie-Salmon

Comparison of PC-PI in MGUS and individual stages of MM according to Durie-Salmon presents significant differences between MGUS and MM st. I, MGUS and MM st. II, MGUS and MM st. III, MM st. I and MM st. II, MM st. I and MM st. III. Difference between MM st. II and MM st. III is not statistically significant.

1 – MGUS (n = 78)

2 – MM st. I (n = 43)

3 – MM st. II (n = 115)

4 – MM st. III (n = 145)

PC-PI = propidium iodide (proliferative) index of plasma cells. MGUS = monoclonal gammopathy of undetermined significance. MM = multiple myeloma. NS = statistically non-significant value.

We decided to question the reliability of both proliferative and apoptotic indices as diagnostic parameters within both MGUS and MM as well as within individual stages of MM and also in a smaller group of patients transforming from MGUS into an overt form of MM. Study of a cohort of more than 300 patients with MGUS and MM confirmed significant differences in proliferation between MGUS and MM (M - 1,9 vs 2,5, p < 0,0001). Similar results were found for the apoptotic index, in a reciprocal relationship (M - 7,0 vs 4,5, p < 0,0001), (figure 18). Significant differences were also between MGUS and individual stages of MM, both according to D-S and IPI staging systems. The individual stages of MM between themselves were not constantly different, although we could trace some significance and a trend of increasing proliferation and decreasing apoptosis with more advanced stages (figures 19-22).

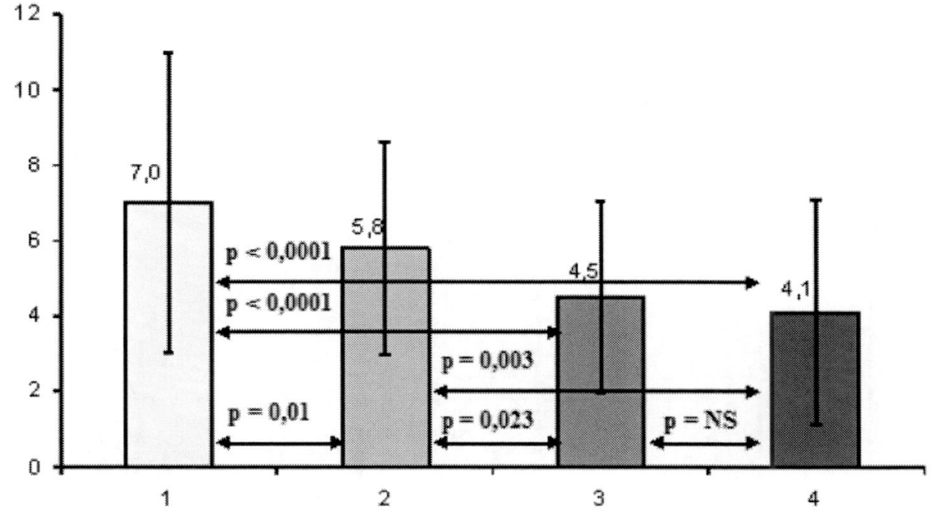

Figure 20. Comparison of apoptotic index in monoclonal gammopathy of undetermined significance and individual stages of multiple myeloma according to Durie-Salmon

Comparison of PC-AI in MGUS and individual stages of MM according to Durie-Salmon presents significant differences between MGUS and MM st. I, MGUS and MM st. II, MGUS and MM st. III, MM st. I and MM st. II, MM st. I and MM st. III. Difference between MM st. II and MM st. III is not statistically significant.

1 – MGUS (n = 78)
2 – MM st. I (n = 43)
3 – MM st. II (n = 115)
4 – MM st. III (n = 145)

PC-AI = annexin-V (apoptotic) index of plasma cells. MGUS = monoclonal gammopathy of undetermined significance. MM = multiple myeloma. NS = statistically non-significant value.

Lack of correlation between individual MM stages and proliferative and apoptotic activity indicates the independence of both the indices on D-S and IPI clinical staging systems. Obviously, patients with more aggressive myeloma were diagnosed at more advanced stages with a greater tumor mass, which could cause the increasing trend of proliferation and decreasing apoptosis. Nevertheless, even in lower stage of MM we could detect individuals with low apoptosis and short overall survival. This finding raises an important issue that indirect parameters such as IPI might be missing the measures of tumor biological properties, i.e. the aggressiveness of the tumor clone. The absolute values of both proliferation and apoptosis, however, varied in a wide range with certain overlap within the different units, i.e. MGUS, SMM and active MM, which substantially limits their diagnostic use.

Possible advances can be made with dynamic evaluation of proliferation and apoptosis. Our preliminary results revealed that a group of 16 patients who underwent transformation from MGUS into symptomatic MM with a need for induction chemotherapy registered significant changes in both the indices, i.e. the increase in proliferative index together with the decrease of apoptosis. In patients with long lasting stable MGUS there was no change in apoptosis and only a small increase in proliferative features (figure 23). These findings support the idea of "multistep pathogenesis" in multiple myeloma where the transformation leads to a gradual increase in proliferative potential [147]. Loss of apoptotic controls belongs to events characterizing the independent neoplastic population. Measurement of proliferation and apoptosis in MGUS thus suggests an easy method for the assessment of a group of patients with a real threat of transformation into overt MM.

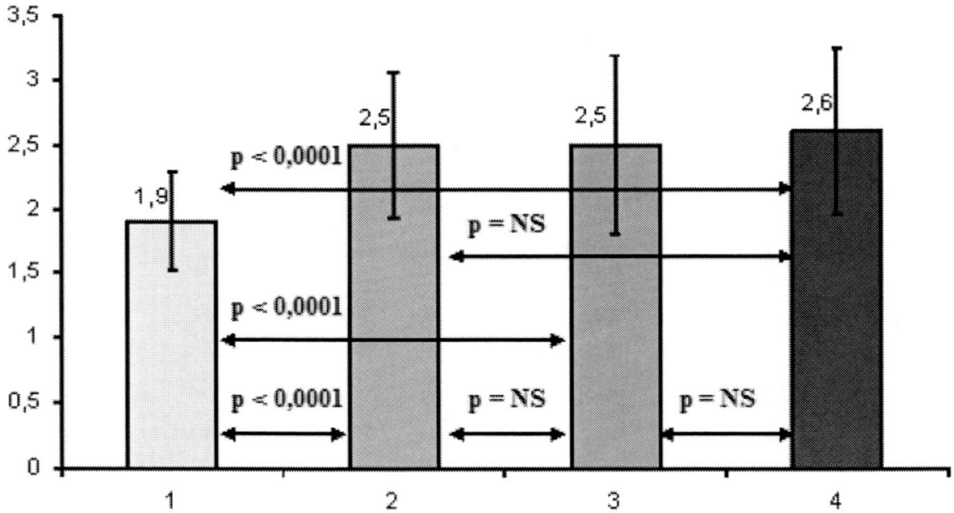

Figure 21. Comparison of proliferative index in monoclonal gammopathy of undetermined significance and individual stages of multiple myeloma according to IPI

Comparison of PC-PI in MGUS and individual stages of MM according to IPI presents significant differences between MGUS and MM IPI I, MGUS and MM IPI II, MGUS and MM IPI III. Differences between individual stages of MM according to IPI are not significant.

1 – MGUS (n = 78)
2 – MM IPI I (n = 62)
3 – MM IPI II (n = 82)
4 – MM IPI III (n = 133)

PC-PI = propidium iodide (proliferative) index of plasma cells. MGUS = monoclonal gammopathy of undetermined significance. MM = multiple myeloma. IPI = International Prognostic Index. NS = statistically non-significant value.

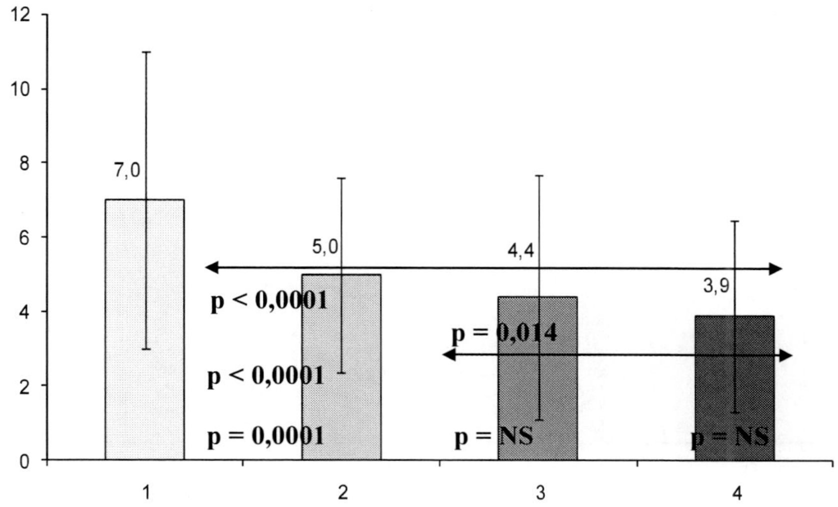

Figure 22. Comparison of apoptotic index in monoclonal gammopathy of undetermined significance and individual stages of multiple myeloma according to IPI

Comparison of PC-AI in MGUS and individual stages of MM according to IPI presents significant differences between MGUS and MM IPI I, MGUS and MM IPI II, MGUS and MM IPI III and MM IPI I and MM IPI III. Differences between stages MM IPI I and MM IPI II as well as MM IPI II and MM IPI III are not statistically significant.

1 – MGUS (n = 78)
2 – MM IPI I (n = 62)
3 – MM IPI II (n = 82)
4 – MM IPI III (n = 133)

PC-AI = annexin-V (apoptotic) index of plasma cells
MGUS = monoclonal gammopathy of undetermined significance
MM = multiple myeloma
IPI = International Prognostic Index
NS = statistically non-significant value

Conclusion

The presented data show that measurement of proliferative index maintains its prognostic potential in patients treated with conventional therapy only, whereas the biological treatment and HD-ASCT suppressed its prognostic strength. Because apoptosis is not only a complementary path for tumor proliferation but it is a different and independent active process itself, its evaluation together with proliferative index could be an important step for a better understanding cellular pathways during the transformation from an asymptomatic variant into a malignant clone. Apoptotic index overcomes the influence of novel drugs and may be, therefore, recommended as a convenient prognostic factor in newly diagnosed patients. Stratification of patients according to different proliferation and apoptosis of myeloma cells provides valuable information about biological features of MM and about the behavior of different populations of plasma cells. Identification of patients with an accumulation of unfavorable prognostic parameters defines a group with very poor prognosis for whom contemporary standard chemotherapy is insufficient, and who need a treatment with more intensive therapeutical approaches.

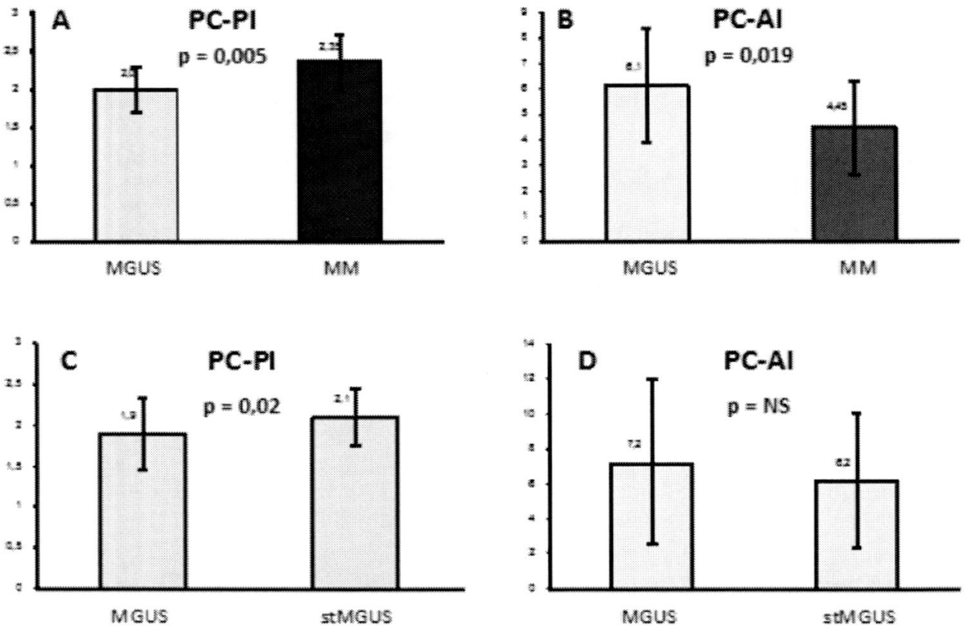

Figure 23. Behavior of proliferative and apoptotic indices in monoclonal gammopathy of undetermined significance and during transformation into multiple myeloma

During the transformation of MGUS into MM (n=16) we can trace simultaneous increase of proliferative index (A) together with a decrease of apoptotic index (B). In long lasting stable MGUS (n=35) there is only a small increase of PC-PI, and apoptosis is without a significant change.

MGUS = monoclonal gammopathy of undetermined significance.

MM = multiple myeloma.

stMGUS = long lasting stable monoclonal gammopathy of undetermined significance.

PC-PI – propidium iodide (proliferative) index of plasma cells.

PC-AI – annexin-V (apoptotic) index of plasma cells.

Longitudinal measurement of proliferation and apoptosis in the course of MM showed significant differences between the active and stable disease. Therefore, it could be used for the detection of progression and/or relapse of the disease as well as for the assessment of the persistence of stable/plateau phase and evaluation of refractory myeloma. Increase in proliferative index and/or decrease of apoptosis should be a clear signal for possible disease activation. Moreover, patients with unfavorable constellation of proliferative and apoptotic features should be considered as candidates for maintenance or consolidation therapy.

Diagnostic use of proliferative and apoptotic index is strongly attenuated by the overlapping of marginal values even though the levels of both proliferation and apoptosis are significantly different in MM and MGUS. On the other hand, being regarded as "kinetic parameters", monitoring of PC-PI and PC-AI in monoclonal gammopathies together with the evaluation of bone marrow involvement can depict a group with a high risk of transformation from MGUS into symptomatic MM.

Presented results display the image of MM as a complex disease with an unusually heterogenous course and prognosis. Our findings supplement the need for sophisticated prognostic parameters and a focus on molecular biology, cytogenetics, gene profiling and other biological markers of the activity of the disease to enhance the knowledge of the tumor´s biology, and to find new alternatives for targeted therapy and, possibly, for a cure.

Proliferation
Key process in MM pathogenesis
Dysregulation of series of enzymatic and non-enzymatic processes
Essential role of IL-6 and other growth factors
Reason for tumor growth - not speed of cell cycle itself but the total number of cells entering cell cycle.
Proliferative index
Prognostic factor in MM patients treated with conventional chemotherapy
HD-ASCT and/or biological based treatment very likely overcome prognostic significance of PI
Significantly increased in active myeloma vs MGUS or stable phase MM
Longitudinal measurement contributes to disease status evaluation (active vs stable disease) and for differentiation of a risk group for transformation or progression
Apoptosis
MM tumor expansion – due to a defect in apoptosis rather than excess proliferation
Loss of apoptotic controls – contributes to both the transformation and accumulation of neoplastic tissue
Multiple apoptotic pathways disrupted in MM pathogenesis
Apoptotic index
Better prognosticator than proliferative index, maintaining its significance even in biological drugs based treatment
Significantly lower values in overt MM than in MGUS or stable phase MM
Decrease in apoptotic index sorts out a high risk group for MM transformation or progression

Acknowledgments

This study was supported by the grant MZ CR NR 9500-3. We would like to acknowledge dr. M. Ordeltova and A. Spidlova, Department of Immunology, University Hospital Olomouc, for flow-cytometry assessment, dr. J. Bacovsky, dr. T. Pika, dr. M. Zemanova, Department of Internal Medicine III, University Hospital Olomouc, for data collection, mgr. K. Langova Department of Statistics and Biophysics, Palacky University, Olomouc, for statistical evaluation and also prof. B. Van Ness, Department of Genetics, Cell Biology and Develepment, University of Minnesota, for assistance and valuable remarks.

References

[1] Ščudla, V. Monoklonální gamapatie. In Indrák, K., et al. *Hematologie*, Triton, Praha/Kroměříž, 2006: 182-195. ISBN 80-7254-868-9.

[2] Davies, F.E., Anderson, K.C. Novel therapeutic targets in multiple myeloma. *Eur. J. Hematol.*, 2000; 64: 359–367.

[3] Kumar, S.K., Rajkumar, S.V., Dispenzieri, A., et al. Improved survival in multiple myeloma and the impact of novel therapies. *Blood,* 2008; 111: 2516-2520.

[4] San Miguel, J.F., Fonseca, R., Greipp, P.R. Prognostic Factors and Classification for Multiple Myeloma (Contribution to Clinical Management). In Malpas, J.S., Bergsagel, D.E., Kyle, R.A., et al. *Myeloma Biology and Management*, third edition, Elsevier Inc., Philadelphia, 2004: 196; ISBN 0-7216-0006-9.

[5] Greipp, P.R., Raymond, N.M., Kyle, R.A., et al. Multiple myeloma: Significance of plasmablastic subtype in morphological classification. *Blood,* 1985; 65: 305-310.

[6] Greipp, P.R., Kyle, R.A. Staging, Kinetics and Prognosis of Multiple Myeloma. In Wiernik, P.H., Canellos, G.P., Dutcher, J.P. et al., *Neoplastic Diseases of the Blood,* Third Edition. Churchill Livingstone, Inc., New York, 1996: 537-559, ISBN 0-443-07600-6.

[7] Calligaris-Cappio, F. Biology of the malignant plasma cell. In Gahrton, G., Durie, B.G.M., Samson, D.M. *Multiple myeloma and related disorders*, Arnold, London, 2004: 58-73; ISBN 0-340-81010-6.

[8] Mrozek, K., Heerema, N.A., Bloomfield, C.D. Cytogenetics in acute leukemia. *Blood Rev*, 2004; 18: 115-136.

[9] Zandecki, M. Multiple myeloma – Almost all patients are cytogenetically abnormal. *Br J. Haematol.,* 1996; 94: 217-227.

[10] Fonseca, R., Harrington, D., Blood, E., et al. A molecular classification of multiple myeloma based on cytogenetic abnormalities detected by interphase FISH, is powerful in identifying discrete groups of patients with dissimilar prognosis. *Blood,* 2001; 98: 733a.

[11] Hájek, R., Kuglík, P., Zaoralová, R., et al. Genetic lesions in multiple myeloma: prognostic and predictive significance in the era of the new drugs. *Blood Rev*, 2007; 21: 74.

[12] Rajkumar, S.V., Fonseca, R., Dewald, G.W., et al. Cytogenetic Abnormalities Correlate with the Plasma Cell Labeling index and Extent of Bone Marrow Involvement in Myeloma. *Cancer Gen. Cytogen*, 1999; 113: 73-77.

[13] Liu, P., Leong, T., Quam, L., et al. Activating mutations of N- and K-ras in multiple myeloma show different clinical associations: Analysis of the Eastern Cooperative Oncology Group Phase III Trial. *Blood,* 1996; 88: 2699-2706.

[14] Alexandrakis, M., Passam, F., Ganotakis, E., et al. Bone marrow microvascular density and angiogenic growth factors in multiple myeloma. *Clin. Chem. Lab. Med.,* 2004; 42: 1122-1126.

[15] Greipp, P.R., Lust, J., O´Fallon, W.M., et al. Plasma Cell Labeling Index and beta-2-Microglobulin Predict Survival Independent of Thymidine Kinase and C-reactive protein in Multiple Myeloma. *Blood,* 1993; 18: 3382-3387.

[16] Greipp, P.R., Katzmann, J.A., O'Fallon, M., et al. Value of Beta-2-Microglobulin Level and Plasma Cell Labeling Indices as Prognostic Factors in Patients With Newly Diagnosed Myeloma. *Blood,* 1988; 72: 219-223.

[17] Greipp, P.R., Kumar, S. Plasma Cell Labeling Index. In Brown, R.D., Ho, P.J. *Methods In Molecular Medicine. Multiple myeloma. Methods and Protocols*. Humana Press, Totowa, NJ, 2005: 25-35; ISBN 978-1-58829-392-3.

[18] Greipp, P.R., Kyle, R.A. Clinical, morphological and cell kinetic differences among multiple myeloma, monoclonal gammopathy of undetermined significance, and smoldering multiple myeloma. *Blood,* 1983; 62: 166-171.

[19] Minařík, J., Ščudla, V., Ordeltová, M., et al. Evaluation of plasma cell propidium-iodide and annexin-V indices: their relation to prognosis in multiple myeloma. *Biomed Pap,* 2005: 81-84.

[20] Scudla, V., Ordeltova, M., Bacovsky, J. et al. The relationship between proliferation and apoptosis in patients with monoclonal gammopathy of undetermined significance or multiple myeloma. *Haematologica,* 2005; 90: 1713-1714.

[21] Scudla, V., Ordeltova, M., Minarik, J., et al. Prognostic significance of plasma cell propidium iodide and annexin-V indices and their mutual ratio in multiple myeloma. *Neoplasma*, 2006; 53: 199-205.

[22] Witzig, T.E., Greipp, P.R., Therneau, T., et al. Measurement of apoptosis and proliferation of bone marrow plasma cells in patients with plasma cell proliferative disorders. *Br. J. Haematol.*, 1999; 104: 131-137.

[23] Chen-Kiang, S. Multiple Myeloma and Plasma Cells: Cell Cycle and Apoptotic Controls. In Malpas, J.S., Bergsagel, D.E., Kyle, R.A., et al. *Myeloma Biology and Management*, third edition, Elsevier Inc., Philadelphia, 2004: 21-33; ISBN 0-7216-0006-9.

[24] Mateos, M.V., Garcia-Sanz, R., Lopez-Perez, R., et al. P16/INK4a gene inactivation by hypermetylation is associated with aggressive variants of monoclonal gammopathies. *Hematol. J.,* 2001; 3: 146-149.

[25] Heinrich, P.C., Behrmann, I., Muller-Newen, G., et al. Interleukin-6 type cytokine signalling through the gp130/Jak/STAT pathway. *Biochem J,* 1998; 334: 297-314.

[26] Hideshima, T., Chauhan, D., Anderson, K.C. Cytokines, Cytokine Receptors, and Signal Transduction in Human Multiple Myeloma. In Malpas, J.S., Bergsagel, D.E., Kyle, R.A., et al. *Myeloma Biology and Management*, third edition, Elsevier Inc., Philadelphia, 2004: 35-57; ISBN 0-7216-0006-9.

[27] Ludwig, H. et al. Interleukin 6 is a prognostic factor in multiple myeloma. *Blood*, 1991; 77: 2794-1795.

[28] Pratt, G. Molecular aspects of multiple myeloma. *J. Clin. Pathol.*, 2002; 55: 273 – 283.

[29] Ščudla, V., Bačovský, J., Budíková, M., et al. Imunoreaktivní interleukin-6 u mnohočetného myelomu: vztah k vybraným charakteristikám nemoci. *Hematol. Transf,* 1995; 5: 49-58.

[30] Ščudla, V., Bačovský, J., Budíková, M., et al. Interleukin-6 v séru u mnohočetného myelomu. II. Vztah k aktivitě a k pokročilosti nemoci. *Vnitř Lék,* 1995; 41: 599-604.

[31] Loffler, D., Brocke-Heidrich, K., Pfeifer, G., et al. Interleukin-6-dependent survival of multiple myeloma cells involves the Stat3-mediated induction of microRNA-21 through a highly conserved enhancer, *Blood,* 2007; 110: 1330-1333.

[32] Billadeau, D., Liu, P., Shah, N., et al. Activating mutations in the N- and K-ras oncogenes differentially affect the growth properties of the IL-6-dependent myeloma cell line ANBL6. *Cancer Res*, 1997; 57: 2268-75.

[33] Croonquist, P.A., Linden, M.A., Zhao, F., et al. Gene profiling of a myeloma cell line reveals similarities and unique signatures among IL-6 response, N-ras-activating mutations, and coculture with bone marrow stromal cells. *Blood*, 2003; 102: 2581-2592.

[34] Shiratsuchi, M., Muta, K., Umemura, T., et al. Telomerase Activity in Myeloma Cells is Closely Related to Cell Cycle status, but not to Apoptotic Signals Induced by Interferon-α. *Leuk Lymph*, 1999; 34: 349-359.

[35] Billedeau, D., Ahmann, G., Greipp, P.R., et al. The Bone marrow of multiple myeloma patients contains B cell populations at different stages of differentation that are clonally related to malignant plasma cell. *J. Exp. Med.*, 1993; 178: 1023-1031.

[36] Vacca, A., Ribatti, D., Roncali, L., et al. Angiogenesis in B Cell Lymphoproliferative Diseases. Biological and Clinical Studies. *Leuk Lymph*, 1995; 20: 27-38.

[37] Vacca, A., Ribatti, D., Roncali, L., et al. Bone marrow angiogenesis and progression in multiple myeloma. *Br. J. Haematol.*, 1994; 87: 503-508.

[38] Adam, Z., Krejčí, M., Vorlíček, J., et al. Hematologie. *Přehled maligních hematologických nemocí,* 2. vydání, Grada Publishing, Praha, 2008: 209-239, ISBN 978-80-247-2502-4.

[39] Bergsagel, P.L., Kuehl, W.M. The Molecular Biology of Multiple Myeloma. In Malpas, J.S., Bergsagel, D.E., Kyle, R.A., et al. *Myeloma Biology and Management*, third edition, Elsevier Inc., Philadelphia, 2004: 35-57; ISBN 0-7216-0006-9.

[40] Ehlert, J.E., Kubbutat, M.H.G. Apoptosis and Its Relevance in Cancer Therapy. *Onkologie*, 2001; 24: 433-440.

[41] Bharti, A.C., Shoshodia, S., Reuben, J.M., et al. Nuclear factor-κB and STAT3 are constitutively active in CD138+ cells derived from multiple myeloma patients, and suppression of these transcription factors leads to apoptosis. *Blood*, 2004; 103: 3175-3184.

[42] Hanahan, D., Weinberg, R.A. The hallmarks of cancer. *Cell*, 2000; 100: 57-70.

[43] Oancea, M., Mani, A., Hussein, M.A., et al. Apoptosis of Multiple Myeloma. *Int. J. Hematol*, 2004; 80: 224–231.

[44] Ziegler, D.S., Kung, A.L. Therapeutic targeting of apoptosis pathways in cancer. *Cur. Opin. Oncol.*, 2008; 20: 97-103.

[45] Dubská, L., Sheard, M.A. Apoptóza zprostředkovaná death receptory: úloha FasL a TRAIL při smrti maligních buněk. *Klin. onkol.*, 2003; 6: 257-264.

[46] Peter, M.E., Krammer, P.H. The CD95 (APO-1/Fas) DISC and beyond. *Cell Death Dif*, 2003; 10: 26–35.

[47] Spets, H., Georgii-Hemming, P., Siljason, J., et al. Fas/APO-1 (CD95)-Mediated Apoptosis Is Activated by Interferon-γ and Interferon-α in Interleukin-6 (IL-6)-

Dependent and IL-6-Independent Multiple Myeloma Cell Lines. *Blood*, 1998, 92: 2914-2923.

[48] De Vos, J., Jourdan, M., Tarte, K., et al. JAK2 tyrosine kinase inhibitor tyrphostin AG490 downregulates the mitogen-activated protein kinase (MAPK) and signal transducer and activator of transcription (STAT) pathways and induces apoptosis in myeloma cells. *Br. J. Hematol.*, 2000; 109: 823-828.

[49] Tai, Y-T., Podar, K., Mitsiades, N., et al. CD40 induces human multiple myeloma cell migration via phosphatidylinositol 3-kinase/AKT/NF-κB signaling. *Blood*, 2003; 101: 2762-2769.

[50] Chen, Q., Ray, S., Hussein, M.A., et al. Apo2L/TRAIL and Bcl-2-family proteins in apoptosis of multiple myeloma. *Leuk Lymph*, 2003; 44: 1209-1214.

[51] Kim, H.J., Kim, S.W., Kim, C.K., et al. Arsenic trioxide induced apoptosis and overcomes trail resistance in multiple myeloma. *Proc Am Soc Clin Oncol*, 2003; 22: 2429.

[52] Shipman, C.M., Rogers, M.J., Apperley, J.F., et al. Bisphosphonates induce apoptosis in human myeloma cell lines: a novel anti-tumour activity. *Brit. J. Haematol.*, 1997, 98: 665–672.

[53] Silvestris, F., Cafforio, P., Tucci, M., et al. Negative regulation of erythroblast maturation by FasL+/TRAIL+ highly malignant plasma cells: a major pathogenetic mechanism of anemia in multiple myeloma. *Blood*, 2002; 99: 1305-1313.

[54] Locklin, R.M., Croucher, P.I., Russell, R.G., et al. Agonists of TRAIL death receptors induce myeloma cell apoptosis that is not prevented by cells of the bone marrow microenvironment. *Leukemia*, 2007; 21: 805-812.

[55] Georgii-Hemming, P., Wiklund, H.J., Ljunggren, O., et al. Insulin-like growth factor I is a growth and survival factor in human multiple myeloma cell lines. *Blood*, 1996; 88: 2250-2258.

[56] Chng, W.J., Gualberto, A., Fonseca, R. IGF-1R is overexpressed in poor-prognostic subtypes of multiple myeloma. *Leukemia*, 2006; 20: 174-176.

[57] Jernberg-Wiklund, H., Nilsson, K. Control of Apoptosis in Human Multiple Myeloma by Insulin-like Growth Factor I (IGF-I). *Adv. Cancer Res.*, 2007; 97: 139-165.

[58] Pene, F., Claessens, Y.E., Muller, O., et al. Role of the phosphatidylinositol 3-kinase/Akt and mTOR/P70S6-kinase pathways in the proliferation and apoptosis in multiple myeloma. *Oncogene*, *2002*; 21: 6587-6597.

[59] Qiang, Y.W., Kopantzev, E., Rudikoff, S. Insulin like growth factor-I signaling in multiple myeloma: downstream elements, functional correlates, and pathway cross-talk. *Blood*, 2002; 99: 4138-4146.

[60] Tu, Y., Gardner, A., Lichtenstein, A. The phosphatidylinositol 3-kinase/AKT kinase pathway in multiple myeloma plasma cells: roles in cytokine-dependent survival and proliferative responses. *Cancer Res.*, 2000; 60: 6763-6770.

[61] Fuchs, O., Neuwirtová, R. Ubikvitiny, proteazomy, sumoylace a použití dnes a zítra v terapii nádorů i jiných chorob I., Ubikvitin-proteazomový systém a transkripční faktor NF-kB. *Vnitř. Lék.*, 2006; 52: 371-378.

[62] Yang, H.H., Ma, M.H., Vescio, R.A., et al. Overcoming Drug Resistance in Multiple Myeloma: The Emergence of Therapeutic Approaches ti Induce Apoptosis. *J. Clin. Oncol.*, 2003; 21: 4239-4247.

[63] Annunziata, C.M., Davis, R.E., Demchenko, Y., et al. Frequent engagement of the classical and alternative NF-kappaB pathways by diverse genetic abnormalities in multiple myeloma. *Cancer Cell*, 2007; 12: 115-130.

[64] Keats, J.J., Fonseca, R., Chesi, M., et al. Promiscuous mutations activate the noncanonical NF-kappaB pathway in multiple myeloma. *Cancer Cell*, 2007; 12: 131-144.

[65] Gomez-Bougie, P., Oliver, L., Le Gouill, S., et al. Melphalan-induced apoptosis in multiple myeloma cells is associated with a cleavage of Mcl-1 and Bim and a decrease in the Mcl-1/Bim complex. *Oncogene*, 2005; 24: 8076-8079.

[66] Pettersson, M., Jernberg-Wiklund, H., Larsson, L.G., et al. Expression of the bcl-2 gene in human multiple myeloma cell lines and normal plasma cells. *Blood*, 1992; 79: 495-502.

[67] Jourdan, M., De Vos, J., Mechti, N., et al. Regulation of Bcl-2-family proteins in myeloma cells by three myeloma survival factors: interleukin-6, interferon-alpha and insulin-like growth factor 1. *Cell Death Differ.*, 2000; 7: 1244-1252.

[68] Jourdan, M., Ferlin, M., Legouffe, E., et al. The myeloma cell antigen syndecan-1 is lost by apoptotic myeloma cells. *Br. J. Haematol.*, 1998; 100: 637-646.

[69] Jourdan, M., Veyrune, J.L., Vos, J.D., et al. A major role for Mcl-1 antiapoptotic protein in the IL-6-induced survival of human myeloma cells. *Oncogene*, 2003; 22: 2950-2959.

[70] Spets, H., Stromberg, T., Georgii-Hemming, P., et al. Expression of the bcl-2 family of pro- and antiapoptotic genes in multiple myeloma and normal plasma cells: regulation during interleukin-6 (IL-6)-induced growth and survival. *Eur. J. Haematol.*, 2002; 69: 76-89.

[71] Xu, F., Sharma, S., Gardner, A., et al. Interleukin-6-Induced Inhibition of Multiple Myeloma Cell Apoptosis: Support for the Hypothesis That Protection Is Mediated Via Inhibition of the JNK/SAPK Pathway. *Blood*, 1998; 92: 241-251.

[72] Pichiorri, F., Suh, S.-S., Ladetto, M., et al. MicroRNAs regulate critical genes associated with multiple myeloma pathogenesis. *PNAS*, 2008; 105: 12885-12890.

[73] Novosad, J., Kodydková, K., Krejsek, J. Apoptóza, její mechanismy a medicínský význam. I. Definice apoptózy a její průběh na buněčné úrovni. *Vnitř. Lék.*, 2001; 47: 381-386.

[74] Roy, N., Deveraux, Q.L., Takahashi, R., et al. The c-IAP-1 and c-IAP-2 proteins are direct inhibitors of specific caspases. *Embo J.*, 1997; 16: 6914-6925.

[75] Shin, S., Sung, B.J., Cho, Y.S., et al. An anti-apoptotic protein human survivin is a direct inhibitor of caspase-3 and -7. *Biochemistry*, 2001; 40: 1117-1123.

[76] Takahashi, R., Deveraux, Q., Tamm, I., et al. A single BIR domain of XIAP sufficient for inhibiting caspases. *J. Biol. Chem.*, 1998; 273: 7787-7790.

[77] Tamm, I., Wang, Y., Sausville, E., et al. IAP-family protein survivin inhibits caspase activity and apoptosis induced by Fas (CD95), Bax, caspases, and anticancer drugs. *Cancer Res.*, 1998; 58: 5315-5320.

[78] Alberts, D.S., Golde, D.W. DNA Synthesis in Multiple Myeloma Cells following Cell Cycle-nonspecific Chemotherapy. *Cancer Res.,* 1974; 34: 2911-2914.

[79] Bednar, O., Magrot, T. Apparatus for rapid determination of the mitotic index. *Plzen Lek. Sb.*, 1964; 23: 97-99.

[80] Fliedner, T.M., Cronkite, E.P., Bond, V.P., et al. The mitotic index of human bone marrow in healthy individuals and irradiated human beings. *Acta Haematol.*, 1959; 22: 65-78.

[81] Hoffman, J.G. Wright's Hypothesis: Its Relation to Volume Growth of Tissue Cells and Mitotic Index. *Science*, 1947; 106: 343-344.

[82] Invernizzi, P., Salera, U. Studies on proliferation of erythroblasts based on mitotic index and on karyokinetic histogram; constitutional hemolytic jaundice. *Haematologica,* 1952; 36: 569-582.

[83] Smith, C.L., Dendy, P.P. Relation between mitotic index, duration of mitosis, generation time and fraction of dividing cells in a cell population. *Nature*, 1962; 193: 555-556.

[84] Boccadoro, M., Gavarotti, P., Ciaiolo, C., et al. Cytokinetic studies in human myeloma. *Bas. Appl. Histochem.*, 1986; 30: 233-237.

[85] Boccadoro, M., Gavarotti, P., Fossati, G. et al. Low plasma cell 3H thymidine incorporation in monoclonal gammopathy of undetermined significance (MGUS), smouldering myeloma and remission phase myeloma: a reliable indicator of patients not requiring therapy. *Brit. J. Haematol.*, 1984; 58: 689-696.

[86] Boccadoro, M., Durie, B.G.M, Frutiger, Y., et al. Lack of Correlation between Plasma Cell Thymidine Labelling Index and Serum Beta-2-Microglobulin in Monoclonal Gammopathies. *Acta Haematol.*, 1987; 78: 239-242.

[87] Büchi, G., Girotto, M., Veglio, M., et al. Kappa/lambda ratio on peripheral blood lymphycytes and bone marrow plasma cell labeling index in monoclonal gammopathies. *Haematologica,* 1990; 75: 132.

[88] Greipp, P.R., Witzig ,T.E, Gonchoroff, N.J., et al. Immunofluorescence labeling indices in myeloma and related monoclonal gammopathies. *Mayo Clin. Proc.*, 1987; 62: 969.

[89] Greipp, P.R., Witzig, T.E., Gonchoroff, N.J. Immunofluorescent Plasma Cell Labeling Indices (LI) Using a Monoclonal Antibody (BU-1), *Am. J. Hematol.*, 1985; 20: 289-292.

[90] Duque, R.E., Andreef, M., Braylan, R.C., et al. Consensus review of the clinical utility of DNA flow cytometry in neoplastic hematopathology. *Cytometry*, 1993; 14: 492-496.

[91] Orfao, A., Ciudad, J., Gonzales, M., et al. Prognostic value of S-phase white blood cell count in B-cell chronic lymphocytic leukemia. *Leukemia*, 1992; 6: 47-51.

[92] Vidriales, M.B., Orfao, A., Lopez-Berges, M.C., et al. Prognostic value of S-phase cells in AML patients. *Br. J. Haematol.*, 1995; 89: 342.

[93] Tafuri, A., Meyers, J., Lee, B.J., et al. DNA and RNA flow cytometric study in multiple myeloma. *Am. J. Clin. Pathol.*, 1991; 97: 322-330.

[94] Trendle, M.C., Leong, T., Kyle, R.A., et al. Prognostic significance of the S-phase fraction of light-chain-restricted cytoplasmic immunoglobulin (cIg) positive plasma cells in patients with newly diagnosed multiple myeloma enrolled on Eastern

Cooperative Oncology Group treatment trial E9486. *Am. J. Hematol.*, 1999; 61: 232-237.

[95] San Miguel, J.F., Garcia-Sanz, R., Gonzales, M., et al. A New Staging System for Multiple Myeloma Based on the Number of S-Phase Plasma Cells. *Blood*, 1995; 85: 448-455.

[96] Maisnar, V., Toušková, M., Tichý, M., et al. The significance of soluble CD138 in diagnosis of monoclonal gammapathies. *Neoplasma*, 2006; 53: 26-29.

[97] Ordeltová, M., Špidlová, A., Ščudla, V. Hodnocení S-fáze buněčného cyklu (CD38/propidium iodidového indexu) myelomových plasmocytů s pomocí průtokové cytometrie. *Diagnoza*, 1999; 1: 11-15.

[98] San Miguel, J.F., Garcia-Sanz, R., Gonzales, M., et al. DNA Cell Content Studies In Multiple Myeloma. *Leuk. Lymph.*, 1996; 23: 33-41.

[99] Joshua, D., Petersen, A., Brown, R., et al. The labeling index of primitive plasma cells determines the clinical behaviour of patients with myelomatosis, *Br. J. Haematol.*, 1996; 94: 76-81.

[100] Kawano, M.M., Huang, N., Harad, H., et al. Identification of immature and mature myeloma cells in the bone marrow of human myelomas. *Blood*, 1993; 82: 564-570.

[101] Drach, J., Gattringer, C., Glassl, H., et al. The Biological and clinical significance of the Ki-67 growth fraction in multiple myeloma. *Hematol. Oncol.*, 1992; 10: 125 –134.

[102] Fabian, P., Křen, L., Nenutil, R. Stanovení proliferační aktivity myelomových buněk z histologického materiálu, *Čes-slov. Patol.*, 2004; 39: 46-49.

[103] Sasaki, K., Matsumura, K., Tsuji, T., et al. Relationship Between Labeling Indices of Ki-67 and BrdUrd in Human Malignant Tumors. *Cancer*, 1988; 62: 989-993.

[104] Skopelitou, A., Tselenis, S., Theocharis, S., et al. Expression of priliferating cell nuclear antigen (PCNA) and nuclear organizer regions (NORs) in multiple myeloma. *Anticancer Res.*, 1994; 14: 787-792.

[105] Usnarska-Zubkiewicz, L. Cytomorphology and proliferating cell nuclear antigen in myeloma plasma cells correlate with serum IL-6 and sIL-6R concentrations in multiple myeloma. *Eur. J. Int. Med.*, 1999; 10: 101-105.

[106] Pich, A., Chiusa, L., Marmont, F., et al. Risk Groups of Myeloma Patients by Histologic Pattern and Proliferative Activity. *Am. J. Surg. Pathol.*, 1997; 21: 339-347.

[107] Brown, R.D., Joshua, D.E., Nelson, M., et al. Serum thymidinekinase as a prognostic indicator for patients with multiple myeloma: results from the MRC (UK) V trial. *Br. J. Haematol.*, 1993; 84: 238-241.

[108] Pellat-Deceunynck, C. Adhesion molecules on human myeloma cells: Significant changes in expression related to malignancy, tumour spreading, and immortalization. *Cancer Res.*, 1995; 55: 3647-3653.

[109] Robillard, N., Jego, G., Pellat-Deceunynck, C., et al. CD28, a marker associated with tumoral expansion in multiple myeloma. *Clin. Cancer Res.*, 1998; 4: 1521-1526.

[110] Shou, Y., Martelli, M.L., Garbea, A., et al. Diverse karyotypic abnormalities of the c-myc locus associated with c-myc dysregulation and tumour progression in multiple myeloma. *Proc. Natl. Acad. Sci. USA*, 2000; 97: 228-233.

[111] Klein, B., Zhang, X.G., Lu, Z.Y., et al. Interleukin-6 in human multiple myeloma. *Blood*, 1995; 85: 863-872.

[112] Bataille, R., Jourdan, M., Zhang, X.G., et al. Serum levels of interleukin 6, a potent myeloma cell growth factor, as a reflection of disease severity in plasma cell dyscrasias. *J. Clin. Invest.*, 1989; 84: 2008-2011.

[113] Hirano, T. Interleukin 6 and its receptor: ten years later. *Int. Rev. Immunol.*, 1998; 154: 4091-4098.

[114] Zhang, B., Fenton R.G. Proliferation of IL-6-independent multiple myeloma does not require the activity of extracellular signal-regulated kinases (ERK1/2). *J. Cell Physiol.*, 2002; 193: 42-54.

[115] Zhang, X.G., Gu, Z.J., Yasukawa, K., et al. Ciliary neutropic factor, interleukin 11, leukemia inhibitory factor and oncostatin M are growth factors for human myeloma cell lines using the interleukin 6 signal transducer gp 130. *J. Exp. Med.*, 1994; 179: 1337-1342.

[116] Pavlovský, Z., Vagunda, V. Apoptóza – vybrané metody detekce apoptózy a asociovaných regulačních faktorů na tkáňových řezech z nádorového materiálu. *Česslov. Patol.*, 2003; 39: 6-10.

[117] Wijsman, J.H., Jonker, R.R., Keijzer, R., et al. A new method to detect apoptosis in paraffin sections: in situ end- labeling of fragmented DNA. *J. Histochem. Cytochem.*, 1993; 41: 7-12.

[118] Saikumar, P., Dong, Z., Mikhailov, V., et al. Apoptosis: Definition, Mechanisms, and Relevance to Disease. *Am. J. Med.*, 1999; 107: 489-506.

[119] Philpott, N.J., Turner, A.J.C., Scopes, J., et al. The use of 7- Amino Actinomycin D Identifying Apoptosis: Simplicity of Use and Broad Spectrum of Application Compared With Other Techniques. *Blood*, 1996; 87: 2244-2251.

[120] Darzynkiewicz,Z., Juan, G., Li, X. et al. Cytometry in cell necrobiology: analysis of apoptosis and accidental cell death (necrosis). *Cytometry*, 1997; 27: 1-20.

[121] Ordeltová, M., Ščudla, V., Špidlová, A., et al. Hodnocení apoptózy myelomových plazmocytů (annexin V/CD138 indexu) metodou průtokové cytometrie. *Hematol. Transf.*, 2002; 2: 499-508.

[122] Koopman, G., Reutelingsperger, C.P.M., Kuijten, G.A.M. et al. Annexin V for flow cytometric detection of phosphatidylserine expression of B cells undergoing apoptosis. *Blood*, 1994; 84: 1415-1420.

[123] Boccadoro, M., Marmont, F., Tribalto, M. et al. Early responder myeloma: kinetic studies identify a patient subgroup characterised by very poor prognosis. *J. Clin. Oncol.*, 1989; 7: 119-125.

[124] Pileri, A., Massaia, M., Dianzani, U., et al. Cytobiological Studies in Multiple Myeloma, *Acta Haematol.*, 1987; 78: 41-42.

[125] Latreille, J., Barlogie, B., Johnston, D., et al. Ploidy and Proliferative Characteristics in Monoclonal Gammopathies, *Blood*, 1981; 58: 471-476.

[126] Schambeck, Ch.M, Bartl, R., Hochtlein-Vollmar, W., et al. Characterisation of Myeloma Cells by Means of Labeling index, Bone Marrow Histology, and Serum B-2-Microglobulin. *Am. J. Clin. Pathol.*, 1996; 106: 64-68.

[127] Boccadoro, M., Tarella, C., Palumbo, A., et al. An analysis of subgroups of multiple myeloma patients, divided according to beta-2- microglobulin and plasma cell labeling

index, benefit from high dose vs conventional chemotherapy. *Haematologica*, 1999; 84: 905-910.

[128] Gertz, M.A., Witzig, T.E., Pineda, A.A., et al. Monoclonal plasma cells in the blood stem cell harvest from patients with multiple myeloma are associated with shortened relapse-free survival after transplantation. *Bone Mar. Transpl.*, 1997; 19: 337-342.

[129] Rajkumar, S.V., Fonseca, R., Dewald, G.W., et al. Cytogenetic Abnormalities Correlate with the Plasma Cell Labeling index and Extent of Bone Marrow Involvement in Myeloma. *Cancer Gen. Cytogen.*, 1999; 113: 73-77.

[130] Winkler, J.M., Dispenzieri, A., Lacy, M., et al. The plasma cell labeling index (PCLI) supercedes the prognostic significance of karyotypic chromosome 13 abnormalities (Δ13) in multiple myeloma (MM) patients undergoing high-dose chemotherapy with stem cell support (HD). *Proc. Am. Soc. Clin. Oncol.*, 2001; 21: 1075.

[131] Schambeck, C.M., Wick, M., Bartl, R. et al. Plasma cell proliferation in monoclonal gammopathies: measurement using BU-I antibody in flow cytometry and microscopy: comparison with serum thymidine kinase. *J. Clin. Pathol.*, 1995; 48: 477-481.

[132] Ščudla, V., Ordeltová, M. Vyšetření proliferačních charakteristik plasmocytů u mnohočetného myelomu. II. Vztah ke klinickým a laboratorním ukazatelům nemoci. *Hematol. Transf.*, 1998; 4: 22-28.

[133] Rajkumar, S.V. Circulating plasma cells, labeling index, and angiogenesis in MGUS and smoldering multiple myeloma. IX International Myeloma Workshop. From MGUS to Myeloma, Focussed symposia: S33.

[134] Steensma, D.P., Gertz, M.A., Greipp, P.R., et al. A high bone marrow plasma cell labeling index in stable plateau-phase multiple myeloma is a marker for early disease progression and death. *Blood*, 2001; 15: 2522-2523.

[135] Attal, M., Harousseau, J.L., Stoppa, A.M., et al. A Prospective, Randomized Trial of Autologous Bone Marrow Transplantation and Chemotherapy in Multiple Myeloma. *N Engl. J. Med.*, 1996; 335: 91-97.

[136] Child, J.A., Morgan, G.J., Davies, F.E., et al. High dose therapy improves the outcome of patients with multiple myeloma: The MRC Myeloma VII randomized study. *New Eng. J. Med.*, 2003; 348: 1875-1883.

[137] Poon, M.L., Chng, W.J. Is complete remission an important therapeutic aim in Multiple Myeloma? *Cancer Ther.*, 2008, 6: 275-284.

[138] Blade, J., Esteve, J., Rives, S., et al. High dose therapy autotransplantation/ intensification vs. continued standard chemotherapy in multiple myeloma in first remission. Results of a non-randomized study from a single institution. *Bone Mar. Transpl.*, 2000; 26: 845-849.

[139] Fermand, J.P., Revaud, P., Katashian, S., et al. High dose therapy (HDT) and autologous blood stem cell (ABSC) transplantation versus conventional treatment in multiple myeloma (MM): results of a randomised trial in 190 patients 55 to 65 years of age. *Blood*, 1999; 94: Abstr 396a.

[140] Garban, F., Attal, M., Michallet, M., et al. Prospective comparison of autologous stem cell transplantation followed by dosereduced allograft (IFM 99-03 trial) with tandem autologous stem cell transplantation (IFM 99-04 trial) in high-risk de novo multiple myeloma. *Blood*, 2006; 107: 3474-3480.

[141] Segeren, C.M., Sonneveld, P., van der Holt, B., et al. Overall and event-free survival are not improved by the use of myeloablative therapy following intensified chemotherapy in previously untreated patients with multiple myeloma: a prospective randomized phase 3 study. *Blood*, 2003; 101: 2144-2151.

[142] Kyle, R.A. et al. Criteria for the classification of monoclonal gammopathies, multiple myeloma and related disorders: a report of the International Myeloma Working Group. *Br. J. Haematol.*, 2003; 121:749-757.

[143] Greipp, P.R., San Miguel, J.F., Durie, B.G.M., et al. International Staging System for Multiple Myeloma. *J. Clin. Oncol.*, 2005; 23: 1-9.

[144] Ščudla, V., Ordeltová, M. Vyšetření proliferačních charakteristik plasmocytů u mnohočetného myelomu. I. Přehled dosavadních metodických přístupů. *Hematol. Transf.*, 1998; 4: 16-21.

[145] Bataille, R. A cellular model for myeloma cell growth and proliferation. *Hematol. J.*, 2002; 3: 48.

[146] Zubian, G.B. Multiple myeloma: clinical evaluation of plasma cell lymphoproliferative disorders and initial management. *Semin. Hematol.*, 1997; 34: 29-39.

[147] Bergsagel, P.L. Individualizing therapy using molecular markers in multiple myeloma. *Clin. Lymphoma Myeloma*, 2007; 7: 170- 174.

In: Multiple Myeloma: Symptoms, Diagnosis and Treatment ISBN 978-1-60876-108-1
Editors: M. Georgiev and Ev. Bachev

Chapter 2

Wnt Signaling Pathways in Multiple Myeloma

***Ya-Wei Qiang*[*1] *and Stuart Rudikoff*[2]**
[1]Myeloma Institute for Research and Therapy,
University of Arkansas for Medical Sciences, Little Rock, AR, 72205, USA
[2]Laboratory of Cellular and Molecular Biology,
National Cancer Institute, NIH, Bethesda, MD 20892, USA

Abstract

Multiple myeloma is a malignancy of terminally differentiated, antibody-secreting plasma cells frequently associated with osteolytic bone lesions. Wnt signaling is critical in normal bone development and homeostasis, and defects in Wnt signaling pathways have been associated with skeletal diseases. Recent identification of activated Wnt signaling and production of Wnt antagonists (e.g. Dkk1) in multiple myeloma (MM) has attracted attention to the importance of this signaling pathway in myeloma pathogenesis and osteolytic bone disease. Functional signaling through two distinct Wnt pathways (Wnt/β-catenin and Wnt/RhoA) has been characterized in MM plasma cells. Additionally, Wnt/β-catenin signaling plays a significant role in directly regulating osteoblast function responsible for bone formation and indirectly controlling osteoclast function leading to bone resorption. The disruption of this pathway by myeloma plasma cell-derived Dkk1 in the bone marrow microenvironment results in suppression of osteoblast differentiation and enhanced osteoclast function via inhibition of production of regulatory molecules, such as osteoprotegerin, normally produced by osteoblasts. Activation of Wnt/RhoA signaling is also associated with myeloma cell adhesion and drug resistance. Increase in Wnt/β-catenin signaling by Wnt ligands or blockage of Dkk1 via specific antibody prevents MM-induced bone disease and inhibits myeloma cell growth *in vivo*. Herein, we review the current understanding of Wnt signaling in

* Correspondence: Ya-Wei Qiang, MD, PhD. Myeloma Institute for Research and Therapy. University of Arkansas for Medical Sciences. 4301 West Markham Street, Slot 776. Little Rock, AR 72205. Email: yqiang@uams.edu Tel: (501) 296 1503 Ext:1467. Fax: (501) 686 6442

myeloma pathogenesis and bone disease and discuss potential therapeutic implications of modulating this pathway in the treatment of MM.

1. Introduction

Multiple myeloma (MM) is characterized by bone marrow infiltration of malignant plasma cells which then interact with osteoblasts and osteoclasts, triggering osteolytic bone lesions [1]. Resulting bone disease is one of the most debilitating clinical complications observed in MM pateints. In an effort to elucidate the mechanisms of bone destruction considerable attention has been focused on enhanced bone resorption due to increased osteoclast formation and activity [2,3] induced by MM cells. Osteoclast mediated bone resorption in turn leads to the release of growth factors, such as insulin-like growth factor (IGF)-1, from the bone matrix which further stimulate myeloma cell growth [4].This reciprocal interaction between MM cells and osteoclasts results in a "vicious cycle" promoting continued disease progression.

Recently, impaired osteoblast function, leading to reduced bone formation has also been suggested to play a role in MM bone lesion development [5,6]. In the context of this hypothesis, a number of studies have reported fewer osteoblasts and decreased bone formation in MM patients with higher levels of plasma cell infiltration [7,8]. Supporting evidence for this hypothesis comes from the observation that bisphosphonates, which inhibit osteoclast activity and bone resorption, fail to enhance bone formation and recovery of osteolytic bone lesions in MM patients [9].

The results of multiple studies have lead to the current view of MM-associated bone disease as uncoupled bone remodeling. This process involves both enhanced osteoclast resorption resulting from increased osteoclast activity and decreased bone formation resulting from MM-mediated suppression of osteoblast differentiation [5,6].The regulation of bone remodeling is an active and dynamic process orchestrated by bone forming osteoblasts and bone-resorbing osteoclasts. The dysregulation of signaling pathways that control osteoblast and osteoclast differentiation or function may lead to uncoupled bone remodeling and disease. Recent identification of activated Wnt signaling in regulation of normal bone remodeling and production of Wnt antagonists (e.g. Dkk1) in MM has attracted attention to the potential importance of this signaling pathway in myeloma pathogenesis and MM-triggered osteolytic bone disease.

An understanding of how this signaling pathway regulates interactions between MM cells and neighboring osteoblasts and osteoblasts may prove critical to a comprehensive assessment of myeloma disease progression and treatment. In this review, we discuss current progress in the study of functional Wnt signaling in myeloma cells, osteoblasts and osteoclasts with particular attention to the molecular mechanism by which MM cells trigger bone disease by disrupting Wnt signaling. We further explore the potential possibility of targeting this pathway for the design of novel therapeutic strategies for treatment of MM and associated bone disease.

2. Wnt Signaling Pathway

2.1. Overview

Wnt family members are defined by sequence homology to *Drosophila* wingless [10,11] and the murine *int*-1 (Wnt) proto-oncogene identified in 1982 by Nusse and Varmus [12]. At least 19 Wnt proteins exhibiting unique expression patterns and distinct developmental functions have been identified in humans to date [13]. Wnts comprise a large family of 39- to 46-kDa, cystein-rich, secreted, lipid-modified glycoproteins which are hydrophobic and are primarily associated with cell membranes and the extracellular matrix [14,15]. Wnts exert their biological functions by binding to cognate surface receptors and activating receptor coupled signal transduction pathways. Wnt signaling is required for embryonic developmental processes related to formation of brain, heart, kidney and lung [16,17]. Wnt signaling further regulates a variety of cellular activities including cell fate determination, proliferation, differentiation, migration, polarity, and gene expression [17-19]. Recently, Wnts have been identified as playing an important role in bone development [20,21] and modulation of this pathway has been suggested to be associated with myeloma pathogenesis and MM-triggered bone destruction [22-26,103].

2.2. Canonical Wnt/β-Catenin Pathway

Wnts activate at least three distinct intracellular signaling cascades: the canonical Wnt or Wnt/β-catenin pathway [13], the calcium flux pathway [27] and the Wnt planar polarity (RhoA) pathway [28]. Activation of the Wnt/β-catenin pathway is initiated when Wnts bind to frizzled (Fz) receptor and co-receptors LRP5/6 (low-density lipoprotein receptor-related protein) [29-32] (Figure 1). In the absence of Wnt ligand binding and pathway activation, β-catenin is phosphorylated by GSK3β in a complex including axin, [33] the adenomatous polyposis coli (APC) protein [34], and casein kinase I alpha (CKIα) [35]. Phosphorylation occurs first at serine 45 and is indispensable for subsequent phosphorylation at serines 33 and 37 [35]. Phosphorylation targets β-catenin for subsequent ubiquitination and transport to the 26S proteasome for degradation [36]. This process prevents the cytosolic accumulation of β-catenin and maintains β-catenin at levels that restrict its function as a potential transcription factor.

Wnt binding to Fz/LRP leads to activation of downstream elements termed Dishevelled (Dvl) proteins, which, in combination with other cellular proteins (FRAT), disrupt the GSK3β/APC/axin complex. As a result, β-catenin is not phosphorylated and degraded, but accumulates in the cytoplasm and subsequently translocates to the nucleus, where it is found in association with members of the T-cell factor (TCF)/lymphocyte enhancer factor (LEF)-1 transcription family [18] (Figure 1). TCF-1 and LEF-1 were originally cloned as T cell–specific genes [37,38] and later shown to function as transcriptional activators in association with β-catenin [39]. LEF-1 was also demonstrated to be expressed in certain B lineage cells [37] but TCF-1 appears to be restricted to T cells in adult animals.

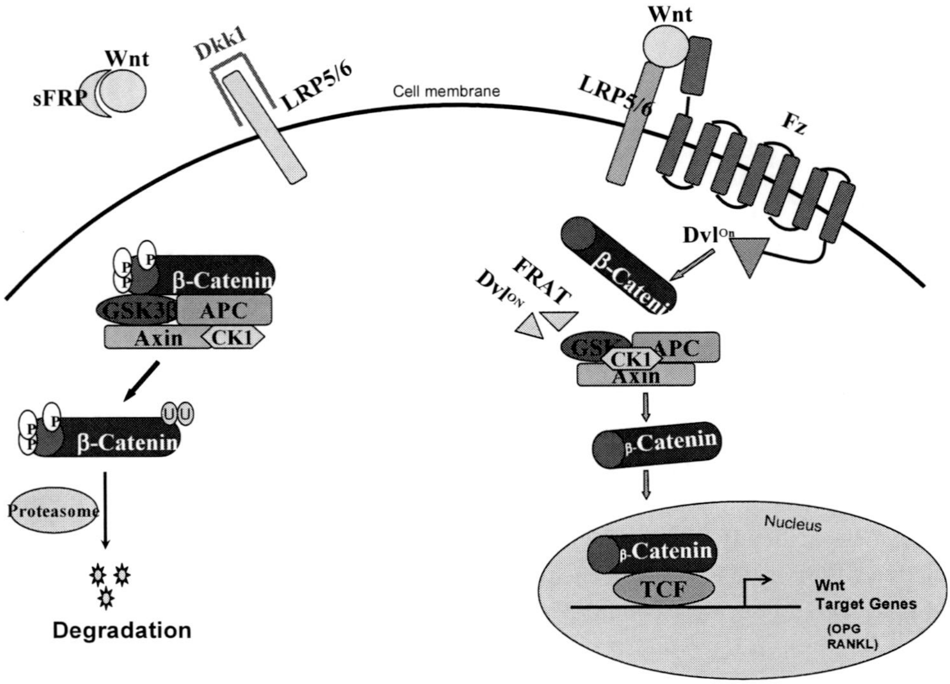

Figure 1. Canonical Wnt signaling pathway. In the absence of Wnt binding to receptors (left side), β-catenin localizes in the cytoplasm in complexes with APC, Axin and GSK3β. In these complexs β-catenin is phosphorylated which 'tags' the protein for subsequent ubiquitination and degradation in the proteasome. Wnt binding to receptors may be blocked either by direct interaction with sFRPs or interference with the LRP5/6 co-receptor by Dkk1. Initiation of Wnt signaling (right side) occurring upon binding of Wnt to Fz and LRP5/6 receptors, leads to activation of downstream elements (Dvl, FRAT) which disrupt the APC, Axin, GSK3β complex leading to an accumulation of non-phosphorylated β-catenin. β-catenin then translocates into the nucleus where, in conjunction with TCF/LEF, functions as a transcription activator regulating expression of specific genes such as OPG and RANKL.

Two other members of this family have been identified in the mouse, TCF-3 and -4, but expression of both is largely restricted to embryonic development and neither is found in lymphoid tissue or cell lines [39,40]. TCF/LEF-1 transcription factors are best characterized as nuclear targets of β-catenin. Upon interaction with TCF/LEF-1, β-catenin displaces co-repressors and recruits transcriptional co-activators resulting in activation of target genes including osteoprotegerin (OPG) and receptor activator of nuclear factor kappa B ligand (RANKL) [41-43]. The Wnt/β-catenin pathway is activated in MM cells [22] although the biological consequences of this activation remain to be clearly defined.

2.3. Wnt/RhoA Pathway

In addition to the Wnt/β-catenin pathway, Wnt/RhoA has been demonstrated to be functional in myeloma cells [23]. Activation of this pathway does not require the LRP co-receptor and results in activation of RhoA and associated downstream kinases [44-48]. RhoA is a member of a family of small guanosine triphosphate (GTP)-ases that includes Rac and Cdc42 [49]. This pathway has been implicated in cell motility and adhesion [50] and several cell types, including melanoma [51] and intestinal epithelial cells [52], have been shown to respond with changes in these properties in response to a variety of Wnts. Wnt mediated migration appears to require activation of both RhoA and, in melanoma cells, members of the protein kinase C (PKC) family of isoenzymes [53] which have also been reported to be involved in other aspects of Wnt signaling [27,54]. Activation of PKCs has been associated with a third Wnt signaling pathway characterized by calcium flux and likely involving G-protein coupled receptors [55,56].

2.4. Wnt Antagonists

Extracellular inhibitors that block Wnt signaling by interruption of receptors and co-receptors have recently been discovered. Two classes of Wnt antagonist have been well studied (Figure 1) and include members of the secreted Frizzled receptor protein (sFRP) family and members of the Dickkopf (Dkk) family [29,57]. Other antagonists, including SOST/Sclerostin [58] and Wnt-inhibitory factor-I (WIF-1) [59] have not been as well characterized.

Five members of the sFRP family have been identified (sFRP-1, -2, -3 (FRZB), -4 and-5 [60-63]) based on homology to the extracellular domains of Fz receptors. This family of secreted proteins acts as decoy receptors and directly binds to Wnts thereby altering the ability of Wnts to bind to the cellular Wnt receptor complex [60-63]. Thus, the sFRP family is proposed to suppress both canonical and non-canonical pathways. It should be noted that sFRP1 potentiates Wnt activity at low concentrations, rather than inhibiting [64].

The Dkk family consists of four members including Dkk-1, -2, -3 and -4. Unlike the sFRP family, Dkk proteins specifically inhibit canonical Wnt signaling by binding to LRP5/6 co-receptors of the Wnt receptor complex rather than Wnt proteins [29,65,66]. To date, Dkk1, Dkk2 and Dkk4 have been shown to function as Wnt antagonists, while Dkk3 has no effect on Wnt signaling [57,67] Dkk1, the most well studied member of this family, was initially cloned as a head inducer in Xenopus embryos [29,68] and later was identified as an antagonist for Wnt/β-catenin signaling. In addition to binding LRP5/6 to block activation of the Wnt signaling pathway [29,66], Dkk1 has been reported to interact with other transmembrane proteins of the Kremen family, Kremen1 (Krm1) and Kremen 2 (Krm2) to function as a Wnt inhibitor [70].

3. Wnt Signaling in MM Plasma Cells

3.1. Activation of Wnt/β-Catenin Pathway in MM Cells

The Wnt/β-catenin signaling pathway is activated in myeloma plasma cells, despite an absence of activation in B-cell lymphoma which reflects the preceding stage to plasma cells in B cell development [22,23,71]. Plasma cell lines express multiple Frizzled receptors (as many as 9 in a single line), and all express either the LRP5 or LRP6 co-receptor. Frizzled and LRP5/6 are also expressed in primary plasma cells from MM pateints. Wnt3a treatment of myeloma cells leads to activation of the Wnt/β-catenin pathway as evidenced by modulation of downstream elements in the pathway including an increase in Dvl-2, an increase and phosphorylation of Dvl-3, and stabilization of β-catenin resulting in transcriptional activation, presumably through an LEF-1-mediated process (LEF-1 is the only member of the TCF/LEF-1 family expressed in these cells) [22,26].

3.2. Biological Effect of Canonical Wnt Signaling in MM Cells

Although Wnt signaling has been shown to be activated in response to Wnt3a stimulation, such activation does not appear to have a direct effect on myeloma cell growth [22]. In *vitro* studies have demonstrated that neither recombinant Wnt3a (rWnt3a) nor Wnt3a containing media had an effect on growth of myeloma cells, and overexpression of Wnt3a in myeloma cells did not confer a growth advantage *in vitro* [23] or when grown subcutaneously in SCID mice [26]. Similarly, inhibition of Wnt signaling, by introduction of rDKK1 or sFRP1 into myeloma cell culture or by transfection of *Dkk1* into myeloma cells [22] had no direct effect on myeloma cell proliferation [22,72]. Conversely, other studies using Wnt3a-conditioned media, rather than purified, rWnt3a, showed that Wnt3a could promote myeloma cell growth *in vitro* [73] and a chemical compound, PKF115-584, which interrupts the interaction of transcriptionally active β-catenin and the TCF complex, induces apoptosis in myeloma cell lines and primary plasma cells from MM patients [74]. Recent observations from this lab suggest that ectopic overexpression of β-catenin induces apoptosis in myeloma cells [69]. Notwithstanding this conflicting data on the effect of activation of canonical Wnt signaling in *in vitro* studies, *in vivo* experiments have demonstrated that increased Wnt signaling in myeloma cells (by expression or administration of Wnt3a [26], by inhibition of Dkk1 activity via neutralizing antibody [75] or by inhibition of GSK3β activity using lithium chloride [76]) suppresses myeloma growth in the bone marrow of myeloma bearing mice. Thus, it is suggested that activation of the Wnt/β-catenin pathway in the bone marrow environment either directly or indirectly affects MM expansion.

3.3. Effect of Activation of Wnt/RhoA Pathway on MM Cells

Activation of the Wnt/Rho A pathway regulates myeloma cell adhesion [22,23] and is responsible for adhesion-mediated drug resistance [77]. In vitro experiments have demonstrated in MM cells that activation of the Wnt/RhoA pathway in response to Wnt3a leads to striking morphological changes resulting in rearrangement of the actin cytoskeleton and adhesion of these normally suspension growing lymphocytes to culture plates [22,23]. Activation of Wnt/RhoA is associated with myeloma adhesion to bone marrow stromal cells and increased adhesion-induced drug resistance (CAM-DR) [77]. High endogenous expression of Wnt3 in myeloma cells resulted in tight adherence to human bone marrow stromal cells compared with low level Wnt3 expression. Silencing Wnt3a expression by small interfering RNA specific to Wnt3a significantly decreased the CAM-DR effect [77].

The morphological changes and increased adhesion associated with Wnt responsiveness strongly suggest enhanced interaction with neighboring mesenchymal stem cells (MSCs) and osteoclasts which is critical for MM progression [78-81]. Furthermore, dysregulation of Wnt signaling via secretion of Wnt antagonists (e.g., Dkk1, sFRPs) by myeloma plasma cells may indirectly (as a result of the effects of these factors on MSCs and osteoclasts) affect disease manifestation. In this context, it is noteworthy that bone lesions are the most common pathological feature of MM, resulting from an imbalance in the normal levels of bone-forming osteoblasts and bone-degrading osteoclasts.

4. Wnt Signaling in Osteoblastogenesis and MM-Triggered Bone Lesions

4.1. Osteoblast Differentiation and Bone Formation

Osteoblasts differentiate (Figure 2) from bone marrow–derived pluripotent MSCs of the colony forming unit-fibroblast (CFU-F) lineage, which also produces fibroblasts, myoblasts, adipocytes, and chondrocytes [82-84]. Osteoblasts are bone-forming cells that synthesize bone matrix by secreting collagen and causing calcium salts and phosphorus to mineralize bone tissue. During new bone layer formation, osteoblasts differentiate into terminal stage osteocytes. The canonical Wnt signaling pathway plays a crucial role in normal bone development [21,85-96] in the regulation of both osteoblasts and osteoclasts (Figure 2). In osteoblasts, Wnt signaling influences three major developmental functions: the commitment of MSCs to an osteoblast stem cell type; stimulation of osteoblast proliferation; and promotion of osteoblast and osteocyte survival [92,97-99].

4.2. Role of Canonical Wnt Signaling in Osteoblastogenesis

A role for Wnt signaling in osteoblast biology was initially suggested by Bradbury [100]. However, seminal discoveries elucidating the importance of the canonical Wnt signaling pathway in osteoblastogenesis stem from observations that inactivating mutations of the *LRP5* Wnt co-receptor gene cause osteoporosis-pseudoglioma syndrome (OPPG) [89]. Subsequently, it was shown that a separate and distinct mutation in the same gene, presumably leading to inhibition of Dkk1 binding, results in high bone density [86,94]. Furthermore, deletion of *Lrp5* in a mouse model inhibited osteoblast differentiation [92]. The importance of Wnt/β-catenin signaling in regulating osteoblastogenesis is further supported by the role of β-catenin in the determination of cell fate between osteoblasts and chondrocytes. β-catenin is required for promoting MSC differentiation toward the osteoblast lineage and away from chondrocytes [87,90]. Activation of this pathway through Wnt10 promotes the development of mesenchymal differentiation into osteoblasts, but inhibits adipocyte formation by suppressing the expression of peroxisome proliferator factor-activated receptor γ, an adipogenic transcriptional factor [101] (Figure 2). Additionally, overexpression of Wnt7b and β-catenin in pluripotent C3H10T1/2 cells induces osteoblast differentiation [91,95].

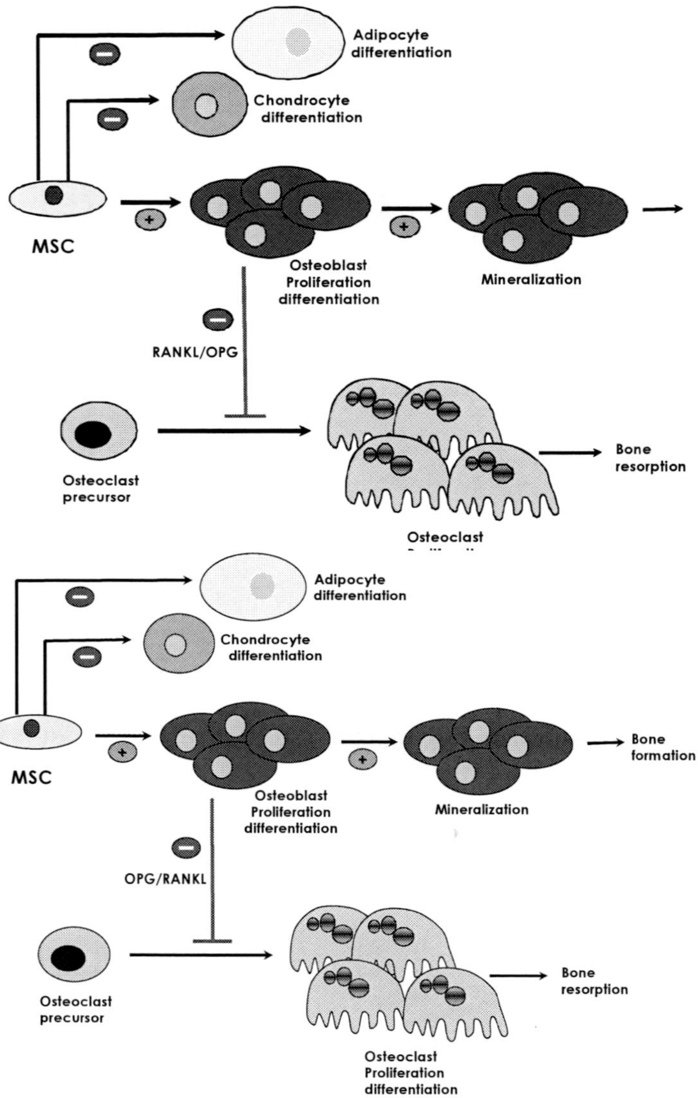

Figure 2. The Wnt pathway directly regulates MSC differentiation into osteoblasts and indirectly regulates osteoclastogenesis. Wnt signaling regulates the commitment of pluripotent MSCs toward osteoblast lineage by inhibiting differentiation into adipocyte and chondrocyte lineages. Signaling in this pathway is also critical to the further proliferation and differentiation of osteoblasts (green plus signs) while, at the same time, regulating osteoclast development (red minus sign) by controlling RANKL/OPG ratios. Inhibition of Wnt signaling increases the RANKL/OPG ratio shifting the balance in favor of osteoclast production and bone destruction.

4.3. Suppression of Osteoblast Differentiation by Wnt Antagonists in MM

4.3.1. Expression of Dkk1 in MM Cells

Suppression of osteoblast differentiation via inhibition of canonical Wnt signaling by MM secreted Wnt antagonists is likely to be one of the most important molecular mechanisms in osteolytic disease associated with MM [102,103] (Figure 3). Initially, gene expression profiling revealed that Dkk1 mRNA expression levels from plasma cells of 173 patients showed a direct correlation with osteolytic lesions [103]. High level expression of Dkk1 mRNA by primary myeloma cells, and correspondingly high Dkk1 protein levels in MM bone marrow plasma, was detected in patients with osteolytic bone lesions [103]. Additional gene expression studies of 171 newly diagnosed MM patients demonstrated that overexpression of Dkk1 mRNA correlated with osteolytic bone disease [104] and, furthermore, with increased Dkk1 protein levels in serum [105,106]. It should be noted that, although Dkk1 is highly expressed in primary plasma cells from patients with bone lesions, it is rarely detected in myeloma cell lines from late stage disease [22,72,107]. Additional studies are needed to ascertain the mechanism responsible for bone disease in this group of late stage patients.

4.3.2. Expression of sFRPs in MM Cells

The sFRP family, comprising the other set of known Wnt antagonists, may also be involved in Wnt-mediated bone disease although the data is more ambiguous. sFRP2 mRNA was found to be expressed in MM cells from pateints with advanced bone lesions and addition of sFRP2 inhibited osteoblast differentiation [108]. However, several other studies indicate that MM cells highly express sFRP3 (FRZB) [109-113]. Gene expression analysis of 351 newly diagnosed MM patients demonstrated increased sFRP2 mRNA in only eight cases, whereas other studies detected only sFRP3 mRNA, but no sFRP3 protein in plasma cells from MM [110,111]. Further studies are obviously required to determine whether sFRP is important in MM-triggered bone disease.

4.3.3. Suppression of Osteoblast differentiation by Dkk1

The molecular mechanism by which MM-derived Dkk1 contributes to bone disease has been suggested to involve suppression of osteoblast differentiation. Canonical Wnt signaling is activated in osteoblastic cell lines and MM-derived Dkk1 is suggested to be responsible for bone destruction via interruption of Wnt signaling in osteoblasts. Multiple Wnt receptors, including Fz-1, 2, 3, 4, 7, 8, and 9 [24], and high levels of TCF1 and TCF4 mRNA are expressed in osteoblast progenitor cells and primary MM-derived MSCs. In response to Wnt3a in these cells, β-catenin accumulates in the cytoplasm, translocates to the nucleus and leads to TCF transcriptional activity [24,25]. Expression of dominant-negative β-catenin attenuated BMP-2–induced alkaline phosphatase activity, an early marker of osteoblast differentiation. Moreover, blocking this pathway by rDkk1 or expression of *Dkk1* mRNA in these cells attenuated osteoblast differentiation. Importantly, cultures of osteoblasts with serum from MM patients containing high concentrations of Dkk1 [24,103] or co-cultures of osteoblasts with *Dkk1*-overexpressing myeloma cells resulted in inhibition of BMP-mediated osteoblast differentiation [24].

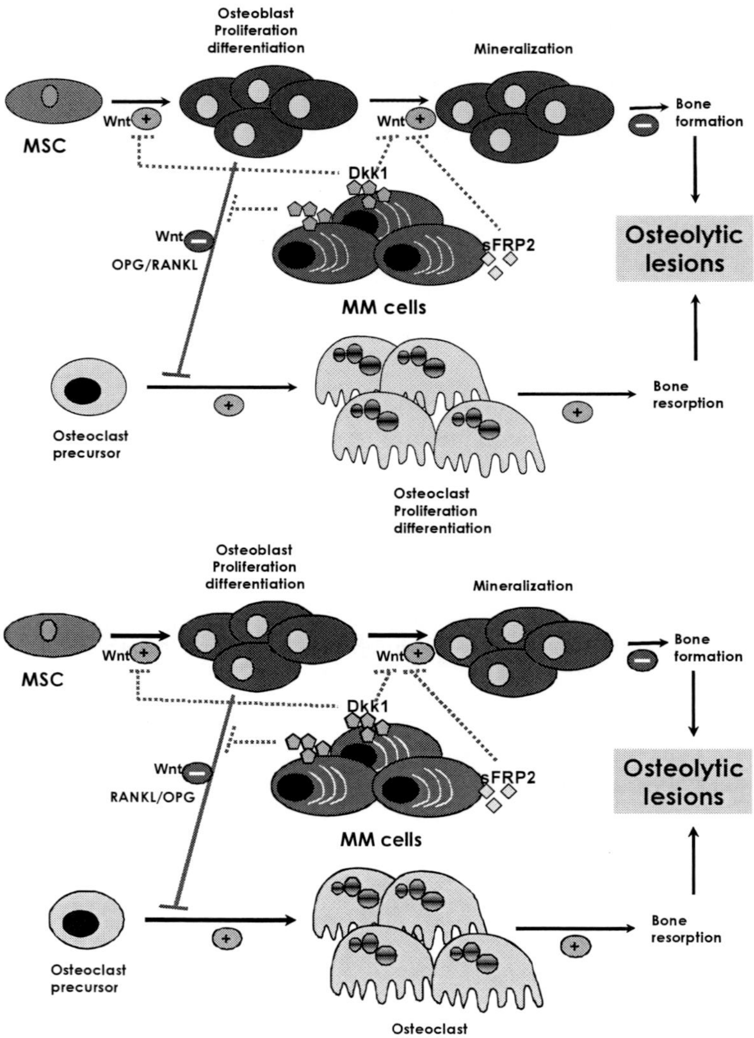

Figure 3. Wnt antagonists attenuate Wnt-promoted osteoblast differentiation and promote osteoclastogenesis. MM cells secrete Dkk1 or sFRP2 which block (red dotted lines) normal Wnt-induced osteoblastogenesis (green positive circles). Furthermore, Dkk1 causes an increase in RANKL/OPG ratio leading to increased osteoclastogenesis. As a result, bone resorption surpasses bone formation leading to net bone destruction and disease.

4.3.4. Inhibition of Dkk1 Increases Osteoblast Numbers in Myeloma Bearing Mice

The restoration of canonical Wnt signaling by inhibition of Dkk1 using neutralizing anti-Dkk1 antibody prevents development of osteolytic bone disease in a myeloma bone disease model using SCID-rab mice. In this model immuno-deficient SCID mice are reconstituted with rabbit bone marrow (in contrast to human fetal bone marrow in the SCID-hu model) prior to introduction of human myeloma cells. Mice were engrafted with primary MM cells from patients expressing varying levels of Dkk1 and treated with control and Dkk1-neutralizing antibodies [75]. Histological examination revealed that myelomatous bones of anti-Dkk1-treated mice had increased numbers of osteocalcin-expressing osteoblasts. Dkk1 inhibition of Wnt-induced osteoblastogenesis was confirmed in studies using the 5T2 murine model of myeloma. Injection of anti-Dkk1 neutralizing antibody into 5T2 MM bearing mice decreased tumor-induced suppression of osteoblast numbers [114]. In support of the suggestion that Dkk1 suppression of Wnt signaling is the cause of impaired osteoblast differentiation, other studies have revealed that an increase in Wnt signaling by administration of Wnt3a to myeloma bearing mice or injection of Wnt3a-expressing myeloma cells into SCID-hu mice increases osteoblast numbers [26]. Inhibition of β-catenin degradation by blocking GSK3β activity using lithium chloride leads to similar results [76].

5. Wnt Signaling in Osteoblast/Osteoclast Crosstalk

5.1. Osteoclast Differentiation and Activity

Osteoblasts maintain bone homeostasis by balancing bone resorption mediated by osteoclasts, with bone formation. Osteoblasts regulate osteoclastogenesis through expression of RANKL and OPG, two key factors critical for osteoclast formation and activity [115-118] in conjunction with other growth factors and chemokines [119-121]. Osteoclasts are activated by binding of RANKL [115,116,122] to its cognate receptor, RANK, while OPG [117] (a soluble member of the tumor necrosis receptor super-family) acts as a naturally occurring decoy receptor that competes with RANK for binding of RANKL [118]. The balance of these two molecules plays a critical role in the control of osteoclastogenesis. MM cells likely stimulate expression of RANKL and suppress expression of OPG by osteoblasts or their progenitors [2,3,123,124,144]. Increased serum levels of RANKL and decreased levels of OPG have been associated with a poor prognosis in MM [125]. Restoring the RANKL/OPG imbalance by RANKL antagonists or recombinant OPG not only reduces MM-associated bone lesions, but halts disease progression in animal models [2,80,126,127].

5.2. Role of Wnt in Regulation of RANKL/OPG Axis

The Wnt signaling pathway has also been reported to indirectly mediate osteoclastogenesis via regulation of RANKL and OPG production in osteoblast cells (Figure 2). Studies of *in vivo* murine models using transgenic mice expressing active β-catenin in osteoblasts, and therefore demonstrating enhanced Wnt signaling, revealed a decrease in osteoclastogenesis [41]. Similarly, it has been shown that deletion of APC, one component of the complex leading to phosphorylation and degradation of β-catenin, leads to increased Wnt signaling and results in reduced osteoclastogenesis [42]. In these mice, osteoblasts with increased Wnt signaling were found to express high levels of OPG, whereas osteoblasts with reduced Wnt signaling had reduced expression of OPG [41,42]. Moreover, increased Wnt signaling in osteoblasts from these mice led to decreased expression of RANKL in the same cells [42]. These data were confirmed by lithium chloride inhibition of GSK3β (an additional component of the APC complex that phosphorylates β-catenin and 'marks' it for degradation), which similarly led to downregulation of RANKL [43]. Additionally, in co-cultures of murine osteoblasts with spleen cells, knockdown of endogenous sFRP1 expression in osteoblast cell lines by transfection of specific siRNA significantly enhanced osteoclast formation [128] and in embryonic carcinoma cells, increased canonical Wnt signaling activity upregulates OPG mRNA expression [129]. Taken together, these data strongly support the concept of a critical role for Wnt signaling in regulation of the RANKL/OPG axis and, correspondingly, osteoblast/osteoclast development and activity (Figure 2).

5.3. MM-Derived Dkk interrupts Wnt Mediated Regulation of RANKL/OPG

Elevated expression of *Dkk1* by myeloma tumor cells and IL-6–dependent myeloma cell lines, as well as Dkk1 protein in serum of MM patients [103-107,109], are associated with bone lesion formation [103]. Dkk1 not only directly inhibits canonical Wnt signaling-mediated osteoblast differentiation in MM, but also indirectly activates osteoclastogesis by interrupting the normal Wnt-regulated RANKL/OPG axis affected by osteoblasts (Figure 3). In vitro studies using human and murine osteoblasts have demonstrated that MM-derived Dkk1 protein deregulates RANKL/OPG production in osteoblasts [25]. Pretreatment with rDkk1 completely abolished Wnt3a-induced OPG mRNA and protein in mouse and human osteoblasts. Additionally, Wnt3a-induced OPG expression is diminished in osteoblasts co-cultured with a Dkk1-expressing MM cell line or primary MM cells. Finally, bone marrow fluid from 21 MM patients significantly suppressed Wnt3a-induced OPG expression in osteoblasts, while enhancing RANKL in a Dkk1-dependent manner. These results suggest that Dkk1 may be a master regulator of MM-associated osteoblastogenesis by directly interrupting Wnt-regulated differentiation of osteoblasts, which, in turn, indirectly leads to increased osteoclastogenesis via a Dkk-1 mediated increase in local RANKL-to-OPG ratios promoting osteolytic bone lesions.

6. Targetingt Wnt Signaling as a Potential Therapeutic Staregy for Treatment of Osteolytic Bone Lesion in MM

6.1. Increase in Wnt Agonists

Although much remains to be learned about the molecular mechanisms of Wnt signaling, it is reasonable to suggest that increasing Wnt activity by specific targeting of this pathway may be a potential therapeutic strategy in treatment of myeloma bone disease (Figure 4). One possible approach to elevated signaling would be direct administration of Wnts. To explore this possibility, in vivo studies have been performed in which myeloma cells were transfected with Wnt3a or empty vector as control and injected into human bone marrow in SCID-hu mice [26].

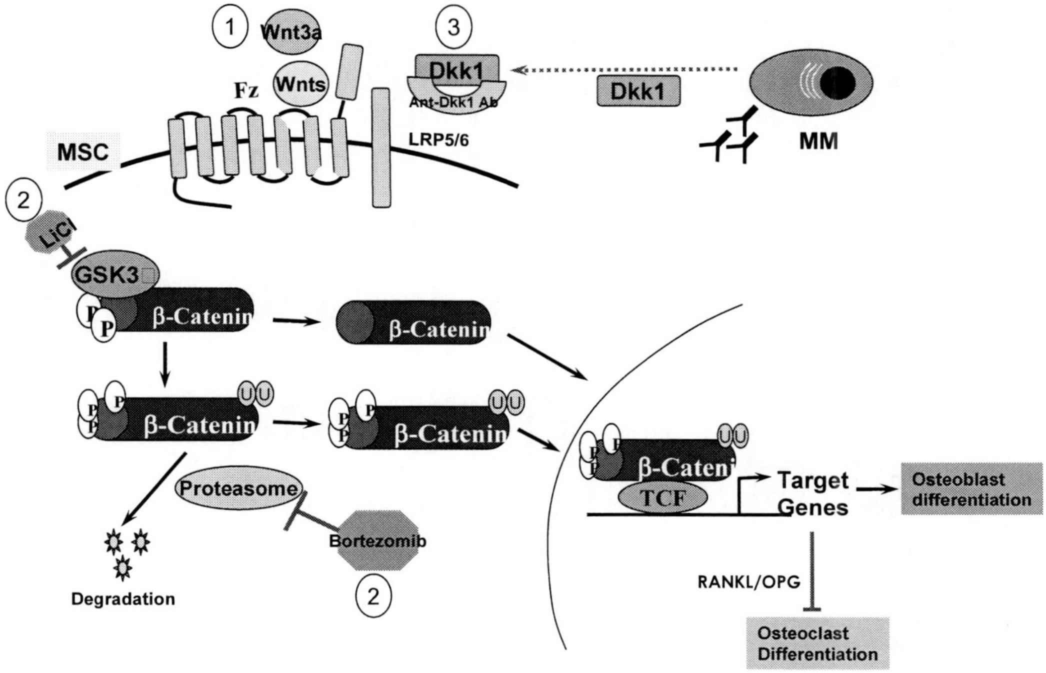

Figure 4. Potential therapeutic strategies for targeting Wnt signaling in the treatment of MM-induced bone disease: 1) Increase in Wnt signaling by administration of Wnts (i.e. Wnt3a) into the bone marrow microenvironment; 2) increase in β-catenin levels by inhibition of β-catenin degradation through suppression of either GSK3β via lithium chloride (LiCl) or proteasome activity via agents such as bortezomib (Bzb); (3) increase in Wnt signaling by blocking inhibitors (Dkk1) using monoclonal antibodies (anti-Dkk1).

While cells stably expressing empty vector grew rapidly and induced a marked reduction in bone mineral density, bones engrafted with Wnt3a-expressing myeloma cells were preserved, exhibited increased osteoblast/osteoclast ratios, and reduced tumor burden. Correspondingly, recombinant Wnt3a treatment of myelomatous SCID-hu mice with primary disease stimulated bone formation and attenuated MM growth [26]. Wnt proteins are extremely difficult to purify and as a result attention has turned to the identification of Wnt agonists. One such candidate is R-spind1 which stimulates Wnt activation by inhibiting internalization of the LRP6 co-receptor. R-spind1 has been shown to induce osteoblast differentiation and promote OPG secretion [130,131] and is a potential candidate for future trials involving the treatment of bone disease.

6.2. Prevention of β-Catenin Degradation

An alternative to the direct delivery of Wnts, or the use of Wnt agonists, to increase Wnt signaling is the identification of agents that prevent degradation of components of the Wnt/β-catenin pathway. As an example, LiCl is a well studied inhibitor of the GSK3β kinase that phosphorylates β-catenin promoting its degradation. Lithium chloride induces increases in β-catenin protein and TCF transcriptional activity in osteoblast cells [132]. Administration of LiCl in myeloma bearing mice inhibits myeloma bone disease and decreases tumor burden in bone [76]. It should be noted, however, that in the 5TGM1 murine myeloma model, LiCl administration increased tumor growth when cells were inoculated subcutaneously. It can be argued that subcutaneous injection is not an accurate reflection of human myeloma disease, but these studies raise a caution for careful evaluation of GSK3β inhibitors before clinical use as bone anabolic agents. An alternate approach to targeting enzymes involved in Wnt/β-catenin processing is the inhibition of proteasomes, the actual sites of β-catenin degradation. In this regard, the proteasome inhibitor Bortezomib has shown efficacy as an anti-myeloma agent. Bortezomib stimulates osteoblast differentiation and induces increases in both free and active forms of β-catenin protein in the cytoplasm and nucleus of mouse and human osteoblast progenitor cell lines, and in primary normal human MSC as well as MSC from MM patients [132]. Bortezomib induces an increase in ubiquitinated β-catenin indicating inhibition of proteasome-mediated degradation (Figure 4) as ubiquitin addition 'marks' proteins for proteasome localization and degradation. Correspondingly, following treatment an increase in TCF transcriptional activity is seen.

Blocking the activation of β-catenin/TCF signaling by expression of dominant negative TCF attenuated bortezomib-induced matrix mineralization indicating that bortezomib induced MSC differentiation into osteoblasts through activation of β-catenin/TCF signaling. These results provide insights into a clinically relevant mechanism of action of bortezomib and as such a rational for its use in the treatment of diseases related to suppression of Wnt/β-catenin/TCF signaling. Indeed, the clinical efficacy of bortezomib, currently used as a frontline treatment of MM, has been linked to an increase in bone anabolic markers in MM patients [133,134] and reduced myeloma induced bone disease in animal models *in vivo* [135,136,145].

6.3. Inhibition of Dkk1

Additional potential therapeutic targets directed toward increasing Wnt signaling as a treatment for MM-triggered bone disease include Dkk1. In an *in vivo* model, SCID-rab mice were engrafted with primary MM cells expressing varying levels of Dkk1 and subsequently treated with control and anti-Dkk1 neutralizing antibodies [75]. Whereas bone mineral density (BMD) of the implanted myelomatous bone in control antibody treated mice was reduced during the experimental period, BMD in mice treated with anti-Dkk1 increased significantly from pretreatment levels. Histological examination revealed that myelomatous bones of anti-Dkk1-treated mice had increased numbers of osteocalcin-expressing osteoblasts and reduced numbers of multinucleated TRAP-expressing osteoclasts. The role of Dkk1 in

MM-triggered bone disease has been confirmed in the 5T2 murine myeloma model. Injection of 5T2 MM cells into appropriate recipient mice leads to the development of osteolytic bone lesions [114], but treatment with anti-Dkk1 neutralizing antibody results in decreased tumor-induced suppression of osteoblast number and increase in bone formation. Efficacy of anti-Dkk1 antibody on myeloma bone disease is currently being assessed in phase I clinical trials.

7. Perspectives (Summary and Future Directions)

Activation of the Wnt/β-catenin pathway is required for normal bone development and osteoblastogenesis. Suppression of osteoblast differentiation and dysregulation of osteoclastogenesis by MM-derived Dkk1 is likely one of the important molecular mechanisms associated with osteolytic bone disease. It remains to be determined if similar mechanisms cause bone lesions in advanced MM as Dkk1 is not expressed in MM cell lines which are derived from late stage patients. It is also unclear if other Wnt inhibitors, in particular sFRP3 which is also highly expressed in MM plasma cells, similarly play a role in osteolytic bone disease. These questions will need to be addressed by studies focusing on the role of the sFRP family in osteoblast differentiation.

β-catenin is highly expressed endogenously in myeloma cell lines and primary myeloma cells, in contrast to lymphoma cells representing the preceding stage of B lymphocyte development. The cause for constitutive accumulation of β-catenin in myeloma cells has not been determined. Although mutations in the adenomatous polyposis coli (APC) and β-catenin (CTNNB1) genes in colorectal cancer are thought to be responsible for β-catenin accumulation in this and other cancers, such mutations are not found in myeloma cell lines and primary myeloma plasma cells [22,73]. In this context, recent studies have reported that methylation occurs in the sFRP1 gene in 42% of myeloma cells and suggests this may, in some way, cause constitutive activation of the Wnt/β-catenin pathway in myeloma [137]. However, this suggestion is difficult to reconcile with the presence of β-catenin in primary myeloma plasma cells where Dkk1 and sFRP3 are readily expressed [103,107,109].

While the Wnt/β-catenin pathway is activated in MM plasma cells, much remains to be learned about the downstream targets of β-catenin/TCF transcriptional activity. In osteoblast progenitor cell lines and primary MSC, OPG and RANKL have been identified as downstream genes regulated by β-catenin/TCF. These two key factors are responsible for regulation of osteoclast maturation and activity by osteoblasts in the orchestration of bone formation and resorption. Other Wnt target genes that have been identified include Myc [138], cyclin D1[139], CD44 [140] and fibronectin [141]. However, expression of these genes is not increased by Wnt3a treatment of myeloma cells as evaluated by microarray analysis (Qiang et al, unpublished data). The basis for TCF failure to regulate growth-related genes in the nucleus of myeloma remains unknown. However, in other systems, CDK8 kinase activity was found necessary for β-catenin-driven transformation and for expression of several β-catenin transcriptional targets [142] and E2F1 represses β-catenin transcription activity [143]. Studies focused on elucidating the role of CDK8 kinase and E2F1 on β-catenin /TCF complex regulation in the nucleus of myeloma cells may provide insights to this question.

Given that activation of the Wnt/β-catenin pathway is required for normal bone development and osteoblastogenesis, important questions remain to be answered regarding this signaling pathway. Which specific Wnts and Wnt receptors in MSCs are functionally important? Multiple Wnts are highly expressed in normal MSCs and, importantly, there are constitutive, high free β-catenin levels in primary MSCs and MSC cell lines. Is Wnt signaling in these cells paracrine or autocrine in nature? While sFRP proteins are thought to directly interact with Wnts, there is no known specificity to interactions between members of these two families so that sFRPs are unlikely to be useful in identifying biologically important Wnts. Similarly, Dkk proteins inhibit Wnts by blocking co-receptors and, therefore, are also unlikely to be useful in analyzing Wnt specificity. However, one possible approach is the use of siRNA technology to 'knockdown' specific Wnts, which may permit an analysis of the effects of each ligand individually.

In summary, activation of the Wnt/β-catenin pathway is necessary for MSC/osteoblast differentiation [24] and maintenance of osteoblast/osteoclast balance by regulation of RANKL/OPG [25]. Suppression of Wnt/β-catenin signaling by myeloma-derived Dkk1 in osteoblasts promotes osteoclastogenesis and myeloma bone disease although direct effects of Wnt/β-catenin on osteoclast maturation and activity remain to be determined. Given this critical role of Wnt signaling in the complex process of bone remodeling, and the ability of myeloma derived proteins to create biologically harmful imbalances, the Wnt pathway would appear to be a prime candidate for therapeutic targeting in the treatment of this, and possibly other, disease(s) with associated bone lesions.

Acknowledgment

The authors would like to thank Drs. John D. Shaughnessy Jr and Bart Barlogie for their continuous support. This work was supported by a Senior Research Grant from the Multiple Myeloma Research Foundation to Y W Q.

References

[1] Kyle RA, Rajkumar SV. Multiple myeloma. *N. Engl. J. Med.* 2004;351:1860-1873.

[2] Pearse RN, Sordillo EM, Yaccoby S, et al. Multiple myeloma disrupts the TRANCE/ osteoprotegerin cytokine axis to trigger bone destruction and promote tumor progression. *Proc. Natl. Acad. Sci. SA.* 2001;98:11581-11586.

[3] Sezer O, Heider U, Zavrski I, Kuhne CA, Hofbauer LC. RANK ligand and osteoprotegerin in myeloma bone disease. *Blood.* 2003;101:2094-2098.

[4] Roodman GD. Pathogenesis of myeloma bone disease. *Blood Cells Mol. Dis.* 2004;32:290-292.

[5] Bataille R, Chappard D, Marcelli C, et al. Recruitment of new osteoblasts and osteoclasts is the earliest critical event in the pathogenesis of human multiple myeloma. *J. Clin. Invest.* 1991;88:62-66.
[6] Roodman GD. Mechanisms of bone metastasis. *N. Engl. J. Med.* 2004;350:1655-1664.
[7] Bataille R, Chappard D, Marcelli C, et al. Mechanisms of bone destruction in multiple myeloma: the importance of an unbalanced process in determining the severity of lytic bone disease. *J. Clin. Oncol.* 1989;7:1909-1914.
[8] Taube T, Beneton MN, McCloskey EV, Rogers S, Greaves M, Kanis JA. Abnormal bone remodelling in patients with myelomatosis and normal biochemical indices of bone resorption. *Eur. J. Haematol.* 1992;49:192-198.
[9] Berenson JR. Zoledronic acid in cancer patients with bone metastases: results of Phase I and II trials. *Semin. Oncol.* 2001;28:25-34.
[10] Nusslein-Volhard C, Wieschaus E. Mutations affecting segment number and polarity in Drosophila. *Nature*. 1980;287:795-801.
[11] Rijsewijk F, Schuermann M, Wagenaar E, Parren P, Weigel D, Nusse R. The Drosophila homolog of the mouse mammary oncogene int-1 is identical to the segment polarity gene wingless. *Cell.* 1987;50:649-657.
[12] Nusse R, Varmus HE. Many tumors induced by the mouse mammary tumor virus contain a provirus integrated in the same region of the host genome. *Cell.* 1982;31:99-109.
[13] Gordon MD, Nusse R. Wnt signaling: multiple pathways, multiple receptors, and multiple transcription factors. *J. Biol. Chem.* 2006;281:22429-22433.
[14] Nusse R. Wnt signaling and stem cell control. Cell Res. 2008;18:523-527.
[15] Willert K, Brown JD, Danenberg E, et al. Wnt proteins are lipid-modified and can act as stem cell growth factors. *Nature*. 2003;423:448-452.
[16] Endo Y, Rubin JS. Wnt signaling and neurite outgrowth: insights and questions. *Cancer Sci.* 2007;98:1311-1317.
[17] Logan CY, Nusse R. The Wnt signaling pathway in development and disease. *Annu. Rev. Cell Dev Biol.* 2004;20:781-810.
[18] Clevers H. Wnt/beta-catenin signaling in development and disease. *Cell.* 2006;127:469-480.
[19] Fuerer C, Nusse R, Ten Berge D. Wnt signalling in development and disease. Max Delbruck Center for Molecular Medicine meeting on Wnt signaling in Development and Disease. *EMBO Rep.* 2008;9:134-138.
[20] Kirstetter P, Anderson K, Porse BT, Jacobsen SE, Nerlov C. Activation of the canonical Wnt pathway leads to loss of hematopoietic stem cell repopulation and multilineage differentiation block. *Nat. Immunol.* 2006;7:1048-1056.
[21] Westendorf JJ, Kahler RA, Schroeder TM. Wnt signaling in osteoblasts and bone diseases. *Gene*. 2004;341:19-39.
[22] Qiang Y, Endo Y, Rubin J, Rudikoff S. Wnt signaling in B-cell neoplasia. *Oncogene.* 2003;22:1536-1545.
[23] Qiang Y, Walsh K, Yao L, et al. Wnts induce migration and invasion of myeloma plasma cells. *Blood.* 2005;106:1786-1793.

[24] Qiang YW, Barlogie B, Rudikoff S, Shaughnessy JD, Jr. Dkk1-induced inhibition of Wnt signaling in osteoblast differentiation is an underlying mechanism of bone loss in multiple myeloma. *Bone*. 2008;42:669-680.

[25] Qiang YW, Chen Y, Stephens O, et al. Myeloma-derived Dickkopf-1 disrupts Wnt-regulated osteoprotegerin and RANKL production by osteoblasts: a potential mechanism underlying osteolytic bone lesions in multiple myeloma. *Blood.* 2008.

[26] Qiang YW, Shaughnessy JD, Jr., Yaccoby S. Wnt3a signaling within bone inhibits multiple myeloma bone disease and tumor growth. *Blood*. 2008;112:374-382.

[27] Kuhl M, Sheldahl L, Malbon C, Moon R. Ca(2+)/calmodulin-dependent protein kinase II is stimulated by Wnt and Frizzled homologs and promotes ventral cell fates in Xenopus. *J. Biol. Chem*. 2000;275:12701-12711.

[28] Habas R, Dawid I, He X. Coactivation of Rac and Rho by Wnt/Frizzled signaling is required for vertebrate gastrulation. *Genes Dev*. 2003;17:295-309.

[29] Mao B, Wu W, Li Y, et al. LDL-receptor-related protein 6 is a receptor for Dickkopf proteins. *Nature*. 2001;411:321-325.

[30] Pinson KI, Brennan J, Monkley S, Avery BJ, Skarnes WC. An LDL-receptor-related protein mediates Wnt signalling in mice. *Nature.* 2000;407(6803):535-538.

[31] Tamai K, Semenov M, Kato Y, et al. LDL-receptor-related proteins in Wnt signal transduction. *Nature.* 2000;407:530-535.

[32] Wehrli M, Dougan ST, Caldwell K, et al. arrow encodes an LDL-receptor-related protein essential for Wingless signalling. *Nature*. 2000;407(6803):527-530.

[33] Willert K, Shibamoto S, Nusse R. Wnt-induced dephosphorylation of axin releases beta-catenin from the axin complex. *Genes Dev*. 1999;13:1768-1773.

[34] Rubinfeld B, Albert I, Porfiri E, Fiol C, Munemitsu S, Polakis P. Binding of GSK3beta to the APC-beta-catenin complex and regulation of complex assembly. *Science.* 1996;272:1023-1026.

[35] Liu C, Li Y, Semenov M, et al. Control of beta-catenin phosphorylation/degradation by a dual-kinase mechanism. *Cell.* 2002;108:837-847.

[36] Aberle H, Bauer A, Stappert J, Kispert A, Kemler R. beta-catenin is a target for the ubiquitin-proteasome pathway. *Embo J.* 1997;16:3797-3804.

[37] Travis A, Amsterdam A, Belanger C, Grosschedl R. LEF-1, a gene encoding a lymphoid-specific protein with an HMG domain, regulates T-cell receptor alpha enhancer function [corrected]. *Genes Dev.* 1991;5:880-894.

[38] van de Wetering M, Oosterwegel M, Dooijes D, Clevers H. Identification and cloning of TCF-1, a T lymphocyte-specific transcription factor containing a sequence-specific HMG box. *Embo J.* 1991;10:123-132.

[39] Behrens J, von Kries JP, Kuhl M, et al. Functional interaction of beta-catenin with the transcription factor LEF-1. *Nature.* 1996;382:638-642.

[40] Arce L, Yokoyama NN, Waterman ML. Diversity of LEF/TCF action in development and disease. *Oncogene.* 2006;25:7492-7504.

[41] Glass DA, 2nd, Bialek P, Ahn JD, et al. Canonical Wnt signaling in differentiated osteoblasts controls osteoclast differentiation. *Dev Cell.* 2005;8:751-764.

[42] Holmen SL, Zylstra CR, Mukherjee A, et al. Essential role of beta-catenin in postnatal bone acquisition. *J. Biol. Chem*. 2005;280:21162-21168.

[43] Spencer GJ, Utting JC, Etheridge SL, Arnett TR, Genever PG. Wnt signalling in osteoblasts regulates expression of the receptor activator of NFkappaB ligand and inhibits osteoclastogenesis in vitro. *J. Cell Sci.* 2006;119:1283-1296.

[44] Strutt D, Weber U, Mlodzik M. The role of RhoA in tissue polarity and Frizzled signalling. *Nature*. 1997;387:292-295.

[45] Winter C, Wang B, Ballew A, et al. Drosophila Rho-associated kinase (Drok) links Frizzled-mediated planar cell polarity signaling to the actin cytoskeleton. *Cell.* 2001;105:81-91.

[46] Habas R, Kato Y, He X. Wnt/Frizzled activation of Rho regulates vertebrate gastrulation and requires a novel Formin homology protein Daam1. *Cell.* 2001;107:843-854.

[47] Zhu S, Liu L, Korzh V, et al. RhoA acts downstream of Wnt5a and Wnt11 to regulat convergence and extension movements by involving effectors Rho kinase and diaphanous: use of zebrafish as an in vivo model for GTPase signaling. *Cell Signal.* 2006;18:359-372.

[48] Kishida S, Yamamoto H, Kikuchi A. Wnt-3a and Dvl induce neurite retraction by activating Rho-associated kinase. *Mol Cell Biol*. 2004;24:4487-4501.

[49] Ridley A, Hall A. The small GTP-binding protein rho regulates the assembly of focal adhesions and actin stress fibers in response to growth factors. *Cell.* 1992;70:389-399.

[50] Nelson W, Nusse R. Convergence of Wnt, beta-catenin, and cadherin pathways. *Science.* 2004;303:1483-1487.

[51] Weeraratna A, Jiang Y, Hostetter G, et al. Wnt5a signaling directly affects cell motility and invasion of metastatic melanoma. *Cancer Cell.* 2002;1:279-288.

[52] Ouko L, Ziegler T, Gu L, Eisenberg L, VW. Y. Wnt11 signaling promotes proliferation, transformation, and migration of IEC6 intestinal epithelial cells. *J. Biol. Chem*. 2004;279:26707-26715.

[53] Mellor H, Parker P. The extended protein kinase C superfamily. *Biochem. J.* 1998;332:281-292.

[54] Kinoshita N, Iioka H, Miyakoshi A, Ueno N. PKC delta is essential for Dishevelled function in a noncanonical Wnt pathway that regulates Xenopus convergent extension movements. *Genes Dev*. 2003;17:1663-1676.

[55] Kuhl M, Sheldahl L, Park M, Miller J, Moon R. The Wnt/Ca2+ pathway: a new vertebrate Wnt signaling pathway takes shape. *Trends Genet*. 2000;16:279-283.

[56] Wang H, Malbon C. Wnt signaling, Ca2+, and cyclic GMP: visualizing Frizzled functions. *Science*. 2003;300:1529-1530.

[57] Kawano Y, Kypta R. Secreted antagonists of the Wnt signalling pathway. *J. Cell Sci.* 2003;116:2627-2634.

[58] Semenov MV, He X. LRP5 mutations linked to high bone mass diseases cause reduced LRP5 binding and inhibition by SOST. *J. Biol. Chem*. 2006;281:38276-38284.

[59] Hsieh JC, Kodjabachian L, Rebbert ML, et al. A new secreted protein that binds to Wnt proteins and inhibits their activities. *Nature*. 1999;398:431-436.

[60] Finch P, He X, Kelley M, et al. Purification and molecular cloning of a secreted, Frizzled-related antagonist of Wnt action. *Proc. Natl. Acad. Sci. USA*. 1997;94:6770-6775.

[61] Hoang B, Moos M, Jr., Vukicevic S, Luyten FP. Primary structure and tissue distribution of FRZB, a novel protein related to Drosophila frizzled, suggest a role in skeletal morphogenesis. *J. Biol. Chem.* 1996;271:26131-26137.

[62] Rattner A, Hsieh JC, Smallwood PM, et al. A family of secreted proteins contains homology to the cysteine-rich ligand-binding domain of frizzled receptors. *Proc. Natl. Acad. Sci. USA*. 1997;94:2859-2863.

[63] Wang S, Krinks M, Lin K, Luyten FP, Moos M, Jr. Frzb, a secreted protein expressed in the Spemann organizer, binds and inhibits Wnt-8. *Cell.* 1997;88:757-766.

[64] Uren A, Reichsman F, Anest V, et al. Secreted frizzled-related protein-1 binds directly to Wingless and is a biphasic modulator of Wnt signaling. *J. Biol. Chem.* 2000;275:4374-4382.

[65] Bafico A, Liu G, Yaniv A, Gazit A, Aaronson SA. Novel mechanism of Wnt signalling inhibition mediated by Dickkopf-1 interaction with LRP6/Arrow. *Nat Cell Biol.* 2001;3:683-686.

[66] Semenov M, Tamai K, Brott B, Kuhl M, Sokol S, He X. Head inducer Dickkopf-1 is a ligand for Wnt coreceptor LRP6. *Curr Biol.* 2001;11:951-961.

[67] Krupnik VE, Sharp JD, Jiang C, et al. Functional and structural diversity of the human Dickkopf gene family. *Gene*. 1999;238:301-313.

[68] Glinka A, Wu W, Delius H, Monaghan AP, Blumenstock C, Niehrs C. Dickkopf-1 is a member of a new family of secreted proteins and functions in head induction. *Nature.* 1998;391:357-362.

[69] Raab MS, Breitkreutz I, Tonon G, et al. Targeting PKC: a novel role for beta-catenin in ER stress and apoptotic signaling. *Blood.* 2009;113:1513-1521.

[70] Mao B, Wu W, Davidson G, et al. Kremen proteins are Dickkopf receptors that regulate Wnt/beta-catenin signalling. *Nature*. 2002;417:664-667.

[71] Qiang Y, Rudikoff S. Wnt signaling in B and T lymphocytes. *Front Biosci* 2004;9:1000-1010.

[72] Colla S, Zhan F, Xiong W, et al. The oxidative stress response regulates DKK1 expression through the JNK signaling cascade in multiple myeloma plasma cells. *Blood.* 2007;109:4470-4477.

[73] Derksen PW, Tjin E, Meijer HP, et al. Illegitimate WNT signaling promotes proliferation of multiple myeloma cells. *Proc. Natl. Acad. Sci. USA*. 2004;101:6122-6127.

[74] Sukhdeo K, Mani M, Zhang Y, et al. Targeting the beta-catenin/TCF transcriptional complex in the treatment of multiple myeloma. *Proc. Natl. Acad. Sci. USA*. 2007;104:7516-7521.

[75] Yaccoby S, Ling W, Zhan F, Walker R, Barlogie B, Shaughnessy JD, Jr. Antibody-based inhibition of DKK1 suppresses tumor-induced bone resorption and multiple myeloma growth in vivo. *Blood.* 2007;109:2106-2111.

[76] Edwards CM, Edwards JR, Lwin ST, et al. Increasing Wnt signaling in the bone marrow microenvironment inhibits the development of myeloma bone disease and reduces tumor burden in bone in vivo. *Blood*. 2008;111:2833-2842.

[77] Kobune M, Chiba H, Kato J, et al. Wnt3/RhoA/ROCK signaling pathway is involved in adhesion-mediated drug resistance of multiple myeloma in an autocrine mechanism. *Mol. Cancer Ther.* 2007;6:1774-1784.

[78] Abe M, Hiura K, Wilde J, et al. Osteoclasts enhance myeloma cell growth and survival via cell-cell contact: a vicious cycle between bone destruction and myeloma expansion. *Blood.* 2004;104:2484-2491.

[79] Roodman GD. Role of the bone marrow microenvironment in multiple myeloma. *J. Bone Miner Res.* 2002;17:1921-1925.

[80] Yaccoby S, Pearse RN, Johnson CL, Barlogie B, Choi Y, Epstein J. Myeloma interacts with the bone marrow microenvironment to induce osteoclastogenesis and is dependent on osteoclast activity. *Br. J. Haematol.* 2002;116:278-290.

[81] Yaccoby S, Wezeman MJ, Henderson A, et al. Cancer and the microenvironment: myeloma-osteoclast interactions as a model. *Cancer Res.* 2004;64:2016-2023.

[82] Caplan AI. Mesenchymal stem cells. *J. Orthop Res.* 1991;9:641-650.

[83] Pittenger MF, Mackay AM, Beck SC, et al. Multilineage potential of adult human mesenchymal stem cells. *Science.* 1999;284:143-147.

[84] Prockop DJ. Marrow stromal cells as stem cells for nonhematopoietic tissues. *Science.* 1997;276:71-74.

[85] Baron R, Rawadi G. Targeting the Wnt/beta-catenin pathway to regulate bone formation in the adult skeleton. *Endocrinology.* 2007;148:2635-2643.

[86] Boyden LM, Mao J, Belsky J, et al. High bone density due to a mutation in LDL-receptor-related protein 5. *N. Engl. J. Med.* 2002;346:1513-1521.

[87] Day TF, Guo X, Garrett-Beal L, Yang Y. Wnt/beta-catenin signaling in mesenchymal progenitors controls osteoblast and chondrocyte differentiation during vertebrate skeletogenesis. *Dev Cell.* 2005;8:739-750.

[88] Glass DA, 2nd, Karsenty G. In vivo analysis of Wnt signaling in bone. *Endocrinology.* 2007;148:2630-2634.

[89] Gong Y, Slee RB, Fukai N, et al. LDL receptor-related protein 5 (LRP5) affects bone accrual and eye development. *Cell.* 2001;107:513-523.

[90] Hill TP, Spater D, Taketo MM, Birchmeier W, Hartmann C. Canonical Wnt/beta-catenin signaling prevents osteoblasts from differentiating into chondrocytes. *Dev Cell.* 2005;8:727-738.

[91] Hu H, Hilton MJ, Tu X, Yu K, Ornitz DM, Long F. Sequential roles of Hedgehog and Wnt signaling in osteoblast development. *Development.* 2005;132:49-60.

[92] Kato M, Patel MS, Levasseur R, et al. Cbfa1-independent decrease in osteoblast proliferation, osteopenia, and persistent embryonic eye vascularization in mice deficient in Lrp5, a Wnt coreceptor. *J. Cell Biol.* 2002;157:303-314.

[93] Krishnan V, Bryant HU, Macdougald OA. Regulation of bone mass by Wnt signaling. *J. Clin. Invest.* 2006;116:1202-1209.

[94] Little RD, Carulli JP, Del Mastro RG, et al. A mutation in the LDL receptor-related protein 5 gene results in the autosomal dominant high-bone-mass trait. *Am. J. Hum. Genet.* 2002;70:11-19.

[95] Rawadi G, Vayssiere B, Dunn F, Baron R, Roman-Roman S. BMP-2 controls alkaline phosphatase expression and osteoblast mineralization by a Wnt autocrine loop. *J. Bone Miner Res.* 2003;18:1842-1853.

[96] Williams B, Insogna K. The Exploding Field of Lrp5 and Lrp6 Signaling in Bone. *J. Bone Miner Res*. 2008:10.1359/JBMR.081235.

[97] Almeida M, Han L, Bellido T, Manolagas SC, Kousteni S. Wnt proteins prevent apoptosis of both uncommitted osteoblast progenitors and differentiated osteoblasts by beta-catenin-dependent and -independent signaling cascades involving Src/ERK and phosphatidylinositol 3-kinase/AKT. *J. Biol. Chem*. 2005;280:41342-41351.

[98] Boland GM, Perkins G, Hall DJ, Tuan RS. Wnt 3a promotes proliferation and suppresses osteogenic differentiation of adult human mesenchymal stem cells. *J. Cell Biochem*. 2004;93:1210-1230.

[99] Kang S, Bennett CN, Gerin I, Rapp LA, Hankenson KD, Macdougald OA. Wnt signaling stimulates osteoblastogenesis of mesenchymal precursors by suppressing CCAAT/enhancer-binding protein alpha and peroxisome proliferator-activated receptor gamma. *J. Biol. Chem*. 2007;282:14515-14524.

[100] Bradbury JM, Niemeyer CC, Dale TC, Edwards PA. Alterations of the growth characteristics of the fibroblast cell line C3H 10T1/2 by members of the Wnt gene family. *Oncogene*. 1994;9:2597-2603.

[101] Bennett CN, Longo KA, Wright WS, et al. Regulation of osteoblastogenesis and bone mass by Wnt10b. *Proc. Natl. Acad. Sci. USA*. 2005;102:3324-3329.

[102] Pinzone JJ, Hall BM, Thudi NK, et al. The role of Dickkopf-1 in bone development, homeostasis, and disease. *Blood.* 2009;113:517-525.

[103] Tian E, Zhan F, Walker R, et al. The role of the Wnt-signaling antagonist DKK1 in the development of osteolytic lesions in multiple myeloma. *N. Engl. J. Med.* 2003;349:2483-2494.

[104] Haaber J, Abildgaard N, Knudsen LM, et al. Myeloma cell expression of 10 candidate genes for osteolytic bone disease. Only overexpression of DKK1 correlates with clinical bone involvement at diagnosis. *Br. J. Haematol*. 2008;140:25-35.

[105] Politou MC, Heath DJ, Rahemtulla A, et al. Serum concentrations of Dickkopf-1 protein are increased in patients with multiple myeloma and reduced after autologous stem cell transplantation. *Int. J. Cancer*. 2006;119:1728-1731.

[106] Kaiser M, Mieth M, Liebisch P, et al. Serum concentrations of DKK-1 correlate with the extent of bone disease in patients with multiple myeloma. *Eur. J. Haematol.* 2008;80:490-494.

[107] Qian J, Xie J, Hong S, et al. Dickkopf-1 (DKK1) is a widely expressed and potent tumor-associated antigen in multiple myeloma. *Blood.* 2007;110:1587-1594.

[108] Oshima T, Abe M, Asano J, et al. Myeloma cells suppress bone formation by secreting a soluble Wnt inhibitor, sFRP-2. *Blood*. 2005;106:3160-3165.

[109] De Vos J, Couderc G, Tarte K, et al. Identifying intercellular signaling genes expressed in malignant plasma cells by using complementary DNA arrays. *Blood.* 2001;98:771-780.

[110] Giuliani N, Morandi F, Tagliaferri S, et al. Production of Wnt inhibitors by myeloma cells: potential effects on canonical Wnt pathway in the bone microenvironment. *Cancer Res*. 2007;67:7665-7674.

[111] Stewart JP, Shaughnessy JD, Jr. Role of osteoblast suppression in multiple myeloma. *J. Cell Biochem*. 2006;98:1-13.

[112] Tarte K, Zhan F, De Vos J, Klein B, Shaughnessy J, Jr. Gene expression profiling of plasma cells and plasmablasts: toward a better understanding of the late stages of B-cell differentiation. *Blood*. 2003;102:592-600.

[113] Zhan F, Hardin J, Kordsmeier B, et al. Global gene expression profiling of multiple myeloma, monoclonal gammopathy of undetermined significance, and normal bone marrow plasma cells. *Blood*. 2002;99:1745-1757.

[114] Heath DJ, Chantry AD, Buckle CH, et al. Inhibiting Dickkopf-1 (Dkk1) removes suppression of bone formation and prevents the development of osteolytic bone disease in multiple myeloma. *J. Bone Miner Res*. 2009;24:425-436.

[115] Kong YY, Yoshida H, Sarosi I, et al. OPGL is a key regulator of osteoclastogenesis, lymphocyte development and lymph-node organogenesis. *Nature*. 1999;397:315-323.

[116] Lacey DL, Timms E, Tan HL, et al. Osteoprotegerin ligand is a cytokine that regulates osteoclast differentiation and activation. *Cell*. 1998;93:165-176.

[117] Simonet WS, Lacey DL, Dunstan CR, et al. Osteoprotegerin: a novel secreted protein involved in the regulation of bone density. *Cell*. 1997;89:309-319.

[118] Suda T, Takahashi N, Udagawa N, Jimi E, Gillespie MT, Martin TJ. Modulation of osteoclast differentiation and function by the new members of the tumor necrosis factor receptor and ligand families. *Endocr Rev*. 1999;20:345-357.

[119] Manolagas SC. Birth and death of bone cells: basic regulatory mechanisms and implications for the pathogenesis and treatment of osteoporosis. *Endocr Rev*. 2000;21:115-137.

[120] Mundy GR, Boyce B, Hughes D, et al. The effects of cytokines and growth factors on osteoblastic cells. *Bone*. 1995;17:71S-75S.

[121] Takahashi N, Yamana H, Yoshiki S, et al. Osteoclast-like cell formation and its regulation by osteotropic hormones in mouse bone marrow cultures. *Endocrinology*. 1988;122:1373-1382.

[122] Anderson DM, Maraskovsky E, Billingsley WL, et al. A homologue of the TNF receptor and its ligand enhance T-cell growth and dendritic-cell function. *Nature*. 1997;390:175-179.

[123] Giuliani N, Bataille R, Mancini C, Lazzaretti M, Barille S. Myeloma cells induce imbalance in the osteoprotegerin/osteoprotegerin ligand system in the human bone marrow environment. *Blood*. 2001;98:3527-3533.

[124] Seidel C, Hjertner O, Abildgaard N, et al. Serum osteoprotegerin levels are reduced in patients with multiple myeloma with lytic bone disease. *Blood*. 2001;98:2269-2271.

[125] Terpos E, Szydlo R, Apperley JF, et al. Soluble receptor activator of nuclear factor kappaB ligand-osteoprotegerin ratio predicts survival in multiple myeloma: proposal for a novel prognostic index. *Blood*. 2003;102:1064-1069.

[126] Vanderkerken K, De Leenheer E, Shipman C, et al. Recombinant osteoprotegerin decreases tumor burden and increases survival in a murine model of multiple myeloma. *Cancer Res.* 2003;63:287-289.

[127] Oyajobi BO, Anderson DM, Traianedes K, Williams PJ, Yoneda T, Mundy GR. Therapeutic efficacy of a soluble receptor activator of nuclear factor kappaB-IgG Fc fusion protein in suppressing bone resorption and hypercalcemia in a model of humoral hypercalcemia of malignancy. *Cancer Res.* 2001;61:2572-2578.

[128] Hausler KD, Horwood NJ, Chuman Y, et al. Secreted frizzled-related protein-1 inhibits RANKL-dependent osteoclast formation. *J. Bone Miner Res.* 2004;19:1873-1881.

[129] Willert J, Epping M, Pollack JR, Brown PO, Nusse R. A transcriptional response to Wnt protein in human embryonic carcinoma cells. *BMC Dev Biol.* 2002;2:8-15.

[130] Binnerts ME, Kim KA, Bright JM, et al. R-Spondin1 regulates Wnt signaling by inhibiting internalization of LRP6. *Proc. Natl. Acad. Sci USA.* 2007;104:14700-14705.

[131] Lu W, Kim KA, Liu J, et al. R-spondin1 synergizes with Wnt3A in inducing osteoblast differentiation and osteoprotegerin expression. *FEBS Lett.* 2008;582:643-650.

[132] Qiang YW, Hu B, Chen Y, et al. Bortezomib induces osteoblast differentiation via Wnt-independent activation of {beta}-catenin/TCF signaling. *Blood.* 2009.

[133] Terpos E, Sezer O, Croucher P, Dimopoulos MA. Myeloma bone disease and proteasome inhibition therapies. *Blood.* 2007;110:1098-1104.

[134] Zangari M, Esseltine D, Lee CK, et al. Response to bortezomib is associated to osteoblastic activation in patients with multiple myeloma. *Br. J. Haematol.* 2005;131:71-73.

[135] Mukherjee S, Raje N, Schoonmaker JA, et al. Pharmacologic targeting of a stem/progenitor population in vivo is associated with enhanced bone regeneration in mice. *J.Clin. Invest.* 2008;118:491-504.

[136] Oyajobi BO, Garrett IR, Gupta A, et al. Stimulation of new bone formation by the proteasome inhibitor, bortezomib: implications for myeloma bone disease. *Br. J. Haematol.* 2007;139:434-438.

[137] Chim CS, Pang R, Fung TK, Choi CL, Liang R. Epigenetic dysregulation of Wnt signaling pathway in multiple myeloma. *Leukemia*. 2007;21:2527-2536.

[138] He TC, Sparks AB, Rago C, et al. Identification of c-MYC as a target of the APC pathway. *Science.* 1998;281:1509-1512.

[139] Tetsu O, McCormick F. Beta-catenin regulates expression of cyclin D1 in colon carcinoma cells. *Nature.* 1999;398:422-426.

[140] Wielenga VJ, Smits R, Korinek V, et al. Expression of CD44 in Apc and Tcf mutant mice implies regulation by the WNT pathway. *Am. J. Pathol.* 1999;154:515-523.

[141] Gradl D, Kuhl M, Wedlich D. The Wnt/Wg signal transducer beta-catenin controls fibronectin expression. *Mol. Cell Biol.* 1999;19:5576-5587.

[142] Firestein R, Bass AJ, Kim SY, et al. CDK8 is a colorectal cancer oncogene that regulates beta-catenin activity. *Nature.* 2008;455:547-551.

[143] Morris EJ, Ji JY, Yang F, et al. E2F1 represses beta-catenin transcription and is antagonized by both pRB and CDK8. *Nature.* 2008;455:552-556.

[144] Pearse RN, Sordillo EM, Yaccoby S, et al. Multiple myeloma disrupts the TRANCE/osteoprotegerin cytokine axis to trigger bone destruction and promote tumor progression. *Proc. Natl. Acad. Sci. USA*. 2001;98:11581-11586.
[145] Pennisi A, Li X, Ling W, Khan S, Zangari M, Yaccoby S. The proteasome inhibitor, bortezomib suppresses primary myeloma and stimulates bone formation in myelomatous and nonmyelomatous bones in vivo. *Am. J. Hematol*. 2009;84:6-14.

In: Multiple Myeloma: Symptoms, Diagnosis and Treatment ISBN 978-1-60876-108-1
Editors: M. Georgiev and Ev. Bachev

Chapter 3

The Activation of Transcription Factor NF-KappaB in Multiple Myeloma and Its Role in Therapy of This Malignancy

Ota Fuchs*
Institute of Hematology and Blood Transfusion,
U Nemocnice 1, 128 20 Prague 2,
Czech Republic and Center of Experimental Hematology,
First Medical Faculty,
Charles University, Prague, Czech Republic

Abstract

Nuclear factor-kappaB (NF-κB) upregulates the transcription of proteins that promote cell survival, stimulate growth and reduce susceptibility to apoptosis. NF-κB signaling pathway is constitutively activated in multiple myeloma (MM). TNF (tumor necrosis factor) receptor associated factor 3 (TRAF3) mutation may account for many cases of constitutive NF-κB activation in MM. TRAF3 is a negative regulator of NF-κB signaling pathway. Three major mammalian inhibitors of NF-κB are IκB (α,β and ε). Two protein kinases with a high degree of sequence similarity, IKKα and IKKβ, mediate phosphorylation of IκB proteins and represent a convergence point for most signal transduction pathways leading to NF-κB activation. NF-κB regulates expression of many proteins that function as MM cell growth factors including interleukin-6 (IL-6), granulocyte-macrophage colony stimulation factor (GM-CSF), B-cell-activating factor (BAFF) and macrophage inflammatory protein-1α (MIP-1α). IL-6 is amajor growth and antiapoptotic cytokine in MM. GM-CSF activates the IL-6 signaling molecule STAT3 (signal transducer and activator of transcription 3) and synergizes with IL-6 to support MM growth. BAFF contributes to MM proliferation and survival. The chemokine MIP-1α mediates bone destruction in MM patients and contibutes to osteolytic bone lesions. MIP-1α acts also as a potential growth and survival factor in MM cells. NF-κB is also

* Corresponding author: Ota Fuchs, PhD. Tel: +420 221977313; Fax: +420 221977370; E- mail: Ota.Fuchs@uhkt.cz

involved in transcriptional regulation of cyclin D and antiapoptotic proteins of the Bcl-2 family. Two members of vascular endothelial growth factor (VEGF) family (VEGF-C and placental growth factor /PLGF/), adhesion molecules (integrin /VLA-4/ and inter-cellular adhesion molecule 1 /ICAM-1/) and matrix metalloproteinases (MMP-1 and MMP-9) are transcriptionally regulated by NF-κB and correlate with bone disease. Upregulated expression of adhesion molecules is involved in the resistance of MM cells to drugs. Several drugs effective for the treatment of MM, including proteasome inhibitors, thalidomide, lenalidomide and arsenic trioxide, block NF-κB activation. These drugs inhibit survival and antiapoptotic pathways in MM cells. Therefore, the treated MM cells are more sensitive to cytotoxic stimuli including chemotherapy used at low doses. New agents with NF-κB inhibitory activity enhance the anti-MM effects of conventional chemotherapeutic agents and reduce different side-effects. Triptolide (diterpenoid triepoxyde), a purified component of a traditional Chinese medicine, extracted from a shrub-like vine named Trypterygium wilfordii Hook F (TWHF) inhibits transcriptional activation of NF-κB and downregulates the expression of various NF-κB-regulated genes, including IL-6, bcl-2, cIAP, XIAP,TNF, VEGF and the adhesion molecules. Triptolide (10-80 ng/ml) induces apoptosis of MM cells and effectively inhibits cell growth of MM cells. NF-κB activation can be also inhibited by IKK inhibitors, for example by PS-1145 dihydrochloride.

Keywords: multiple myeloma; NF-κB, IκBα, apoptosis.

Introduction

Multiple myeloma (MM) remains incurable disease due to both intrinsic and acquired drug resistance [1, 2]. The bone marrow (BM) microenvironment induces growth, survival, and drug resistance in MM cells via different mechanisms. Adhesion of MM cells to fibronectin is the cause of cell adhesion-mediated drug resistance [3, 4]. Cytokines (interleukin /IL/-6, insulin-like growth factor /IGF/-1, and vascular endothelial growth factor /VEGF/) in the BM milieu induce phosphatidylinositol 3-kinase (PI3K)/Akt (proteinase B)/mTOR (phosphoprotein mammalian target of rapamycin) and JAK-STAT pathway (Janus kinase 2 -signal transducer and activator of transcription 3 /STAT3/ signaling cascades [5-11]. Akt signaling has been shown to mediate multiple myeloma cell resistance to conventional therapeutics [3-8]. Many other signaling pathways and proteins are associated with multiple myeloma pathogenesis including transforming growth factor (TGF)-β [12, 13], wingless (*Drosophila*)-type (Wnt) [14, 15], Notch [16, 17], insulin-like growth factor-1 (IGF-1) [18, 19], pleiotrophin [20], Ras/Raf/MAPK [21, 22] and IκB kinase (IKK)/nuclear factor (NF)-κB signaling pathway [23-26].

In this review, the role of IKK/NF-κB signaling pathway in the pathogenesis of MM and the development of agents specifically targeting this pathway as candidates for MM treatment are discussed. The interplay between intrinsically activated NF-κB and another antiapoptotic transcription factor STAT3 may contribute to MM pathogenesis [27]. NF-κB upregulates the expression of interleukin (IL)-6, which in turn activates STAT3 [28-30]. The expression of Bcl-X_L, a prominent antiapoptotic Bcl-2 homolog, is induced by both STAT3 and NF-κB, and Bcl-X_L overexpression has been demonstrated in MM cells at the protein level [27]. The expression of Bcl-X_L is negatively correlated with chemotherapy responses in MM.

Gene expression profiling data from 606 multiple myeloma samples identified a promiscuous array of abnormalities contributing to the dysregulation of NF-κB in approximately 20% of MM patients [25, 26]. Mutations in ten genes causing the inactivation of *TRAF2, TRAF3, CYLD, cIAP1/cIAP2,* and activation of *NFKB1, NFKB2, CD40, LTBR, TAC1, and NIK* that result primarily in constitutive activation of both, the canonical and the noncanonical NF-κB pathways, with the single most common abnormality being inactivation of *TRAF3*. These genetic together with epigenetic alterations further demonstrate the critical importance of the NF-κB pathway in the pathogenesis of MM and suggest that this pathway can be promised target for the treatment of this disease.

NF-κB Multigene Family of Proteins and Their Activation

NF-κB exists as a multigene family of proteins that can form stable homo- and heterodimeric complexes that vary in their DNA-binding specificity and transcriptional activation potential. Five proteins belonging to the NF-κB family have been identified in mammalian cells: RelA (p65), c-Rel, RelB, NF-κB1 (p50 and its precursor p105), and NF-κB2 (p52 and its precursor p100) [31-36]. NF-κB/Rel proteins share a highly conserved 300-amino-acid N-terminal Rel homology domain (RHD) responsible for DNA binding, dimerization, and association with the IκB inhibitory proteins. The prototype NF-κB complex is comprised of p50 and p65, but a variety of NF-κB/Rel – containing dimers are also known to exist. The p50/p65 complex displays strong transcriptional activation, whereas the p50/p50 and p52/p52 homodimers function to repress transcription of NF-κB target genes. Thus, the existence of a multigene family provides one way of regulation by which the cell can regulate NF-κB-mediated gene expression. Knock-out mice lacking distinct NF-κB subunits display distinct phenotypes. Thus, specific NF-κB dimers act as activators of different sets of NF-κB target genes [37-39].

NF-κB/Rel dimers are retained in an inactive state in the cytoplasm of several cell types by inhibitors of the IκB family. Cell stimulation by a broad range of signals activates the IκB kinase (IKK) complex, which is composed of two catalytic subunits (IKK-α and IKK-β) and a regulatory subunit (IKK-γ/NEMO) [40-42]. Activated IKK phosphorylates NF-κB-bound IκB proteins, and targets them for polyubiquitination and rapid degradation by creating a binding site for the SCF (Skp1/Cullin/F-box protein) - type E3 ubiquitin ligase complex [31, 43, 44]. Freed NF-κB dimers translocate to the nucleus where they bind to specific promoters and coordinate the transcriptional activation of several hundred target genes, many of which also depend on other transcription factors [45-48]. A variety of other signaling events, including phosphorylation of NF-κB, hyperphosphorylation of IKK, induction of IκB synthesis, and the processing of NF-κB precursors, provide additional mechanisms that modulate the level and duration of NF-κB activity.

NF-κB proteins transactivate target genes encoding regulators of the cell cycle (e.g., cyclins D_1 and cyclin D_2, c-myc and c-myb), survival factors (e.g., Bcl-2, Bcl-X_L, Bfl-1, c-

FLIP, c-IAP1/2 and survivin), inflammatory and immunoregulatory molecules (e.g., IL-2, IL-6, CD40L, TLR2 and ICAM1), signaling molecules (e.g., TRAFs), microRNAs (miRNAs, e.g., miR-146), angiogenesis regulators (e.g., VEGF) and drug efflux pumps (MDR1).

Two main pathways exist for activation of NF-κB proteins, the classical, also called the canonical pathway and the second alternative or noncanonical pathway (Figures 1 and 2).

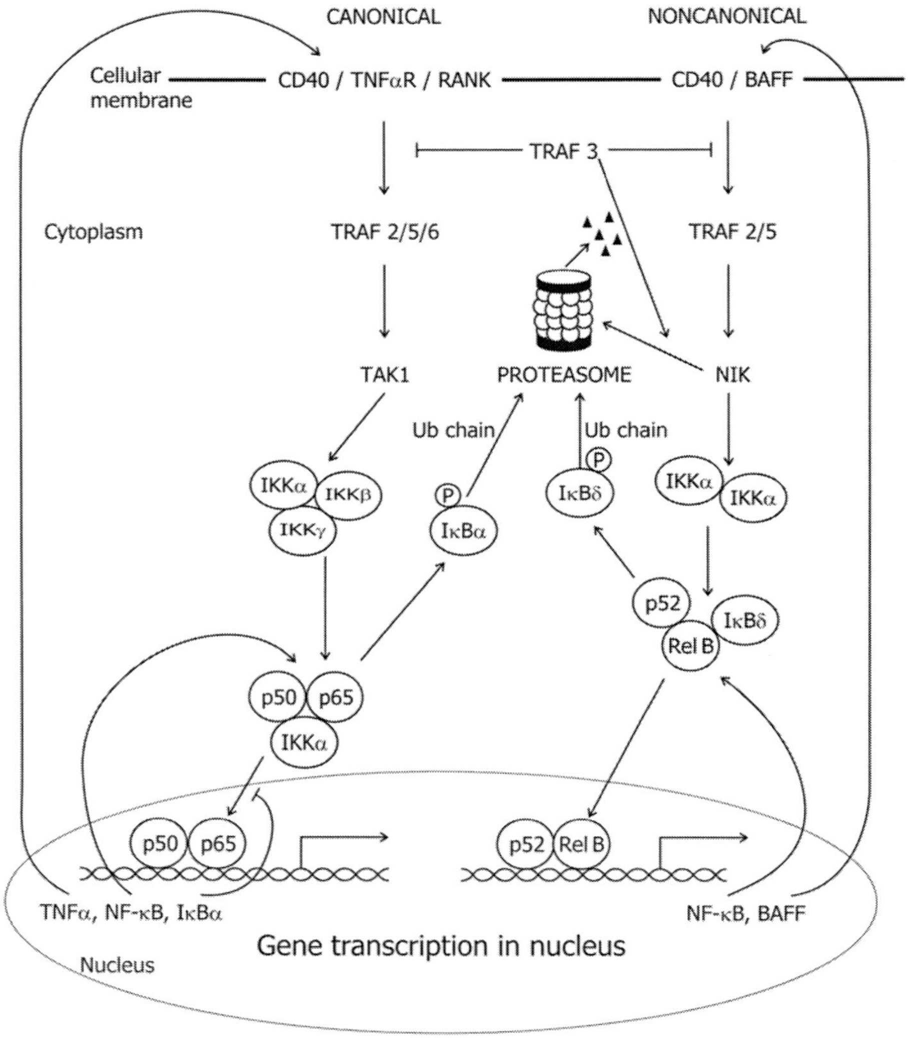

Figure 1. Schematic representation of components of the classical or canonical and of the alternative or noncanonical of NF-κB activation signal transduction pathways in multiple myeloma cells. NF-κB activators in MM cells such as CD40, tumor necrosis factor receptor (TNFR), RANK and B-cell-activating factor (BAFF) are shown. Tumor necrosis factor receptor associated factors (TRAFs) are both positive (TRAF2/5/6) and negative (TRAF3) regulators of NF-κB signaling. Some NF-κB-regulated molecules that are involved in positive (TNFα, BAFF and NF-κBs) or negative (IκBα) feedback are indicated. P100 was shown as p52 and IκBδ, the C-terminal portion of p100. The canonical pathway is mostly dependent on IKKγ-regulated IKKβ activation. The noncanonical pathway is controlled by IKKα phosphorylation of p100 to form a heterodimer with RelB.

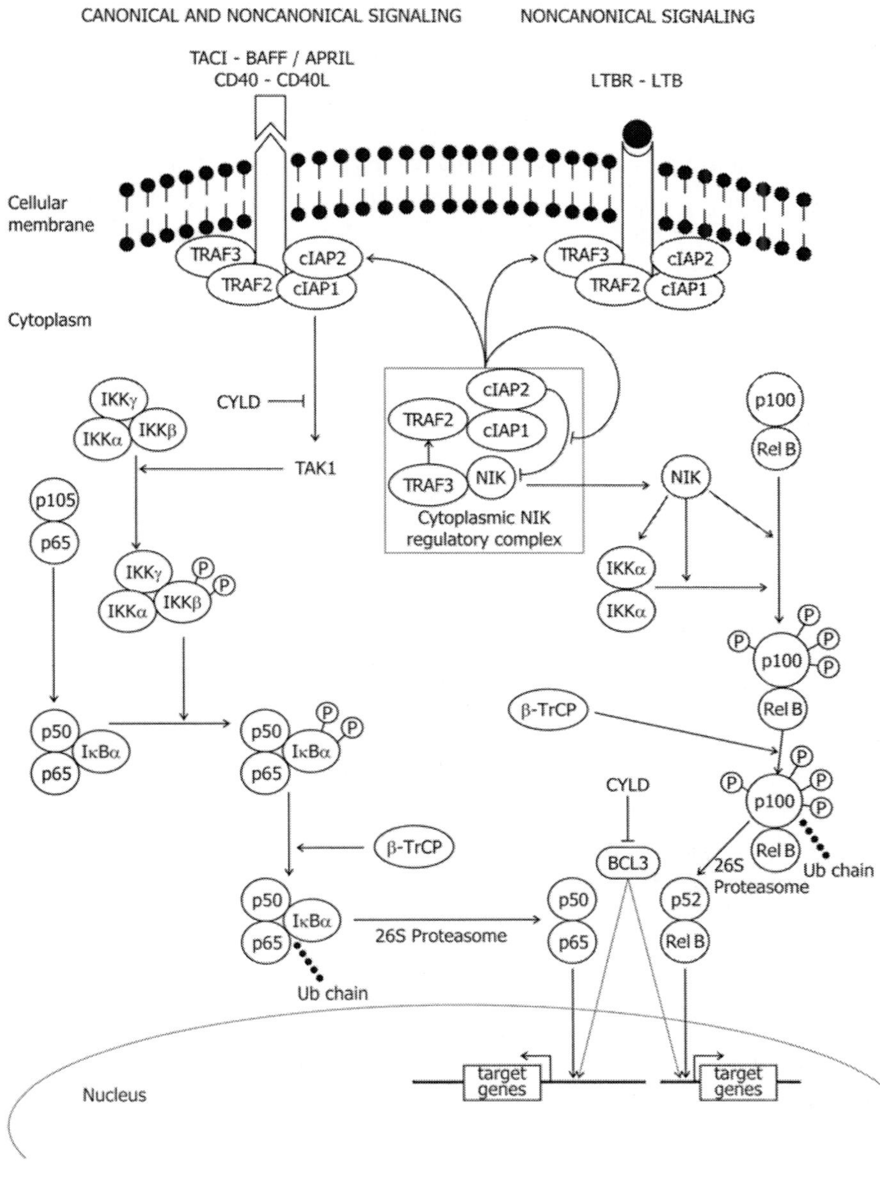

Figure 2. Proposed model from the effect of inactivating abnormalities of genes for components of NF-κB activation signal transduction pathways on NF-κB signaling. The regulation of the noncanonical NF-κB activation signal transduction pathway is absolutely dependent on the presence of NF-κB – inducing kinase (NIK) that, although constitutively transcribed, is normally undetectable in the absence of receptor engagement, which sequesters the normally cytoplasmic localized TRAF2, TRAF3, and cIAP1/cIAP2 proteins to plasma membrane. Cytoplasmic complex regulating the co-translational degradation of NIK is dependent on the presence of TRAF2, TRAF3, and cIAP1 and/or cIAP2. In the absence of stimuli, cytoplasmic TRAF3 scavenges the cytoplasm for NIK, which is then recruited to complexes containing TRAF2, cIAP1, and cIAP2 for degradation. Upon receptor engagement, these regulators are sequestered to the plasma membrane, leading to NIK stabilization. Any mutation in these regulators affecting this mechanism would result in NIK stabilization.

The canonical pathway is mostly dependent on IKK-γ-regulated IKK-β activation. The noncanonical pathway, the alternative pathway, results in specific activation of p52-RelB and it is based on IKK-α homodimers, the preferred substrate of which is the precursor of p52-p100/NF-κB2 [49, 50]. IKK-α is therefore a pivotal component of a second, noncanonical NF-κB activation pathway based on regulated NF-κB2 processing rather than IκB degradation. This pathway is not required for activation of the more ubiquitous p50-RelA dimers used in canonical pathway [51]. The canonical pathway is more generic and it is directly involved in innate immunity and inflammation. The noncanonical pathway is required for the generation of secondary lymhoid organs, and for B-cell maturation and survival [51].

The third or atypical pathway that can lead to NF-κB activation is independent of IKK and, instead, is based on activation of casein kinase 2 (CK2), which induces IκBα degradation through the phosphorylation of carboxy-terminal sites [52]. This pathway has only a minor role in physiological NF-κB activation, although it might contribute to skin carcinogenesis because it is activated by ultraviolet radiation.

CD40 as a Typical NF-κB Activator in Multiple Myeloma Cells

CD40 — a type I glycosilated phosphoglycoprotein with the molecular weight of 48 kDa belongs to the superfamily of type I tumor necrosis factor (TNF)α receptors. This molecule was firstly identified on normal and transformed B-lymphocytes, and also on the cells of bladder tumor as early as at 80_{th} of last century [53, 54].

The discovery of CD40 molecules on normal B-lymphocytes has encouraged the researches aimed on the estimation of their role in immunologic response that began after identification of the ligand for this molecule on T-lymphocytes — CD40L (CD154). As a result, it has been shown that CD40 and CD40L play a key role in intercellular interactions of the abovementioned two main populations of cells of immune system [55]. Later it has been revealed that CD40 is expressed also by a number of antigen-presenting cells (dendritic cells, monocytes, macrophages) eosinophils, basophils and also by keratinocytes, epithelial, neural and other types of cells, and its expression possesses pronounced co-stimulatory properties [56–58]. The structure of CD40 includes extracellular, transmembrane and intracellular parts. The patterns of CD40 structure allow to suppose that the molecule can act as a trimeric receptor able to activate different messengers, and its functional activity is manifested at the highest degree when CD40 acts as a trimeric receptor complex.

CD40 plays an important role in different forms of immunologic response, because it is taking part in activation, proliferation, differentiation of different types of cells of immune system [57, 59–61].

CD40 activation has a functional role in MM cell homing and migration. Cross-linking CD40, using either soluble CD40L (sCD40L) or anti-CD40 monoclonal antibody (mAb), induces phosphatidylinositol 3-kinase (PI3K) activity and activates its downstream effector Akt in MM.1S cells. CD40 activation also activates the mitogen-activated protein (MAP) kinase MEK. MEK is a dual-specificity kinase that phosphorylates the tyrosine and threonine residues on extracellular signal-regulated mitogen-activated protein kinase (ERK), but not c-jun amino-terminal kinase (JNK) or p38, in a dose- and time-dependent manner. Using pharmacologic inhibitors of PI3K and MEK, as well as adenoviruses expressing dominant-negative and constitutively expressed Akt, we demonstrate that PI3K and Akt activities are required for CD40-induced MM cell migration. In contrast, inhibition of ERK/MEK phosphorylation only partially (10%-15%) prevents migration, suggesting only a minor role in regulation of CD40-mediated MM migration. We further demonstrate that CD40 induces NF-κB activation as a downstream target of PI3K/Akt signaling, and that inhibition of NF-κB signaling using specific inhibitors PS1145 and SN50 completely abrogates CD40-induced MM migration. CD40-induced MM cell migration is primarily mediated via activation of PI3K/Akt/NF-κB signaling, and further suggest that novel therapies targeting this pathway may inhibit MM cell migration associated with progressive MM [62].

Both, canonical and noncanonical pathways of NF-κB activation signaling are related to the pathogenesis of MM (Figure 2). CD40L is a NF-κB activator that utilizes both these pathways. CD40 is known to recruit TNF receptor associated factor (TRAF) 6 for canonical NF-κB activation [63], whereas in response to CD40L stimulation, TRAF 2 and TRAF 5 activate NF-κB through both pathways [64]. TRAF 6 is also known to be involved in the canonical NF-κB activation in multiple myeloma cells [65].

Mutations of NF-κB Signaling Molecules Activated NF-κB Signaling

Two research groups studied mutations of NF-κB signaling molecules [25, 26]. Annunziata et al. [25] analyzed the activity of the NF-κB pathway in gene expression profiles of 451 purified MM samples from newly diagnosed patients. Each of the 11 NF-κB signature genes was significantly correlated in expression with the others in the primary MM samples. NF-κB signature levels in MM were next compared with those in normal plasma cells. 82% of MM samples expressed high levels of NF-κB activation signature molecules. Keats et al. [26] on the other hand, collaborated with Agilent Technologies in Santa Clara, Calif., to undertake a broad search for copy number abnormalities in myeloma cell lines and MM patient samples, using a technique called array comparative genomic hybridization to look genomewide for copy number abnormalities (and ultimately mutations). This method compares tumor DNA to normal DNA on the basis of the intensity of fluorescent labels. Finding an unusual number of two-copy deletions in NF-κB pathway genes, Keats et al. [26] focused on NF-κB. Keats et al. [26] used a low expression level for an NF-κB signaling protein called TRAF3 as a proxy for NF-κB pathway activation (they identified in that report TRAF3 as a tumor-suppressor gene in myeloma). He concluded that 20% of myeloma patients have TRAF3 mutations and estimates that 40% have NF-κB activation via other mechanisms—60% in all. The two groups also disagree on whether the mutations affect mainly the canonical or classical pathway, which is important for inflammation, or the noncanonical or alternative NF-κB signaling pathway, which is involved in B-cell development. Keats et al. [26] placed most of the mutations in the alternative pathway but acknowledged some effect on the classical pathway. Annunziata et al. [25], on the other hand, saw more effect of the genes on the classical pathway—an important distinction because there are drugs in development specific for the classical pathway but not the noncanonical or alternative pathway. For example, several companies, including Millennium, are developing drugs to block IKKß in the classical pathway.

Both groups now report many of the same mutations, derived from completely separate patient populations. A mutation in a single molecule, TRAF 3, may account for many cases of constitutive NF-κB activation in MM by both, canonical and noncanonical pathways. TRAF 3, a putative ubiquitin ligase, is a negative regulator of both the canonical and noncanonical NF-κB signaling pathways (Figure 1) by mediating NF-κB – inducing kinase (NIK) degradation through direct binding to NIK [66] or by affecting other TRAF family members [64].

NIK is necessary for noncanonical NF-κB signaling pathway initiated by various members of the TNF receptor (TNFR) superfamily [67-70]. However, NIK is required for signaling to the classical, canonical pathway by certain TNF family members, such as CD40 ligand and B-cell-specific growth factor BAFF [70]. When overexpressed, NIK can activate the canonical pathway, with resultant IκB degradation and nuclear translocation of p50/p65 [71, 72]. Besides TRAF 3, another negative regulator of TRAF2 and of NF-κB activation pathway is the tumor suppressor CYLD (Cylindromatosis). CYLD has deubiquitinating activity that is directed towards non-Lys-48-linked polyubiquitin chains. The inhibition of NF-κB activation is mediated at least in part, by the deubiquitination and inactivation of the IKK-γ subunit, TRAF2 and, to a lesser extent, TRAF6 and Bcl-3 [73-77]. The ubiquitin ligase cIAP1, a member of the inhibitor of apoptosis protein (IAP) family, can atenuate NF-κB signaling via TNFR family members [78, 79].

Genetic and functional data [25, 26] highlight the critical importance of the NF-κB signaling pathway in the pathogenesis of multiple myeloma and are basis for the rational development of NF-κB pathway inhibitors for the therapy of multiple myeloma.

Role of NF-κB Activation in Multiple Myeloma Pathogenesis

Many studies have reported growth and anti-apoptotic roles of NF-κB in normal and malignant cells. As a transcription factor NF-κB regulates expression of numerous genes (coding cytokines, chemokines, growth factors, cell cycle regulators, antiapoptotic molecules, telomerase catalytic subunit, angiogenic factors, adhesion molecules and matrix proteases) involved in MM pathogenesis in many ways.

Cytokines, Chemokines and Growth Factors

NF-κB regulates expression of IL-6, GM-CSF, BAFF and MIP-1α. IL-6 is a major growth and antiapoptotic cytokine for MM cells. The importance of IL-6 as an autocrine growth factor for MM cells is widely accepted, yet very little is known about the mechanisms at the basis of deregulated IL-6 expression in MM cells. The in vivo chromatin organization of the IL-6 gene is different in MM cells, that constitutively express IL-6 (U266), as compared to MM cells, in which the IL-6 promoter is inactive (L363) [80]. Enhanced nuclease accessibility of the AP-1- and, especially, the Sp1-responsive elements in the IL-6 promoter in U266 cells was desribed. Interestingly, Sp1 was eliminated from the IL-6 promoter after treatment with the ERK inhibitor U0126. The importance of ERK and Sp1 in regulating IL-6 transcription was, furthermore, supported by the observation that treatment of U266 cells with U0126 or mithramycin, an antibiotic that prevents Sp1-DNA binding, abrogated constitutive IL-6 transcription [80]. Importantly, the finding that both U0126 and mithramycin were more potent inhibitors of U266 cell viability than the synthetic glucocorticoid drug, dexamethasone, indicates that targeting the Sp1 transcription factor might have therapeutic value in treatment of autocrine MM [80].

Bone marrow stromal cells (BMSCs) upregulate IL-6 secretion [81]. The serum levels of IL-6 and IL-6R are prognostic factors for MM patients [82, 83]. Moreover, IL-6 transgenic mice develop myeloma kidney [84].

Cytokine GM-CSF is also regulated by transcription factor NF-κB [85] and contributes to MM cell growth synergistically with IL-6 [85, 87]. However, Portier et al. [88] found no detectable GM-CSF levels in the peripheral or bone marrow blood of MM patients. It is probable that GM-CSF, produced locally by the tumoral environment, enhances the IL-6 responsiveness of myeloma cells in vivo in a way similar to that reported in vitro [88].

BAFF modulates MM cell proliferation and survival [89]. Tai et al. [90] characterized the functional significance of BAFF in the interaction between multiple myeloma and BMSCs and further defined the molecular mechanisms regulating these processes. BAFF is detected on BMSCs derived from multiple myeloma patients as evidenced by flow cytometry. BAFF secretion is 3- to 10-fold higher in BMSCs than in multiple myeloma cells, and tumor cell adhesion to BMSCs augments BAFF secretion by 2- to 5-fold, confirmed by both ELISA and immunoblotting. Adhesion of MM1S and MCCAR multiple myeloma cell lines to KM104 BMSC line transfected with a luciferase reporter vector carrying the BAFF gene promoter (BAFF-LUC) significantly enhanced luciferase activity, suggesting that NF-κB activation induced by multiple myeloma adhesion to BMSCs mediates BAFF up-regulation. Moreover, BAFF (0-100 ng/mL) increases adhesion of multiple myeloma lines to BMSCs in a dose-dependent manner; conversely, transmembrane activator and calcium modulator and cyclophylin ligand interactor-Ig or B-cell maturation antigen/Fc blocked BAFF stimulation. Using adenoviruses expressing dominant-negative and constitutively expressed Akt as well as NF-κB inhibitors, we further showed that BAFF-induced multiple myeloma cell adhesion is primarily mediated via activation of Akt and NF-κB signaling. Importantly, BAFF similarly increased adhesion of CD138-expressing patient multiple myeloma cells to BMSCs. These studies establish a role for BAFF in localization and survival of multiple myeloma cells in the bone marrow microenvironment and strongly support novel therapeutics, targeting the interaction between BAFF and its receptors in human multiple myeloma [90].

The chemokines, MIP-1α, monocyte chemotactic protein-1 (MCP-1), IL-8, and stromal cell–derived factor–1 (SDF-1), and their receptors play important roles in homing of MM cells, tumor growth, and bone destruction in myeloma. They are attractive therapeutic targets for treating myeloma patients [91]. Addition of chemokine antagonists to current treatment regimens for myeloma should result in better therapeutic responses because of the loss of both the protective effect of the marrow microenvironment on the MM cells and the induction of osteoclast activity [91].

Multiple myeloma cell adhesion to stromal cells via very late antigen (VLA)-4 and vascular cell adhesion molecule (VCAM)-1 interaction causes enhanced secretion of osteoclastogenic activity by MM cells. Abe et al. [92] reported that MM cell-derived macrophage inflammatory protein MIP-1α and MIP-1β are responsible for most of the osteoclastogenic activity in MM. Thus, adhesion-mediated osteoclastogenesis may be caused by enhanced production of MIP-1 via VLA-4-VCAM-1 interaction. Adhesion of MM cells to VCAM-1 upregulated MIP-1α and MIP-1β production from MM cells and enhanced production of osteoclastogenic activity by MM cells. Blockade of MIP-1α and MIP-1β actions not only abrogated elaboration of osteoclastogenic activity, but also suppressed spontaneous MM cell adhesion to VCAM-1. These results demonstrate that MM cell adhesion to VCAM-1 upregulates MIP-1 production by MM cells to cause enhancement of osteoclastogenesis. In addition, the results suggest that the increased production of MIP-1 further enhances MM cell binding to stromal cells via stimulation of VLA-4-VCAM-1 adhesion, forming a vicious cycle between MM cell adhesion to stromal cells and MIP-1 production via VLA-4-VCAM-1 interaction.

Cell Cycle Regulators

NF-κB regulates expression of cell cycle regulators, such as c-Myc, cyclinDs, cyclin E, Cdk6 and E2F3α, that cause insensitivity of MM cells to cell cycle arrest [93-98]. Cyclin D1, D2, or D3 expression appears to be increased and/or dysregulated in virtually all MM tumors despite their low proliferative capacity [99].

Antiapoptotic Molecules

NF-κB regulates expression of many antiapoptotic molecules (Bcl-2, Bcl-X_L, Bcl-2 homologue A1, the zinc-finger protein A20, cIAP, X-linked IAP /XIAP/ and c-FLICE) involved in MM pathogenesis [100-105]. Inhibition of NF-κB caused growth arrest, apoptosis and downregulation of IAPs, Bcl-X_L, c-FLIP and other antiapoptotic molecules in MM cells [106, 107].

Telomerase

NF-κB regulates telomerase reverse transcriptase (TERT), the catalytic subunit of telomerase [108] and may contribute to immortalization of premalignant cells. Human telomerase extends the life span of a cell by adding telomeric repeats to chromosome ends, is expressed in most cancer cells but not in the majority of normal somatic cells. Sustained proliferation of cancer cells requires telomerase to maintain telomeres that regulate chromosomal stability and cellular mitosis. Expression of human telomerase reverse transcriptase (hTERT) catalytic subunit, which modulates telomerase activity, is regulated at both the transcriptional level and via phosphorylation by Akt kinase. Moreover, nuclear localization of hTERT is required to promote elongation of telomere sequences. Akiyama et al. [108] showed for the first time that hTERT protein interacts directly with nuclear factor NF-κB p65 in MM.1S cells. Importantly, TNFα modulates telomerase activity by inducing translocation from the cytoplasm to the nucleus of hTERT protein bound to NF-κB p65. Conversely, a specific IκB kinase (IKK) inhibitor PS-1145, and a specific NF-κB nuclear translocation inhibitor SN-50, both block TNFα-induced hTERT nuclear translocation. These studies suggest that NF-κB p65 plays a pivotal role in regulating telomerase by modulating its nuclear translocation.

Inhibition of telomerase therefore holds great promise as anticancer therapy. Shammas et al. [109] synthesized a novel telomerase inhibitor GRN163L, a lipid-attached phosphoramidate oligonucleotide complementary to template region of the RNA subunit of telomerase. GRN163L was efficiently taken up by human myeloma cells without any need of transfection and was resistant to nucleolytic degradation. The exposure of myeloma cells to GRN163L led to an effective inhibition of telomerase activity, reduction of telomere length and apoptotic cell death after a lag period of 2-3 weeks [109].

Angiogenic Factors

Two vascular endothelial factor (VEGF) family members, VEGF-C and PLGF, are transcriptionally regulated by NF-κB [110, 111]. VEGF is known to be one of the most important if not the main regulator of physiologic and pathologic angiogenesis which triggers growth, survival and migration of myeloma cells. It has been shown that circulating mature or bone marrow driven endothelial precursor cells play an important role in neovascularisation. In accordance with these observations, current therapeutic approaches to myeloma include VEGF inhibitors. Stifter [112] established that by blocking NF-κB production monocyte chemotactic protein-1(MCP-1) secretion was reduced up to 60%. MCP-1 upregulates VEGF and IL-6 production. Angiogenesis could be induced by myeloma cells themselves through NF-κB activation pathway and by inhibiting its activation we might prevent myeloma expansion in bone marrow and progression of the disease by decreased MCP-1 secretion.

Adhesion Molecules and Matrix Proteases

NF-κB regulates expression of VLA-4 [113], the major adhesion molecule in MM cells which was described together with chemokine MIP-1 above. The integrin VLA-4 plays a major role in mediating myeloma cell adhesion to the stroma, by interacting with its ligands VCAM-1 and fibronectin. VLA-4, as well as other integrins, can be expressed in different states of activation, which convey different levels of adhesion [114]. NF-κB also regulates other adhesion molecules frequently expressed in MM cells, VLA-5 and ICAM (Inter-Cellular Adhesion Molecule 1) also known as CD54 [113].

Two proteases, matrixmetalloproteinase 1 and 9 (MMP-1 and MMP-9) are under transcriptional control by NF-κB [115-117]. The mechanisms behind myeloma-mediated bone destruction are not completely understood. Osteoclastic activities depend on matrix metalloproteinases (MMPs) [118].

NF-κB as a Therapeutic Target in Multiple Myeloma

Several established or novel anti-multiple myeloma agents, such as dexamethasone, thalidomide and its immunomodulatory derivatives (IMiDs), proteasome inhibitors and arsenic trioxide As_2O_3, inhibit NF-κB activity as part of their diverse actions (Figure 3). More specific IκB kinase (IKK) inhibitors PS-1145, MLN120B, Bay 11-7082, BMS-345541 and anilinopyrimidine derivative AS602868, and a specific NF-κB nuclear translocation inhibitor SN-50 were also used in preclinical studies with the aim to find novel MM therapeutics [36, 119-125]. These agents may harbor less of the undesired side effects associated with the current anti-MM drugs which affect multiple other proteins and signaling pathways. Specific NF-κB activity inhibitors has been also used in combination with conventional chem0otherapeutics [119, 120, 122, 124, 125] and other drugs [121, 123] and synergistical effects have been found. The inhibition of NF-κB strongly potentiates the anticancer effects of traditional anti-MM chemotherapy [119, 120, 122, 124, 125].

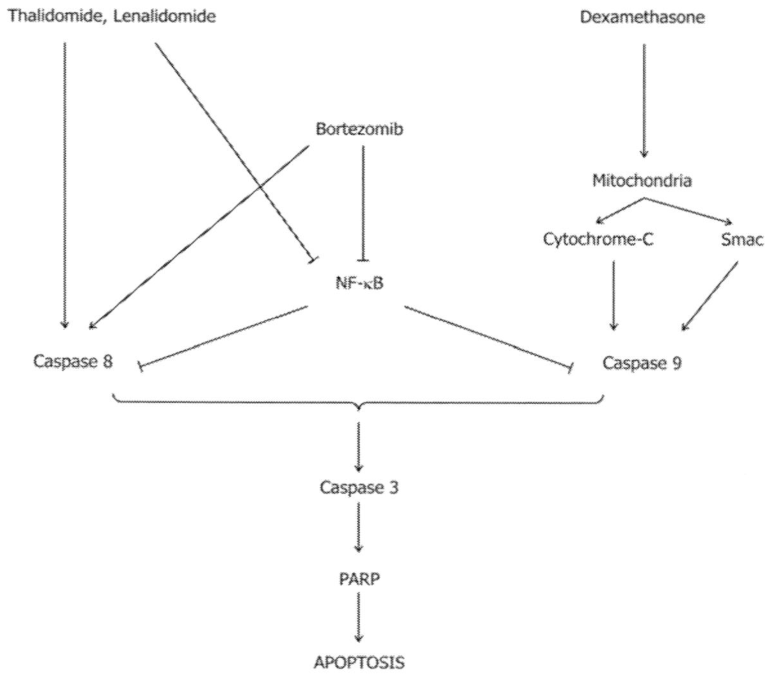

Figure 3. The role of NF-κB in the effects of anti-MM drugs. Apoptosis dependent on caspases is induced by anti-MM drugs (bortezomib, thalidomide, lenalidomide) that inhibit NF-κB activity.

Triptolide (diterpenoid triepoxyde), a purified component of a traditional Chinese medicine, extracted from a shrub-like vine named Trypterygium wilfordii Hook F (TWHF) inhibits transcriptional activation of NF-κB and downregulates the expression of various NF-κB-regulated genes, including IL-6, bcl-2, cIAP, XIAP,TNF, VEGF and the adhesion molecules. Triptolide (10-80 ng/ml) induces apoptosis of MM cells and effectively inhibits cell growth of MM cells [126]. Triptolide also induced chemosensitivity to doxorubicin and suppressed cell proliferation of the mononuclear cell fraction obtained from three MM patients BM aspirates [126]. Triptolide may exert its anticancer effects by initiating apoptosis through both death-receptor- and mitochondria-mediated pathways [127, 128]. Natural triterpenoid, pristimerin also inhibits NF-κB activity and is also a potent inhibitor of proteosome chymotrypsin-like activity [129].

Conclusion and Perspectives

NF-κB is a pleiotropic transcription factor involved in the regulation of diverse cellular processes, including survival, proliferation, differentiation, and inflammatory responses, among numerous others. NF-κB regulates osteoclast formation, function, and survival [130]. The finding that the deletion of both NF-κB p50 and p52 subunits resulted in osteopetrosis due to the absence of osteoclasts was followed by the observation that NF-κB is essential for RANK-expressing osteoclast precursors to differentiate into osteoclasts with tartrate-resistant acid phosphatase (TRAP) activity in response to RANKL and other osteoclastogenic cytokines. Thus, inhibitors of NF-κB should prevent osteoclast formation induced directly or indirectly by RANKL or TNF [130]. Bortezomib, while often effective in myeloma, is not the ideal anti–NF-κB drug. More specific drugs are needed to fully capitalize on the new findings. Besides Millennium, biotech companies Nereus Pharmaceuticals and Reata Pharmaceuticals have reported developing IKK inhibitors. Meanwhile, such inhibitors have already been developed by many major pharmaceutical companies and are going to go into clinical trials in one setting or another. Millennium's IKKβ inhibitor (MLN120B) is now being tested in humans with rheumatoid arthritis, and Dr.Shaughnessy's group from University of Arkansas plans to test it in mouse models of myeloma in preparation for a possible human trial. Because of the promiscuity of NF-κB signaling in human biology, these drugs will have side effects, but Dr.Staudt from Center for Cancer Research, NCI, Bethesda and others hope that myeloma cells will be especially dependent on NF-κB, creating a therapeutic window.

Because of the myeloma field's success in generating new treatments, other cancer researchers are beginning to look to it as a model for translational research. The NF-κB work and other recent advances in myeloma treatment are due partly to the relative ease of obtaining cancer cells from patients as opposed to from solid tumors. But myeloma research has succeeded because cancer cells are studied in the context of the tumor microenvironment, not in isolation. Bone marrow connective tissue from patients can be grown in laboratory dishes for 3–6 weeks before myeloma cells are added, allowing researchers to identify genes in the tumor microenvironment (like NF-κB) that confer a survival advantage or drug resistance to tumor cells. Mouse models of myeloma incorporating the human tumor microenvironment have also been developed.

Acknowledgments

This work was supported by the research intention VZ 00023736 from the Ministry of Health of the Czech Republic (MZO UHKT 2005), and grant LC 06044 from Ministry of Education, Youth and Sport of the Czech Republic.

References

[1] Schwarzenbach, H. Expression of MDR1/P-glycoprotein, the multidrug resistance protein MRP, the lung-resistance protein LRP in multiple myeloma. *Med. Oncol.* 2002, 19, 87-104.

[2] Kastritis, E.; Mitsiades, CS.; Dimopoulos, MA.; Richardson, PG. Management of relapsed and relapsed refractory myeloma. *Hematol. Oncol. Clin. N. Am.* 2007, 21, 1175-1215.

[3] Damiano, JS.; Cress, AE.; Hazlehurst, LA.; Shtil, AA.; Dalton, WS. Cell adhesion mediated drug resistance (CAM-DR): role of integrins and resistance to apoptosis in human myeloma cell lines. *Blood* 1999, 93, 1658-1667.

[4] Hazlehurst, LA.; Damiano, JS.; Buyuksal, I; Pledger, WU.; Dalton, WS. Adhesion to fibronectin via β1 integrins regulates p27kip1 levels and contributes to cell adhesion mediated drug resistance (CAM-DR). *Oncogene* 2000, 19, 4319-4327.

[5] Tu, Y.; Gardner, A.; Lichtenstein A. The phosphatidylinositol 3-kinase/AKT kinase pathway in multiple myeloma plasma cells: roles in cytokine-dependent survival and proliferative responses. *Cancer Res.* 2000, 60, 6763-6770.

[6] Hideshima, T.; Nakamura, N.; Chauhan, D.; Anderson, KC. Biologic sequelae of interleukin-6 induced PI3K/Akt signaling in multiple myeloma. *Oncogene* 2001, 20, 5991-6000.

[7] Mitsiades, CS.; Mitsiades, N.; Poulaki, V.; Schlossman, R.; Akiyama, M.; Chauhan, D. et al. Activation of NF-kappaB and upregulation of intracellular anti-apoptotic proteins via the IGF-1/Akt signaling in human multiple myeloma cells: therapeutic implications. *Oncogene* 2002, 21, 5673-5683.

[8] Hideshima, T.; Anderson, KC. Molecular mechanisms of novel therapeutic approaches for multiple myeloma. *Nat. Rev. Cancer* 2002, 2, 927-937.

[9] Younes, H.;, Leleu, X.; Hatjiharissi, E.; Moreau, AS.; Hideshima, T.; Richardson, P. et al. Targeting the phosphatidylinositol 3-kinase pathway in multiple myeloma. *Clin. Cancer Res* 2007, 13, 3771-3775.

[10] Ferrajoli, A.; Faderl, S.;, Ravandi, F.; Estrov, Z. The JAK-STAT pathway: a therapeutic target in hematological malignancies. *Curr. Cancer Drug Targets* 2006, 6, 671-679.

[11] Sagawa, M.; Nakazato, T.; Uchida, H.; Ikeda, Y.; Kizaki, M. Cantharidin induces apoptosis of human multiple myeloma cells via inhibition of the JAK/STAT pathway. *Cancer Sci.* 2008, 99, 1820-1826.

[12] Hayashi, T.; Hideshima, T.; Nguyen, AN.; Munoz, O.; Podar, K.; Hamasaki, M. et al. Transforming growth factor beta receptor I kinase inhibitor down-regulates cytokine secretion and multiple myeloma cell growth in the bone marrow microenvironment. *Clin. Cancer Res.* 2004, 10, 7540-7546.

[13] Urashima, M.; Ogata, A.; Chauhan, D.; Hatziyanni, M.; Vidriales, MB., Dedera, DA. et al. Transforming growth factor-beta1: differential effects on multiple myeloma versus normal B cells. *Blood* 1996, 87, 1928-1938.

[14] Tian, E.; Zhan, F.; Walker, R.; Rasmussen, E.;, Ma, Y.; Barlogie, B.; Shaughnessy, JD. Jr. The role of the Wnt-signaling antagonist DKK1 in the development of osteolytic lesions in multiple myeloma. *N. Engl. J. Med.* 2003, 349, 2483-2494.

[15] Pearse, RN. Wnt antagonism in multiple myeloma: a potential cause of uncoupled bone remodeling. *Clin. Cancer Res.* 2006, 12 (20,Pt 2), 6274s-6278s.

[16] Jundt, F.; Pröbsting, KS.; Anagnostopoulos, I.; Muehlinghaus, G.; Chatterjee, M.; Mathas, S. et al. Jagged1-induced Notch signaling drives proliferation of multiple myeloma cells. *Blood* 2004, 103, 3511-3515.

[17] Nefedova Y, Cheng P, Alsina M, Dalton WS, Gabrilovich DI. Involvement of Notch-1 signaling in bone marrow stroma-mediated de novo drug resistance of myeloma and other malignant lymphoid cell lines. *Blood* 2004, 103, 3503-3510.

[18] Freund, GG.; Kulas, DT.; Mooney, RA. Insulin and IGF-1 increase mitogenesis and glucose metabolism in the multiple myeloma cell line, RPMI 8226. *J. Immunol.* 1993, 151, 1811-1820.

[19] Mitsiades, CS.; Mitsiades, NS.; McMullan, CJ.; Poulaki, V.; Shringarpure, R.; Akiyama, M. et al. Inhibition of the insulin-like growth factor receptor-1 tyrosine kinase activity as a therapeutic strategy for multiple myeloma, other hematologic malignancies, and solid tumors. *Cancer Cell* 2004, 5, 221-230.

[20] Chen, H.; Gordon, MS.; Campbell, RA.; Li, M.; Wang, CS.; Lee, HJ. et al. Pleiotrophin is highly expressed by myeloma cells and promotes myeloma tumor growth. *Blood* 2007, 110, 287-295.

[21] Intini, D.; Agnelli, L.; Ciceri, G.; Ronchetti, D.; Fabris, S.; Nobili, L. et al. Relevance of Ras gene mutations in the context of the molecular heterogeneity of multiple myeloma. *Hematol. Oncol.* 2007, 25, 6-10.

[22] Bezieau, S.; Devilder, MC.; Avet-Loiseau, H.; Mellerin, MP.; Puthier, D.; Pennarun, E. et al. High incidence of N and K-Ras activating mutations in multiple myeloma and primary plasma cell leukemia at diagnosis. *Hum. Mutat.* 2001, 18, 212-224.

[23] Berenson, JR.; Ma, HM.; Vescio, R. The role of nuclear factor-kappaB in the biology and treatment of multiple myeloma. *Semin. Oncol.* 2001, 28, 626-633.

[24] Feinman, R.; Siegel, DS.; Berenson, J. Regulation of NF-kB in multiple myeloma: therapeutic implications. *Clin. Adv. Hematol. Oncol.* 2004, 2, 162-166.

[25] Annunziata, CM.; Davis, RE.; Demchenko, Y.; Bellamy, W.; Gabrea, A.; Zhan, F. et al. Frequent engagement of the classical and alternative NF-kappaB pathways by diverse genetic abnormalities in multiple myeloma. *Cancer Cell* 2007, 12, 115-130.

[26] Keats, JJ.; Fonseca, R.; Chesi, M.; Schop, R.; Baker, A.; Chng, WJ. et al. Promiscuous mutations activate the noncanonical NF-kappaB pathway in multiple myeloma. *Cancer Cell* 2007, 12, 131-144.

[27] Bharti, AC.; Shishodia, S.; Reuben, JM.; Weber, D.; Alexanian, R.; Raj-Vadhan, S. et al. Nuclear factor-kappaB and STAT3 are constitutively active in CD138+ cells derived from multiple myeloma patients, and suppression of these transcription factors leads to apoptosis. *Blood* 2004, 103, 3175-3184.

[28] Bhardwaj, A.;, Sethi, G.; Vadhan-Raj, S.; Bueso-Ramos, C.; Takada, Y.; Gaur U. et al. Resveratrol inhibits proliferation, induces apoptosis, and overcomes chemoresistance through down-regulation of STAT3 and nuclear factor-kappaB-regulated antiapoptotic and cell survival gene products in human multiple myeloma cells. *Blood* 2007, 109, 2293-2302.

[29] Malara, N.; Focà, D.; Casadonte, F.; Sesto, MF.; Macrina, L.; Santoro, L. et al. Simultaneous inhibition of the constitutively activated nuclear factor kappaB and of the interleukin-6 pathways is necessary and sufficient to completely overcome apoptosis resistance of human U266 myeloma cells. *Cell Cycle* 2008, 7, 3235-3245.

[30] Khong, T.; Sharkey, J.; Spencer, A. The effect of azacitidine on interleukin-6 signaling and nuclear factor-kappaB activation and its in vitro and in vivo activity against multiple myeloma. *Haematologica* 2008, 93, 860-869.

[31] Hayden, MS.; Ghosh S. Signaling to NF-κB. *Genes Dev.* 2004, 15, 2195-2224.

[32] Gilmore, TD. Introduction to NF-kappa B: players, pathways, perspectives. *Oncogene* 2006, 25, 6680-6684.

[33] Ghosh, S.; Karin, M. Missing pieces in the NF-κB puzzle. *Cell* 2002, 109 (suppl.), S81-S96.

[34] Hayden, MS.; Ghosh, S. Shared principles in NF-kappaB signaling. *Cell* 2008, 132, 344-362.

[35] Turco, MC.; Romano, MF.; Petrella, A.; Bisogni, R,; Tassone, P.; Venuta, S. NF-kappaB/Rel-mediated regulation of apoptosis in hematologic malignancies and normal hematopoietic progenitors. *Leukemia* 2004, 18, 11-17.

[36] Li, ZW.; Chen, H.; Campbell, RA.; Bonavida, B.; Berenson, JR. NF-kappaB in the pathogenesis and treatment of multiple myeloma. *Curr. Opin. Hematol.* 2008, 15, 391-399.

[37] Sha, WC.; Liou, HC.; Tuomanen, EI.; Baltimore, D. Targeted disruption of the p50 subunit of NF-kappa B leads to multifocal defects in immune responses. *Cell* 1995, 80, 321-330.

[38] Köntgen, F.; Grumont, RJ.; Strasser, A; Metcalf, D.; Li, R.; Tarlinton, D.; Gerondakis, S. Mice lacking the c-rel proto-oncogene exhibit defects in lymphocyte proliferation, humoral immunity, and interleukin-2 expression. *Genes Dev.* 1995, 9, 1965-1977.

[39] Franzoso, G.; Carlson, L.; Poljak, L.; Shores, EW.; Epstein, S.; Leonardi, A. et al. Mice deficient in nuclear factor (NF)-kappa B/p52 present with defects in humoral responses, germinal center reactions, and splenic microarchitecture. *J. Exp. Med.* 1998, 187, 147-159.

[40] Yamaoka, S.; Courtois, G.; Bessia, C.; Whiteside, ST.; Weil, R.; Agou, F. et al. Complementation cloning of NEMO, a component of the IkappaB kinase complex essential for NF-kappaB activation. *Cell* 1998, 93, 1231-1240.

[41] Rothwarf, DM.; Zandi, E.; Natoli, G.; Karin, M. IKK-gamma is an essential regulatory subunit of the IkappaB kinase complex. *Nature* 1998, 395, 297-300.

[42] Mercurio, F.; Murray BW.; Shevchenko, A.; Bennett, BL.; Young, DB.; Li, JW. et al. IkappaB kinase (IKK)-associated protein 1, a common component of the heterogeneous IKK complex. *Mol. Cell. Biol.* 1999, 19, 1526-1538.

[43] Maniatis, T. A ubiquitin ligase complex essential for the NF-κB, Wnt/Wingless, and Hedgehog signaling pathways. *Genes Dev.* 1999, 13, 505-510.

[44] Karin, M.; Ben-Neriah, Y. Phosphorylation meets ubiquitination: the control of NF-[kappa]B activity. *Annu. Rev. Immunol.* 2000, 18, 621-663.

[45] Werner, SL.; Barken, D.; Hoffmann, A. Stimulus specificity of gene expression programs determined by temporal control of IKK activity. *Science* 2005, 309, 1857-1861.

[46] Park, JM.; Greten, FR.; Wong, A.; Westrick, RJ.; Arthur, JS.; Otsu, K. et al. Signaling pathways and genes that inhibit pathogen-induced macrophage apoptosis--CREB and NF-kappaB as key regulators. *Immunity* 2005, 23, 319-329.

[47] Covert, MW.; Leung, TH.; Gaston, JE.; Baltimore, D. Achieving stability of lipopolysaccharide-induced NF-kappaB activation. *Science.* 2005, 309, 1854-1857.

[48] Hoffmann, A.; Natoli, G.; Ghosh, G. Transcriptional regulation via the NF-kappaB signaling module. *Oncogene* 2006, 25, 6706-6716.

[49] Senftleben, U.; Cao, Y.; Xiao, G.; Greten, FR.; Krähn, G.;, Bonizzi, G. et al. Activation by IKKalpha of a second, evolutionary conserved, NF-kappa B signaling pathway. *Science* 2001, 293, 1495-1499.

[50] Bonizzi, G.; Bebien, M.; Otero, DC.; Johnson-Vroom, KE.; Cao, Y.; Vu, D. et al. Activation of IKKalpha target genes depends on recognition of specific kappaB binding sites by RelB:p52 dimers. *EMBO J.* 2004, 23, 4202-4210.

[51] Bonizzi, G.; Karin, M. The two NF-kappaB activation pathways and their role in innate and adaptive immunity. *Trends Immunol.* 2004, 25, 280-288.

[52] Kato, T. Jr.; Delhase, M.; Hoffmann, A.; Karin, M. CK2 Is a C-Terminal IkappaB Kinase Responsible for NF-kappaB Activation during the UV Response. *Mol. Cell* 2003, 12, 829-839.

[53] Paulie, S.; Rosen, A.; Ehlin-Henriksson, B.; Braesch-Andersen, S.; Jakobson, E.; Koho, H.; Perlmann, P. The human B lymphocyte and carcinoma antigen, CDw40, is a phosphoprotein involved in growth signal transduction. *J. Immunol.*1989, 142, 590–595.

[54] Ledbetter, JA.; Shu, G.; Gallagher, M.; Clark, EA. Augmentation of normal and malignant B-cell proliferation by monoclonal antibody to the B-cell-specific antigen BP50 (CDW40). *J. Immunol.* 1987, 138, 788–794.

[55] Nowak, AK.; Robinson, BW.; Lake, RA. Synergy between chemotherapy and immunotherapy in the treatment of established murine solid tumors. *Cancer Res.* 2003, 63, 4490–4496.

[56] Pirozzi, G.; Lombari, V.; Zanzi, D.; Ionna, F.; Lombardi, ML.; Errico, S. et al. CD40 expressed on human melanoma cells mediates T-cell co-stimulation and tumor cell growth. *Int. Immunol.* 2000, 12, 787–795.

[57] Ottaiano, A.; Pisano, C.; De Chiara, A.; Ascierto, PA.; Botti, G.; Barletta, E. et al. CD40 activation as potential tool in malignant neoplasms. *Tumori* 2002, 88, 361–366.

[58] Villarroel Dorrego, M.; Whawell, SA.; Speight, PM.; Barrett, AW. Transfection and ligation of CD40 in human oral keratinocytes affect proliferation, adhesion and migration but not apoptosis *in vitro*. *Clin. Exp. Dermatol.* 2006, 31, 266–271.

[59] Pinzon-Charry, A.; Schmidt, CW.; Lopez, JA. The key role of CD40 ligand in overcoming tumor-induced dendritic cell dysfunction. *Breast Cancer Res*. 2006, 8, 402.

[60] Noelle, RJ.; Erickson, LD. Determinations of B cell fate in immunity and autoimmunity. *Curr. Dis. Autoimmun.* 2005, 8, 1–24.

[61] Koppold, B.; Sauer, G.; Buening, H.; Hallek, M.; Kreienberg, R.; Deissler, H.; Kurzeder, C. Chemotherapeutic agents enhance AAV2-mediated gene transfer into breast cancer cells promoting CD40 ligand-based immunotherapy. *J. Cancer Res. Clin. Oncol*. 2006, 132, 787–794.

[62] Bereznaya, NM.; Chekhun, VF. Expression of CD40 and CD40L on tumor cells: the role of their interaction and new approach to immunotherapy. *Exp. Oncol.* 2007, 29, 2-12.

[63] Lomaga, MA.; Yeh, WC.; Sarosi, I,; Duncan, GS.; Furlonger, C.; Ho, A. et al. TRAF6 deficiency results in osteopetrosis and defective interleukin-1, CD40, and LPS signaling. *Genes Dev.* 1999, 13, 1015-1024.

[64] Hauer, J.; Püschner, S.; Ramakrishnan, P.; Simon, U.; Bongers, M.; Federle, C.; Engelmann, H. TNF receptor (TNFR)-associated factor (TRAF) 3 serves as an inhibitor of TRAF2/5-mediated activation of the noncanonical NF-kappaB pathway by TRAF-binding TNFRs. *Proc. Natl. Acad. Sci. USA* 2005, 102, 2874-2879.

[65] Chen, H.; Li, M.; Campbell, RA.; Burkhardt, K.; Zhu, D.; Li, SG. et al. Interference with nuclear factor kappa B and c-Jun NH2-terminal kinase signaling by TRAF6C small interfering RNA inhibits myeloma cell proliferation and enhances apoptosis. *Oncogene* 2006, 25, 6520-6527.

[66] Liao, G.; Zhang, M.; Harhaj, EW.; Sun, SC. Regulation of the NF-kappaB-inducing kinase by tumor necrosis factor receptor-associated factor 3-induced degradation. *J. Biol. Chem*. 2004, 279, 26243-26250.

[67] Yin, L.; Wu, L.; Wesche, H.; Arthur, CD.; White, JM.; Goeddel, DV.; Schreiber, RD. Defective lymphotoxin-beta receptor-induced NF-kappaB transcriptional activity in NIK-deficient mice. *Science* 2001, 291, 2162-2165.

[68] Claudio, E.; Brown, K.; Park, S.; Wang, H.; Siebenlist, U. BAFF-induced NEMO-independent processing of NF-kappa B2 in maturing B cells. *Nat. Immunol.* 2002, 3, 958-965.

[69] Coope, HJ.; Atkinson, PG.; Huhse, B.; Belich, M.; Janzen, J.; Holman, MJ. et al. CD40 regulates the processing of NF-kappaB2 p100 to p52. *EMBO J.* 2002, 21, 5375-5385.

[70] Ramakrishnan, P; Wang, W.; Wallach, D. Receptor-specific signaling for both the alternative and the canonical NF-kappaB activation pathways by NF-kappaB-inducing kinase. *Immunity* 2004, 21, 477-489.

[71] Woronicz, JD.; Gao, X.; Cao, Z.; Rothe, M.; Goeddel, DV. IkappaB kinase-beta: NF-kappaB activation and complex formation with IkappaB kinase-alpha and NIK. *Science* 1997, 278, 866-869.

[72] O'Mahony, A.; Lin, X.; Geleziunas, R.; Greene, WC. Activation of the heterodimeric IkappaB kinase alpha (IKKalpha)-IKKbeta complex is directional: IKKalpha regulates IKKbeta under both basal and stimulated conditions. *Mol. Cell. Biol.* 2000, 20, 1170-1178.

[73] Brummelkamp, TR.; Nijman, SM.; Dirac, AM.; Bernards, R. Loss of the cylindromatosis tumour suppressor inhibits apoptosis by activating NF-kappaB. *Nature* 2003, 424, 797-801.

[74] Kovalenko, A.; Chable-Bessia, C.; Cantarella, G.; Israël, A.; Wallach, D.; Courtois, G. The tumour suppressor CYLD negatively regulates NF-kappaB signalling by deubiquitination. *Nature* 2003, 424, 801-805.

[75] Regamey, A.; Hohl, D.; Liu, JW.; Roger, T.; Kogerman, P.; Toftgard, R.; Huber, M. The tumor suppressor CYLD interacts with TRIP and regulates negatively nuclear factor kappaB activation by tumor necrosis factor. *J. Exp. Med.* 2003, 198, 1959-1964.

[76] Trompouki, E.; Hatzivassiliou, E.; Tsichritzis, T.; Farmer, H.; Ashworth, A.; Mosialos, G. CYLD is a deubiquitinating enzyme that negatively regulates NF-kappaB activation by TNFR family members. *Nature* 2003, 424, 793-796.

[77] Massoumi, R.; Chmielarska, K.; Hennecke, K.; Pfeifer, A.; Fässler, R. Cyld inhibits tumor cell proliferation by blocking Bcl-3-dependent NF-kappaB signaling. *Cell* 2006, 125, 665-677.

[78] Rothe, M.; Pan, MG.; Henzel, WJ.; Ayres, TM.; Goeddel, DV. The TNFR2-TRAF signaling complex contains two novel proteins related to baculoviral inhibitor of apoptosis proteins. *Cell* 1995, 83, 1243-1252.

[79] Li, X.; Yang, Y.; Ashwell, JD. TNF-RII and c-IAP1 mediate ubiquitination and degradation of TRAF2. *Nature* 2002, 416, 345-347.

[80] Gerlo, S.; Haegeman, G.; Vanden Berghe, W. Transcriptional regulation of autocrine IL-6 expression in multiple myeloma cells. *Cell Signal.* 2008, 20, 1489-1496.

[81] Chauhan, D.; Uchiyama, H.; Akbarali, Y.; Urashima, M.; Yamamoto, K.; Libermann, TA.; Anderson, KC. Multiple myeloma cell adhesion-induced interleukin-6 expression in bone marrow stromal cells involves activation of NF-kappa B. *Blood* 1996, 87, 1104-1112.

[82] Pelliniemi, TT.; Irjala, K.; Mattila, K.; Pulkki, K.; Rajamäki, A.; Tienhaara, A. et al. Immunoreactive interleukin-6 and acute phase proteins as prognostic factors in multiple myeloma. Finnish Leukemia Group. *Blood* 1995, 85, 765-771.

[83] Pulkki, K.; Pelliniemi, TT.; Rajamäki, A.; Tienhaara, A.; Laakso, M.; Lahtinen, R. Soluble interleukin-6 receptor as a prognostic factor in multiple myeloma. Finnish Leukaemia Group. *Br. J. Haematol.* 1996, 92, 370-374.

[84] Fattori, E.; Della Rocca, C.; Costa, P.; Giorgio, M.; Dente, B.; Pozzi, L.; Ciliberto, G. Development of progressive kidney damage and myeloma kidney in interleukin-6 transgenic mice. *Blood 1*994, 83, 2570-2579.

[85] Schreck, R.; Baeuerle, PA. NF-kappa B as inducible transcriptional activator of the granulocyte-macrophage colony-stimulating factor gene. *Mol. Cell. Biol.* 1990, 10, 1281-1286.

[86] Zhang, XG.; Bataille, R.; Jourdan, M.; Saeland, S.; Banchereau, J.; Mannoni, P.; Klein B. Granulocyte-macrophage colony-stimulating factor synergizes with interleukin-6 in supporting the proliferation of human myeloma cells. *Blood* 1990, 76, 2599-2605.

[87] Villunger, A.; Egle, A.; Kos, M.; Egle, D.; Tinhofer, I.; Henn, T. et al. Functional granulocyte/macrophage colony stimulating factor receptor is constitutively expressed on neoplastic plasma cells and mediates tumour cell longevity. *Br. J. Haematol.* 1998, 102, 1069-1080.

[88] Portier, M.; Zhang, XG.; Ursule, E.; Lees, D.; Jourdan, M.; Bataille, R.; Klein, B. Cytokine gene expression in human multiple myeloma. *Br. J. Haematol.* 1993, 85, 514-520.

[89] Novak, AJ.; Darce, JR.; Arendt, BK.; Harder, B.; Henderson, K.; Kindsvogel, W. et al. Expression of BCMA, TACI, and BAFF-R in multiple myeloma: a mechanism for growth and survival. *Blood* 2004, 103, 689-694.

[90] Tai, YT.; Li, XF.; Breitkreutz, I.; Song, W.; Neri, P.; Catley, L. et al. Role of B-cell-activating factor in adhesion and growth of human multiple myeloma cells in the bone marrow microenvironment. *Cancer Res.* 2006, 66, 6675-6682.

[91] Aggarwal, R.; Ghobrial, IM.; Roodman, GD. Chemokines in multiple myeloma. *Exp. Hematol.* 2006, 34, 1289-1295.

[92] Abe, M.; Hiura, K.; Ozaki, S.; Kido, S.; Matsumoto, T. Vicious cycle between myeloma cell binding to bone marrow stromal cells via VLA-4-VCAM-1 adhesion and macrophage inflammatory protein-1alpha and MIP-1beta production. *J. Bone Miner. Metab.* 2009, 27, 16-23.

[93] Lee, H.; Arsura, M.; Wu, M.; Duyao, M.; Buckler, AJ.; Sonenshein, GE. Role of Rel-related factors in control of c-myc gene transcription in receptor-mediated apoptosis of the murine B cell WEHI 231 line. *J. Exp. Med.* 1995, 181, 1169-1177.

[94] Guttridge, DC.; Albanese, C.; Reuther, JY.; Pestell, RG.; Baldwin, AS. Jr. NF-kappaB controls cell growth and differentiation through transcriptional regulation of cyclin D1. *Mol. Cell. Biol.* 1999, 19, 5785-5799.

[95] Hinz, M.; Krappmann, D.; Eichten, A; Heder, A.; Scheidereit, C.; Strauss, M. NF-kappaB function in growth control: regulation of cyclin D1 expression and G0/G1-to-S-phase transition. *Mol. Cell. Biol.* 1999, 19, 2690-2698.

[96] Joyce, D.; Bouzahzah, B.; Fu, M.; Albanese, C.; D'Amico, M.; Steer, J. et al. Integration of Rac-dependent regulation of cyclin D1 transcription through a nuclear factor-kappaB-dependent pathway. *J. Biol. Chem.* 1999, 274, 25245-25249.

[97] Joyce, D.; Albanese, C.; Steer, J.; Fu, M.; Bouzahzah, B.; Pestell, RG. NF-kappaB and cell-cycle regulation: the cyclin connection. *Cytokine Growth Factor Rev.* 2001, 12, 73-90.

[98] Ogasawara, T.; Katagiri, M.; Yamamoto, A.; Hoshi, K.; Takato, T.; Nakamura, K. et al. Osteoclast differentiation by RANKL requires NF-kappaB-mediated downregulation of cyclin-dependent kinase 6 (Cdk6). J. Bone Miner. Res. 2004, 19, 1128-1136.

[99] Bergsagel PL.; Kuehl, WM.; Zhan, F.; Sawyer, J.; Barlogie, B.; Shaughnessy, J. Jr. Cyclin D dysregulation: an early and unifying pathogenic event in multiple myeloma. Blood 2005, 106, 296-303.

[100] Lee, HH.; Dadgostar, H.; Cheng, Q.; Shu, J.; Cheng, G. NF-κB-mediated up-regulation of Bcl-x and Bfl-1/A1 is required for CD40 survival signaling in B lymphocytes. Proc. Natl. Acad. Sci. U S A 1999, 96, 9136-9141.

[101] Stehlik, C.; de Martin, R.; Kumabashiri, I.; Schmid, JA.; Binder, BR.; Lipp, J. Nuclear factor (NF)-kappaB-regulated X-chromosome-linked iap gene expression protects endothelial cells from tumor necrosis factor alpha-induced apoptosis. *J. Exp. Med.* 1998, 188, 211-216.

[102] Hu, X.; Yee, E.; Harlan, JM.; Wong, F.; Karsan, A. Lipopolysaccharide induces the antiapoptotic molecules, A1 and A20, in microvascular endothelial cells. *Blood* 1998, 92, 2759-2765.

[103] Wang, CY.; Mayo, MW.; Korneluk, RG.; Goeddel, DV.; Baldwin, AS. Jr. NF-kappaB antiapoptosis: induction of TRAF1 and TRAF2 and c-IAP1 and c-IAP2 to suppress caspase-8 activation. *Science* 1998, 281, 1680-1683.

[104] Panwalkar, A.; Verstovsek, S.; Giles, F. Nuclear factor-kappaB modulation as a therapeutic approach in hematologic malignancies. *Cancer* 2004, 100, 1578-1589.

[105] Benayoun, B.; Baghdiguian, S.; Lajmanovich, A.; Bartoli, M.; Daniele, N.; Gicquel, E. et al. NF-kappaB-dependent expression of the antiapoptotic factor c-FLIP is regulated by calpain 3, the protein involved in limb-girdle muscular dystrophy type 2A. *FASEB J.* 2008, 22, 1521-1529.

[106] Watanabe, M.; Dewan, MZ.; Okamura, T.; Sasaki, M.; Itoh, K.; Higashihara, M. et al. A novel NF-kappaB inhibitor DHMEQ selectively targets constitutive NF-kappaB activity and induces apoptosis of multiple myeloma cells in vitro and in vivo. *Int. J. Cancer* 2005, 114, 32-38.

[107] Nakagawa, Y.; Abe, S.; Kurata, M.; Hasegawa, M.; Yamamoto, K.; Inoue, M. et al. IAP family protein expression correlates with poor outcome of multiple myeloma patients in association with chemotherapy-induced overexpression of multidrug resistance genes. *Am. J. Hematol.* 2006, 81, 824-831.

[108] Akiyama M, Hideshima T, Hayashi T, Tai YT, Mitsiades CS, Mitsiades N. et al. Nuclear factor-kappaB p65 mediates tumor necrosis factor alpha-induced nuclear translocation of telomerase reverse transcriptase protein. *Cancer Res.* 2003, 63, 18-21.

[109] Shammas MA, Koley H, Bertheau RC, Neri P, Fulciniti M, Tassone P. et al. Telomerase inhibitor GRN163L inhibits myeloma cell growth in vitro and in vivo. *Leukemia.* 2008, 22, 1410-1418.

[110] Kiriakidis, S.; Andreakos, E.; Monaco, C.; Foxwell, B.; Feldmann, M.; Paleolog, E. VEGF expression in human macrophages is NF-kappaB-dependent: studies using adenoviruses expressing the endogenous NF-kappaB inhibitor IkappaBalpha and a kinase-defective form of the IkappaB kinase 2. *J. Cell Sci.* 2003, 116, 665-674.

[111] Cramer, M.; Nagy, I.; Murphy, BJ.; Gassmann, M.; Hottiger, MO.; Georgiev, O.; Schaffner, W. NF-kappaB contributes to transcription of placenta growth factor and interacts with metal responsive transcription factor-1 in hypoxic human cells. *Biol. Chem.* 2005, 386, 865-872.

[112] Stifter S. The role of nuclear factor kappaB on angiogenesis regulation through monocyte chemotactic protein-1 in myeloma. *Med. Hypotheses* 2006, 66, 384-386.

[113] Tatsumi, T.; Shimazaki, C.; Goto, H.; Araki, S.; Sudo, Y.; Yamagata, N. et al. Expression of adhesion molecules on myeloma cells. *Jpn. J. Cancer Res.* 1996, 87, 837-842.

[114] Sanz-Rodríguez, F.; Teixidó, J. VLA-4-dependent myeloma cell adhesion. *Leuk. Lymphoma* 2001, 41, 239-245.

[115] Bond, M.; Fabunmi, RP.; Baker, AH.; Newby, AC. Synergistic upregulation of metalloproteinase-9 by growth factors and inflammatory cytokines: an absolute requirement for transcription factor NF-kappa B. *FEBS Lett.* 1998, 435, 29-34.

[116] Vincenti, MP.; Coon, CI.; Brinckerhoff, CE. Nuclear factor kappaB/p50 activates an element in the distal matrix metalloproteinase 1 promoter in interleukin-1beta-stimulated synovial fibroblasts. *Arthritis Rheum.* 1998, 41, 1987-1994.

[117] Hecht, M.; von Metzler, I.; Sack, K.; Kaiser, M.; Sezer, O. Interactions of myeloma cells with osteoclasts promote tumour expansion and bone degradation through activation of a complex signalling network and upregulation of cathepsin K, matrix metalloproteinases (MMPs) and urokinase plasminogen activator (uPA). *Exp. Cell Res.* 2008, 314, 1082-1093.

[118] Delaissé, JM.; Andersen, TL.; Engsig, MT.; Henriksen, K.; Troen, T.; Blavier, L. Matrix metalloproteinases (MMP) and cathepsin K contribute differently to osteoclastic activities. *Microsc. Res. Tech.* 2003, 61, 504-513.

[119] Hideshima, T.; Chauhan, D.; Richardson, P.; Mitsiades, C.; Mitsiades, N.; Hayashi, T. et al. NF-kappa B as a therapeutic target in multiple myeloma. *J. Biol. Chem.* 2002, 277, 16639-16647.

[120] Mitsiades, N.; Mitsiades, CS.; Poulaki, V.; Chauhan, D.; Richardson, PG.; Hideshima, T. et al. Biologic sequelae of nuclear factor-kappaB blockade in multiple myeloma: therapeutic applications. *Blood* 2002, 99, 4079-4086.

[121] Dai, Y.; Pei, XY.; Rahmani, M.; Conrad, DH.; Dent, P.; Grant, S. Interruption of the NF-kappaB pathway by Bay 11-7082 promotes UCN-01-mediated mitochondrial dysfunction and apoptosis in human multiple myeloma cells. *Blood* 2004, 103, 2761-2770.

[122] Hideshima, T.; Neri, P.; Tassone, P.; Yasui, H.; Ishitsuka, K.; Raje, N. et al. MLN120B, a novel IkappaB kinase beta inhibitor, blocks multiple myeloma cell growth in vitro and in vivo. *Clin. Cancer Res.* 2006, 12, 5887-5894.

[123] Romagnoli, M.; Desplanques, G.; Maïga, S.; Legouill, S.; Dreano, M.; Bataille, R.; Barillé-Nion, S. Canonical nuclear factor kappaB pathway inhibition blocks myeloma cell growth and induces apoptosis in strong synergy with TRAIL. *Clin. Cancer Res.* 2007, 13, 6010-6018.

[124] Jourdan, M.; Moreaux, J.; Vos, JD.; Hose, D.; Mahtouk, K.; Abouladze, M. et al. Targeting NF-kappaB pathway with an IKK2 inhibitor induces inhibition of multiple myeloma cell growth. *Br. J. Haematol.* 2007, 138, 160-168.

[125] Malara, N.; Focà, D.; Casadonte, F.; Sesto, MF.; Macrina, L.; Santoro, L. et al. Simultaneous inhibition of the constitutively activated nuclear factor kappaB and of the interleukin-6 pathways is necessary and sufficient to completely overcome apoptosis resistance of human U266 myeloma cells. *Cell Cycle* 2008, 7, 3235-3245.

[126] Yinjun, L.; Jie, J.; Yungui, W. Triptolide inhibits transcription factor NF-kappaB and induces apoptosis of multiple myeloma cells. *Leuk. Res.* 2005, 29, 99-105.

[127] Wang, X, Matta R, Shen G, Nelin LD, Pei D, Liu Y. Mechanism of triptolide-induced apoptosis: Effect on caspase activation and Bid cleavage and essentiality of the hydroxyl group of triptolide. *J. Mol. Med.* 2006, 84, 405-415.

[128] Bao X, Cui J, Wu Y, Han X, Gao C, Hua Z, Shen P. The roles of endogenous reactive oxygen species and nitric oxide in triptolide-induced apoptotic cell death in macrophages. *J. Mol. Med.* 2007, 85, 85-98.

[129] Tiedemann, RE.; Schmidt, J.; Keats, JJ.; Shi, CX.; Zhu, YX.; Palmer, SE. et al. Identification of a potent natural triterpenoid inhibitor of proteosome chymotrypsin-like activity and NF-{kappa}B with anti-myeloma activity in vitro and in vivo. *Blood.* 2009, 113, 4027-4037.

[130] Soysa, NS.; Alles, N. NF-kappaB functions in osteoclasts. *Biochem. Biophys. Res. Commun.* 2009, 378, 1-5.

In: Multiple Myeloma: Symptoms, Diagnosis and Treatment ISBN 978-1-60876-108-1
Editors: M. Georgiev and Ev. Bachev

Chapter 4

Proteasome Inhibition as a Therapeutic Strategy in Patients with Multiple Myeloma

*Ota Fuchs**
Institute of Hematology and Blood Transfusion,
U Nemocnice 1, 128 20 Prague 2,
Czech Republic and Center of Experimental Hematology,
First Medical Faculty, Charles University,
Prague, Czech Republic

Abstract

Multiple myeloma (MM) is the second most frequent hematological malignancy and remains fatal despite all available therapies, because of chemotherapeutic resistance. Novel targeted drugs for the treatment of MM are therefore needed to improve outcome of MM patients. Bortezomib (PS-341, Velcade; Millennium Pharmaceuticals, Cambridge MA), a dipeptidyl boronic acid that reversibly inhibits the chymotrypsin-like activity in the 20S core of the 26S mammalian proteasome, is the first proteasome inhibitor that was approved by the US Food amd Drug Administration (FDA) and the European Agency for the Evaluation of Medicinal Products (EMEA) for patients with relapsed and refractory MM who had received at least one prior therapy and who had already undergone or are unsuitable for the transplantation of bone marrow. Phase I-III trials based on previous preclinical studies showed very good antimyeloma activity. Bortezomib acts by disrupting various cell signaling pathways, thereby leading to cell cycle arrest, apoptosis, and inhibition of angiogenesis. The main action of bortezomib is the inhibition of the key transcription factor, nuclear factor-kappaB (NF-κB) activation. Activation of NF-κB has been noted in MM cells. Bortezomib interferes with NF-κB-mediated cell survival, tumor growth and angiogenesis. Several studies have shown that cancer cells are more sensitive than normal cells to the proapoptotic effects of bortezomib, perhaps due to their loss of

* Corresponding author: Ota Fuchs, PhD. Tel: +420 221977313; Fax: +420 221977370; E- mail: Ota.Fuchs@uhkt.cz

checkpoint mechanisms for DNA repair. The accumulation of misfolded proteins in the endoplasmic reticulum (ER) leads to the induction of the unfolded protein response, provoking apoptosis. Proteasome inhibitors induce ER-mediated apoptosis. The increased susceptibility of MM cells to ER stress is caused by the large amounts of immunoglobulins produced by MM cells. The clinical success of bortezomib is encouraging. Bortezomib is relatively well tolerated, causing manageable nonhematologic and hematologic toxicity. However, the overall response rate was 40-50% and bortezomib resistance was also observed. Response rates may be improved with combination therapy (bortezomib with dexamethasone, thalidomide, lenalidomide, arsenic trioxide, cisplatin, doxorubicin, cyclophosphamide, etoposide or with melphalan and prednisone). Clinical evaluation of additional proteasome inhibitors of the next generation with greater efficacy is also needed. Three such proteasome inhibitors (carfilzomib, salinosporamide A and threonine boronic acid-derived proteasome inhibitor CEP-18770) have been recently tested in preclinical models of MM. Carfilzomib (PR-171; Proteolix), an epoxyketone related to epoxomicin inhibits the chymotrypsin-like proteasome activity as bortezomib does. However, carfilzomib is an irreversible inhibitor of all three proteasome proteolytic sites. Salinosporamide A (NPI-0052), a compound related to lactacystin binds irreversibly to the 20S proteasome and acts predominantly through caspase-8 activation. CEP-18770 is a reversible inhibitor of the chymotrypsin-like proteasome activity as bortezomib but it inhibits also the tryptic and peptidyl glutamyl activities of the proteasome.

Keywords: multiple myeloma; proteasome; proteasome inhibitor; bortezomib; apoptosis

Introduction

Multiple myeloma (MM) is a hematologic tumor characterized by the clonal expansion of monoclonal immunoglobulin-secreting plasma cells in the bone marrow (BM). MM is associated with lytic bone lesions, anemia, immunodeficiency, and renal impairtment. MM accounts for more than 10% of all hematologic malignancies and about 1% of all cancers. In the USA, it is estimated that approximately 19, 920 new cases are diagnosed per year with about 10, 790 deaths [1]. MM remains incurable despite conventional intensive high dose chemotherapy followed by hematopoietic stem cell transplant.

The costs associated with MM are among the highest. The median age at MM diagnosis is 70 years, and myeloma occurs in men (7 per 100, 000) at a rate 56% higher than women (4.5 per 100, 000). There has been a significant improvement in overall 5-year survival in patients with MM since the 1960s; 12% from 1960 to 1963 to 34% from 1996 to 2003.

The increasing knowledge of MM biology is already contributing to more specific drug designs. Recently we have learned that, in the pathogenesis of MM, as important as the malignant cells themselves is their interaction with the microenvironment [2]. Discoveries in the genetic abnormalities associated with MM [3.4] and better understanding of the bone marrow [5,6] microenvironment have led to new diagnostic, prognostic and treatment strategies. Therefore, drugs with a dual effect on the plasma cells and their bone marrow millieu in MM could be particularly valuable. Novel agents, such as thalidomide, the immunoregulatory drug lenalidomide (also known as CC-5013, IMID-3 or Revlimid^{TM}) and proteasome inhibitors (bortezomib, also known as PS-341 or Velcade^{TM}) can achieve responses in patients who have relapsed and refractory MM [7-11]. However, the median survival remains at 6 years, with only 10% of MM patients surviving at 10 years.

Ubiquitin-Dependent Proteolysis

Ubiquitin-dependent proteolysis regulates the stability and function of key regulatory proteins that regulate the cell cycle, gene transcription, receptor endocytosis, intracellular trafficking, response to extracellular signal, signal transduction, antigen presentation, and control cell growth. Ubiquitin is a highly conserved protein of 76 amino acids that is covalently attached to substrate proteins through an energy-dependent enzymatic mechanism and polyubiquitinated proteins are degraded by a multicompartmentalized protease called the 26S proteasome [12-15]. For the discovery of ubiquitin and its function in non-lysosomal pathway of protein degradation, the 2004 Nobel Prize in Chemistry was awarded to Drs. Avram Hershko, Aaron Ciechanover and Irwin Rose [16-19].

Schematic representation of the ubiquitin conjugation (ubiquitination, also referred to as ubiquitylation or ubiquitinylation) and of the the ubiquitin-proteasome system is shown in Figure 1. Ubiquitination is a posttranslational modification of proteins. Ubiquitin is activated in an ATP-dependent manner by a ubiquitin –activating enzyme known as an enzyme-1 (E1). Subsequently, ubiquitin is transferred to a ubiquitin-conjugating enzyme-2 (E2). E2, with the help of a ubiquitin-protein ligase (E3) and in some cases in the presence of an accessory factor (E4) [20], specifically attaches ubiquitin to the protein substrate. Only ten E1 enzymes, but about 100 E2 enzymes and 1000 E3 enzymes exist in human cells [21]. E3 ubiquitin ligases determine the specificity of protein substrates and are targets for pharmaceutical intervention. There are two major types of E3 ligases: the RING (really interesting new gene) domain-containing E3s and the Hect (homologous to E6-associated protein carboxyl terminus) domain-containing E3s. RING E3s bring the E2 enzyme in close proximity of the target protein, allowing the E2 to directly ubiquitinate the substrate. However, in the case of Hect E3s, ubiquitin is first transferred onto a conserved cysteine in the Hect domain. Consequently, Hect E3 enzyme ubiquitinates the substrate protein. Polyubiquitin chain formation results from a linkage between the C terminus of one ubiquitin and a lysine side chain in another. Generated polyubiquitin chain (at least four attached ubiquitins) functions as signal for the subsequent degradation of protein substrates in the 26S proteasome.

Eukaryotic proteasomes, model of a barrel-like structure in Figure 2 consist of two outer α-rings and of two inner β-rings, each assembled from seven similar, but distinct, subunits. 19S regulatory complex caps both ends of the 20S proteasome to form 26S proteasome. 19S subunits are involved in the recognition of proteins designated for degradation. Each 19S regulatory complex contains at least seventeen different subunits and is assembled from two main subcomplexes-a base that contains six ATPases (Rpt) plus three non-ATPase subunits (Rpn), and a lid subcomplex that sits on top of the base and consist at least eight non-ATPase regulatory particles (Rpn). 19S regulatory complex recognizes the polyubiquitin proteolytic signal and unfoldes substrates [15]. The 19S regulatory complex also takes a role in recycling ubiquitin as it contains deubiquitinating enzymes.

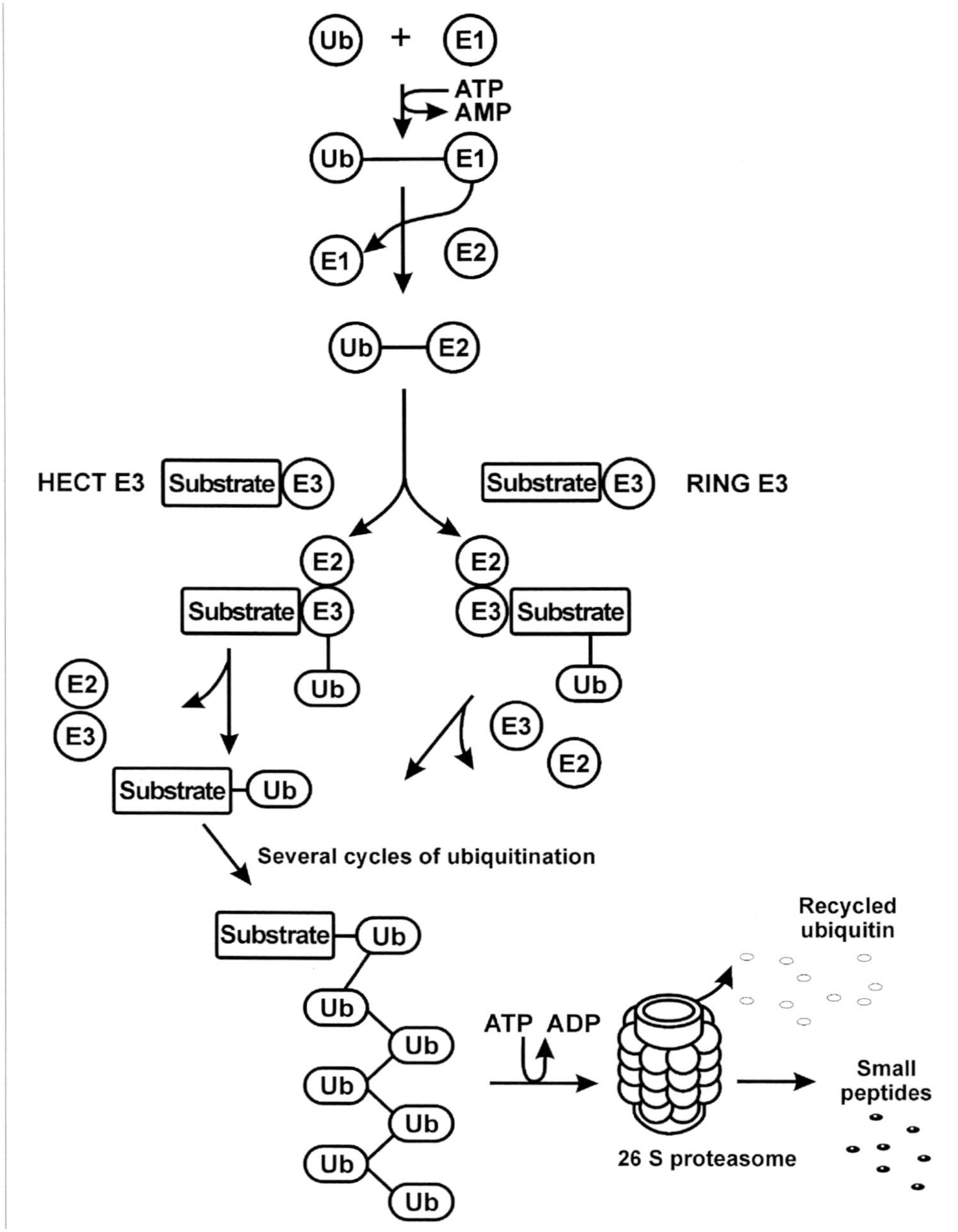

Figure 1. The ubiquitin-proteasome system. Attachment of ubiquitin to the target protein requires three enzymatic steps. Ubiquitin-activating enzymes activate ubiquitin by forming a high energy thiol ester bond between an E1 active site-located cystine residue and the C-terminal glycine residue of ubiquitin. This reaction requires energy provided by the hydrolysis of ATP and forms an activated thiol ester bond to ubiquitin-conjugating enzymes that serve as carrier proteins. Ubiquitin-protein ligases catalyze the covalent attachment of ubiquitin to the target proteinby the formation of isopeptide bonds. Multiple cycles of ubiquitination finally result in the synthesis and attachment of polyubiquitin chains that serve as a recognition signal for the degradation of the target protein by the 26S proteasome.

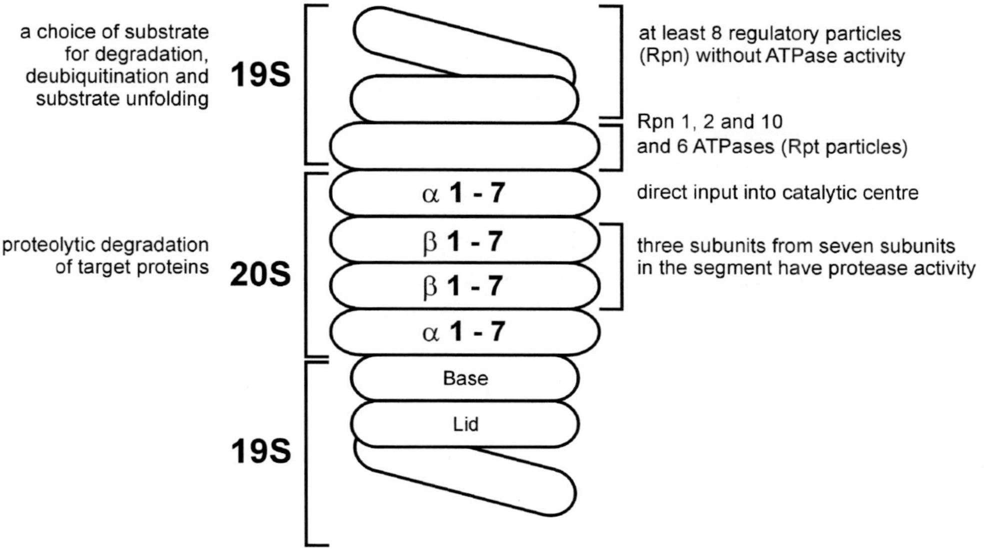

Figure 2. The structure of the 26S proteasome. The 26S proteasome consists of the 20S catalytic core complex and two 19S regulatory complexes capping the 20S complex at both ends. The 20S complex is composed of four axially stacked rings. Each of the outer rings consists of seven polypeptide α subunits that serve as the gates through which proteasome substrates enter, whereas each of the two inner rings is formed by seven proteolytic β subunits, and only three of them, β1,β2, and β5, are proteolytically active and harbor proteolytic sites that face the central cavity of the 20S complex. The 19S complex consists of the base and lid subcomplex. The base subcomplex contains six nonredundant ATPases. The lid subcomplex contains at least eight subunits including deubiquitinating enzymes and receptors for ubiquitinated proteins. The polyubiquitinated target protein enters the 19S regulatory complex and is recognized, deubiquitinated, unfolded, and translocated into the central cavity of the 20S catalytic core complex, where it is degraded by different hydrolytic activities. Ubiquitin is recycled by the ubiquitin carboxy terminal hydrolase. Peptides as a product of degradation are released from the 26S proteasome by diffusion and are used for major histocompatibility class I antigen presentation or are further degraded to single amino acids by cytosolic peptidases.

The 20S core exhibits three enzymatic activities (chymotrypsin-like, trypsin-like, and peptidyl-glutamyl peptide-hydrolyzing also named caspase-like) in the inner β-rings. Many proteins degraded by proteasome are implicated in important cell processes: cell-cycle-regulatory proteins (cyclins A,B,C,D and E, inhibitors of cyclin-dependent kinases -proteins $p21^{WAF1/CIP1}$ and $p27^{KIP1}$, the tumor suppressor p53, inhibitor of NF-κB- protein IκB, intercellular adhesion molecule-1 (ICAM-1) and vascular cell adhesion molecule-1 (VCAM-1).

Proteasome Inhibitors

Proteasomes belong to proteolytic enzymes called threonine proteases. Proteasome inhibitors were first synthesized as tools to probe the function and proteolytic activity specificity of the proteasome [22,23]. Most of the proteasome inhibitors address the chymotryptic activity of the 20S proteasome core via adduct formation with N-terminal threonine hydroxyl group as part of the catalytically active center.

Results of both preclinical and clinical studies suggest that transformed cells are more sensitive to proteasome inhibition than normal cells [24-26]. Similarly, MM cell lines were more sensitive to apoptosis induced by proteasome inhibitors than were peripheral blood mononuclear cells from healthy individuals [27]. The biologic basis for the enhanced susceptibility of cancer cells to proteasome inhibitors has not been fully elucidated. Several hypotheses have been proposed. One from them is the loss of checkpoint mechanisms for DNA repair by cancer cells. Other hypotheses are a greater sensitivity of rapidly proliferating tumor cells to proteasome inhibitors and more efficient uptake and slower inactivation of proteasome inhibitors by tumor cells [28-30]. Thus, the possibility that proteasome inhibitors could be drug candidates appeared as a new hope for cancer therapy.

Several classes of proteasome inhibitors were developed and several proteasome inhibitors are shown in Figure 3. There are six major classes of proteasome inhibitors: peptide aldehydes, peptide semicarbazones, peptide vinyl sulfones, peptide boronates, peptide epoxyketones (epoxomycin and eponomycin) and β-lactones (lactacystin and its derivatives), based on the pharmacophore that reacts with the threonine residue in the active site of the proteasome. In leukemia, three classes of proteasome inhibitors entered clinical trials (peptide boronates /bortezomib/, β-lactones /NPI-0052/ and epoxomycin derivatives /PR-171/). Toxicity profiles of other three classes of proteasome inhibitors (peptide aldehydes, peptide semicarbazones and peptide vinyl sulfones) prevent their use in clinical trials.

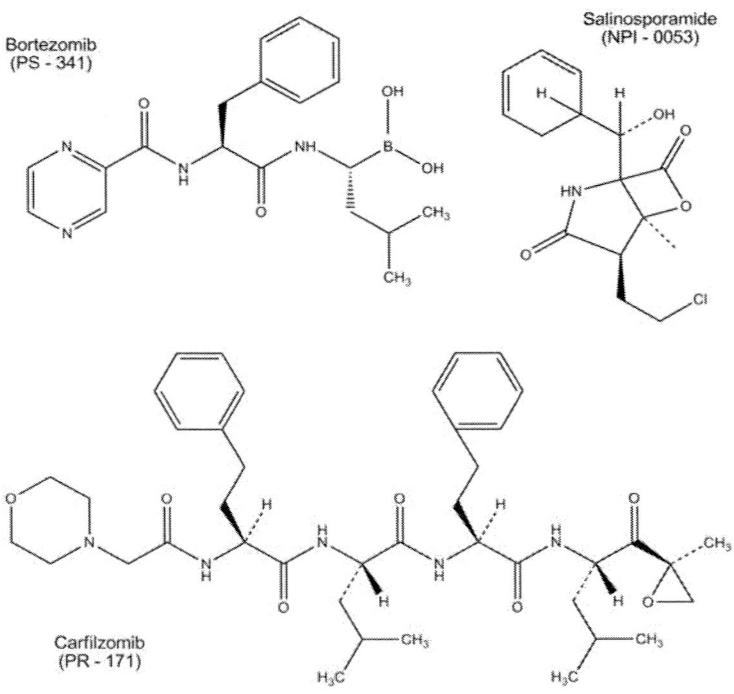

Figure 3. Chemical structures of several selected proteasome inhibitors.

Resistance to apoptosis and enhanced proliferation is characteristic feature of cancer cells. Proteasome inhibitors induce cell cycle arrest by interfering with timely degradation of cyclins and cyclin-dependent kinases inhibitors. Proteasome inhibitors function as apoptosis inducers by inhibition of transcription factor NF-κB and by endoplasmic reticulum stress and subsequent generation of reactive oxygen species. Proteasome inhibitors stabilize proapoptotic proteins, such as p53, Bax, Bik and Bim while reduce levels of some antiapoptotic proteins, such as Bcl2.

The first developed proteasome inhibitors were peptide aldehydes, which mimic a protein substrate [31-33]. The peptide aldehydes form a reversible covalent hemiacetal intermediate between the aldehyde group of the inhibitor and the hydroxyl group of the amino terminal threonine. MG115 (N-benzoyloxycarbonyl(Z)-1-L-leucinyl-L-leucinyl-L-norvalinal), MG132 (N-benzoyloxycarbonyl (Z)-Leu-Leu-leucinal) and PSI (N-benzyloxycarbonyl (Z) -Ile-Glu(O-t-Bu)-Ala-leucinal) are members of this group of proteasome inhibitors. However, many peptide aldehydes, for example MG132 and others, cause significant neurotoxicity and therefore they were not used in clinical trials.

Bortezomib

Boronate inhibitors of the proteasome are more potent than structurally similar peptide aldehydes [34]. Bortezomib (VELCADE, formerly known as PS-341, pyrazinylcarbonyl-Phe-Leu-boronate) inhibits proteasome by binding reversibly to the chymotrypsin-like site in the 20S core of the proteasome [35]. Bortezomib is the first proteasome inhibitor approved by the US Food and Drug Administration for the treatment of relapsed or relapsed and refractory multiple myeloma (MM) and some forms of non-Hodgkin´s lymphoma, mantle cell lymphoma [36-44]. Cellular mechanisms responsible for the clinical efficacy of bortezomib include inhibition of tumor cell adhesion to stroma and disruption cytokine-dependent survival pathways, in part through suppression of the transcription nuclear factor-κB (NF-κB) activity, inhibition of angiogenesis, induction of aggresome (aggregates of ubiquitin-conjugated proteins) formation, endoplasmic reticulum stress, and the unfolded protein response [45-51].

Adhesion of tumor cells to extracellular to extracellular matrix proteins and bone marrow stromal cells (BMSCs) plays a major role in the MM pathogenesis [52]. The most important factors for the development of osteoclasts are macrophage colony-stimulating factor (*M-CSF*) and receptor activator of nuclear factor – kappa B ligand (RANKL). M-CSF expands the pool of osteoclast precursors and subsequently RANKL stimulates osteoclast precursors to develop into mature osteoclasts (Figure 4). Myeloma cells induce RANKL expression and downregulate the expression of osteoprotegerin (OPG), a soluble RANKL decoy receptor. RANKL is responsible for osteoclast-mediated bone resorption in a broad range of conditions and plays a key role in establishment and propagation of skeletal disease in MM. The candidates for the stimulation of osteoclast activity are interleukin (IL)-6, macrophage inflammatory protein-1 alpha (MIP-1α), RANKL, and interleukin-1 beta (IL-1β) (Figure 5). Adhesion of MM cells to extracellular matrix proteins confers cell adhesion-mediated drug resistance and binding of MM cells to BMSCs triggers transcription and secretion of cytokines, primarily NF-κB-dependent secretion of IL-6 [53-55].

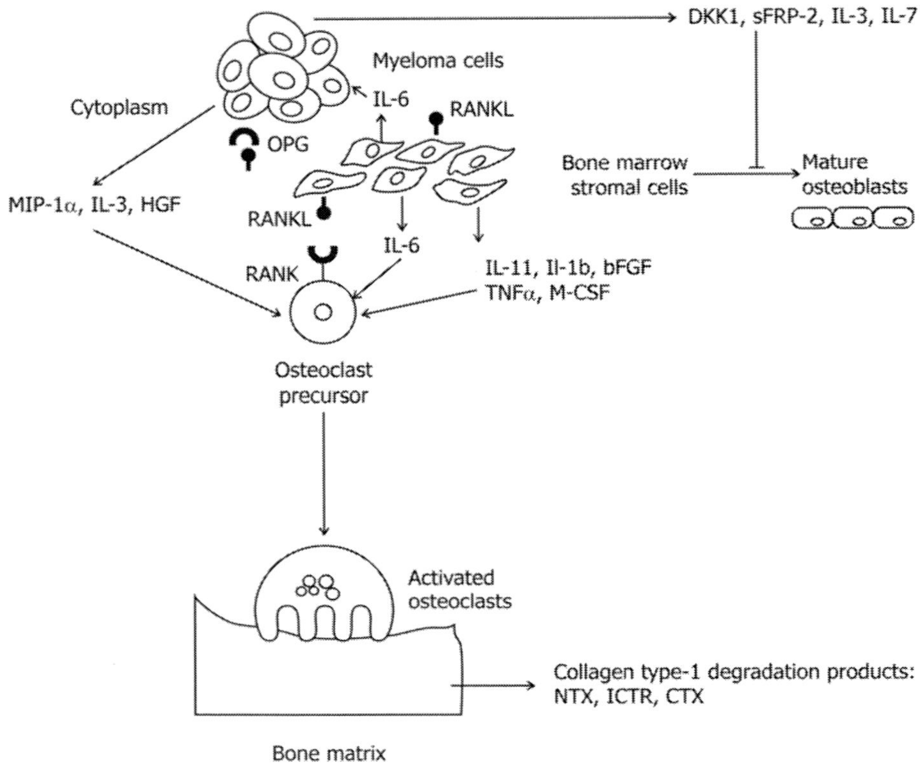

Figure 4. The role of the myeloma microenvironment in pathophysiology of multiple myeloma (MM) bone disease. MM is characterized by extensive bones loss and osteolytic lesions. MM cells bind to bone marrow stromal cells through the interaction of VCAM-1 and integrin α4b1. Myeloma cells produce RANKL and cause bone marrow stromal cells to overexpress RANKL and IL-6. Binding of RANKL to RANK on the surface of osteoclast precursors induces NF-κB activation, which leads to osteoclast differentiation and bone resorption. IL-6 acts as a growth factor for myeloma cells. RANKL and IL-6 induce differentiation of osteoclast precursors into mature osteoclasts. OPG is is the soluble RANKL antagonist. Myeloma cells inhibit OPG. MM cells secrete factors that alter the biology of bone remodeling. Wnt signaling is essential for maintenance of osteoblast and osteoclast homeostasis. Production of Wnt signaling inhibitors dickopf-1 (DKK1) and sFRP2 contributes to osteolytic lesions through the direct inhibition of osteoblast differentiation. Myeloma cells express MIP-1α, which recruits osteoclast precursors and enhances osteoclast activity. The resulting enhanced bone resorption releases collagen type-1 degradation products, cytokines and growth factors that in turn promote myeloma cell proliferation and survival.

This in turn triggers the proliferation of MM cells, promotes both tumor cells survival and upregulation of anti-apoptotic molecules [56, 57]. IL-6 mediates autocrine and paracrine growth of MM cells within the BM millieu. It also confers to tumor cells further resistance to conventional therapy and induces vascular endothelial growth factor (VEGF) expression and secretion [52]. The important role of BM microenvironment in MM pathogenesis is now well established [5, 6, 58]. The balanced homeostasis between the cellular, the extracellular, and the liquid compartments within the BM is disrupted. The results of this disruption are immune suppression, cytopenias and lytic bone lesions.

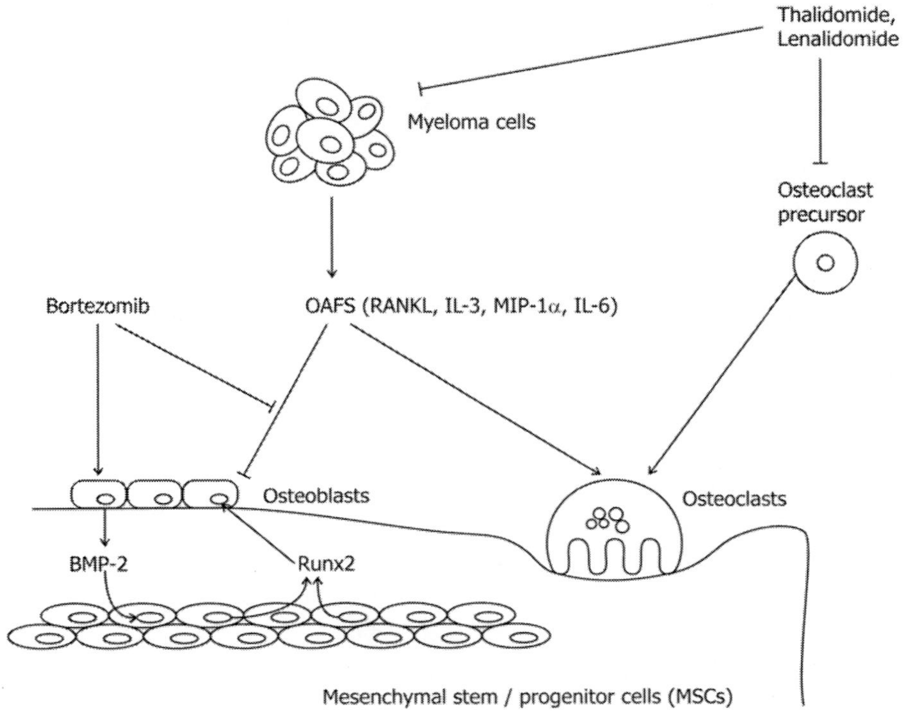

Figure 5. The sites of bortezomib, thalidomide and lenalidomide action in the pathophysiology of MM bone disease. Bortezomib directly inhibits osteoclast formation and function. Bortezomib enhances new bone formation and inhibits DKK1 expression and induces osteoblast differentiation. Bortezomib also increases the mumber of Runx2/Cbfa1-positive osteoblasts of responding MM patients, but not in those who did not respond. Bortezomib reduces serum receptor activator of nuclear NF-κB ligand (RANKL) levels. Thus, bortezomib prevents NF-κB activation, which leads to the prevention of bone resorption. Thalidomide and lenalidomide inhibit osteoclast development by affecting the lineage commitment of osteoclast precursors. These drugs, aside from their antiangiogenic effects, also activate apoptosis of MM cells.

All these effects are caused by the impact of tunor cells on the BM and other cells within the BM millieu. Tumor cell growth, survival, migration, and drug resistance are promoted by these effects. The therapeutic success of proteasome inhibitors, thalidomide and lenalidomide in relapsed refractory disease is associated with targeting interactions between MM cells and BM cells (Figure 5), including tumor angiogenesis and or cytokines or growth factors in the BM microenvironment (also called "niches").

Bortezomib in Preclinical Studies on Human Myeloma Cell Lines and Primary Patient Multiple Myeloma Cells

In these studies bortezomib inhibited the proliferation in human myeloma cell lines, which were both sensitive and refractory to conventional chemotherapeutic agents (melphalan, doxorubicin, mitoxantrone and dexamethasone). Bortezomib induced caspase-dependent apoptosis of myeloma cell lines and primary patient MM cells [55]. MM cell lines were up to 40 times more sensitive to the proapoptotic effects of bortezomib than were peripheral blood mononuclear cells from healthy individuals [55]. Bortezomib also inhibited NF-κB activation in tumor necrosis factor (TNF)-α-treated MM cells by blocking the degradation of the inhibitor protein IκBα and overcame the resistance to apoptosis in MM cells conferred by IL-6 [55, 59, 60]. Proapoptotic regulators upregulation and antiapoptotic proteins downregulation were observed [59, 61]. Bortezomib stabilizes proapoptotic proteins, such as p53, Bax, Bik and Bim while reduce levels of some antiapoptotic proteins, such as Bcl-2. Bortezomib responses are also linked to the upregulation of the proapoptotic Bcl-2 protein family member Noxa [62] and this effect is independent of constitutive activity of the phosphoinositide 3-kinase/AKT (protein kinase B) and NF-κB pathways. Bortezomib induces Noxa and the cleavage of antiapoptotic protein Mcl-1. The myeloid cell leukemia-1 (*Mcl-1*) protein is an antiapoptotic member of the Bcl-2 family. Noxa induction allows the displacement of the direct apoptosis activator Bim, which is able to activate Bax/Bak by a "hit and run" mechanism, triggering mitochondrial dysfunction and apoptosis (Figure 6).

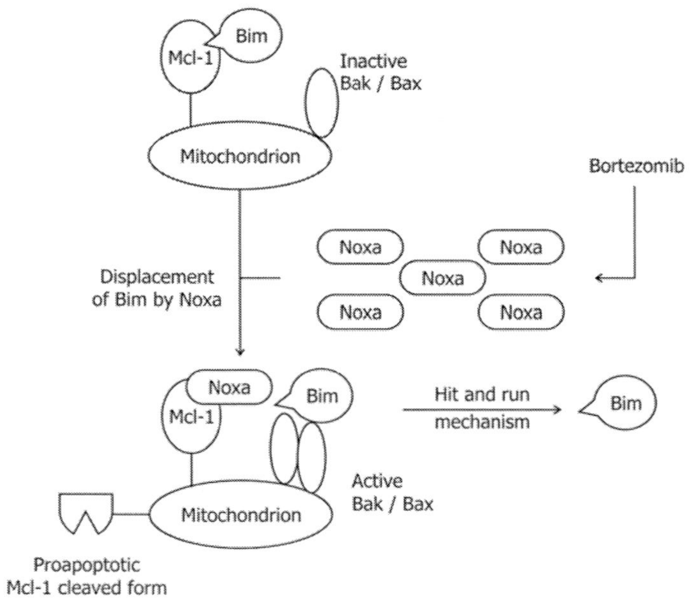

Figure 6. Effect of bortezomibe treatment on the interplay between antiapoptotic and proapoptotic members of the Bcl-2 family in myeloma cells. Myeloma cell death is totally dependent on Mcl-1/Bim complex disruption. Noxa induced by bortezomib is involvrd in the displacement of Bim from Mcl-1 binding. Released Bim triggers Bax/Bak activation and through this it induces apoptosis.

Bortezomib-mediated proteasome inhibition affect multiple signaling pathways, including cell cycle, growth arrest, stress response, microenvironment and apoptosis. Disruption of multiple cellular signaling by bortezomib initiates and maintains an active cell death pathway and causes apoptosis as we show in Figure 7.

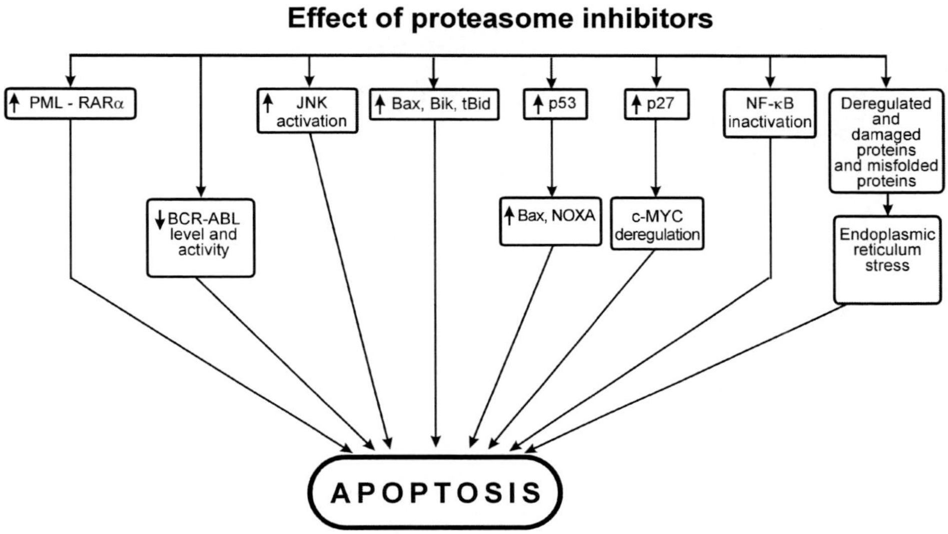

Figure 7. Molecular targets of proteasome inhibitors in the process of apoptosis induction.

Binding of MM cells to BMSCs and abrogation of the NF-κB-dependent transcription and secretion of IL-6 in BMSCs were also inhibited by bortezomib [55]. Molecular mechanisms of the antimyeloma activity of bortezomib was studied by analysis of gene expression profiles of bortezomib-treated MM cells in comparison with nontreated MM cells. Bortezomib also induced the phosphorylation of c-Jun NH_2-terminal kinase (JNK), activating caspase-8 and, subsequently, caspase-3. The activated caspase-3 cleaved DNA protein kinase catalytic subunit and ATM/ATR proteins, and ultimately resulted in impaired DNA repair in MM cells [63]. DNA damage induced by activated caspase-3 was also observed. Subsequent phosphorylation of p53 and the degradation of Mdm2 (the product of expression of murine double minute oncogene that represses p53 transcriptional activity) are in a time and dose-dependent on the level of bortezomib which is comparable with the serum level of bortezomib used in clinical practice [63].

Bortezomib increases osteoblast number, function, and gene expression [64-66] through targeting of a multipotent population of mesenchymal stem progenitor cells (MSCs). Bortezomib induces MSCs to preferentially undergo osteoblastic differentiation, in part by modulation of the bone-specifying transcription factor runt-related transcription factor 2 (Runx-2) [67]. Bortezomib promotes bone formation in myelomatous and nonmyelomatous bones by simultaneously inhibiting osteoclastogenesis and stimulating osteoblastogenesis. As clinical and experimental studies indicate that bone disease is both a consequence and necessity of MM progression our results suggest and that bortezomib's effects on bone remodeling contribute to the antimyeloma efficacy of this drug [68].

Three other studies [69-71] showed an inhibitory effect of bortezomib on osteoclastic bone resorption in MM patients with a significant reduction in serum dickkopf-1 (DKK1) and RANKL levels. DKK1 is an inhibitor of the Wnt signaling pathway (wingless in *Drosophila*) that is important in the growth , development , and function of osteoblasts [72].

Bortezomib in Relapsed and/or Refractory Multiple Myeloma - Clinical Studies

Based on preclinical studies and promising phase 1 trial, two pivotal phase 2 studies, SUMMIT [73] and CREST [74] were performed in relapsed and/or refractory MM patients. Patients were treated with bortezomib 1.3 mg/m^2 on days 1,4,8, and 11 every 3 weeks. Dexamethasone was allowed in patients with suboptimal responses to bortezomib alone. The overall response rate was 35%, including 10% complete or near complete responses with an overall survival of 17 months. The randomized CREST study [74], comparing two dosages of bortezomib (1.3 versus 1,0 mg/m^2) showed that a reduced dose was able to produce responses in up to one third of patients and it was accompanied with a lower toxicity. The addition of dexamethasone in patients with suboptimal responses to bortezomib alone resulted again in an improvement in the response degree [75].

A subsequent randomized phase 3 trial "the Assessment of Proteasome Inhibition for Extending Remissions" (APEX) including 669 patients with relapsed MM has shown that bortezomib is more effective than high dose dexamethasone as demonstrated by a significant improvement in response rate (43% vs 18%), median time to progression (6.2 vs 3.4 months) and 1-year survival rate (80% vs 67%, respectively) [76]. In the updated APEX analysis (median follow-up: 22 months), survival was assessed in both arms (single-agent bortezomib versus high-dose dexamethasone), and efficacy updated for the bortezomib arm. Median survival was 29.8 months for bortezomib versus 23.7 months for dexamethasone, a 6-month benefit, despite substantial crossover from dexamethasone to bortezomib. Overall and complete response rates with bortezomib were 43% and 9%, respectively; among responding patients, 56% improved response with longer therapy beyond initial response, leading to continued improvement in overall quality of response. Higher response quality was associated with longer response duration; response duration was not associated with time to response. These data confirm the activity of bortezomib and support extended treatment in relapsed multiple myeloma patients tolerating therapy [77].

Bortezomib therapy has become an important part of the standard of care for patients with relapsed multiple myeloma, and preliminary clinical evidence suggests that bortezomib retreatment in patients previously treated with the drug may prolong disease control. The retrospective study [78] was designed to clarify the utility of bortezomib as a repeat therapy. Records from 3 major cancer centers that had participated in the phase 2 (SUMMIT or CREST) or phase 3 (APEX) registration studies were used to identify patients who were subsequently retreated off protocol with bortezomib-based therapy. 22 patients who received bortezomib retreatment following a 60 or more day gap between bortezomib treatments were found. Twelve patients had intervening therapy between initial bortezomib treatment and bortezomib retreatment. During retreatment, 14 of 22 patients received bortezomib in combination with another antineoplastic agent. The overall response rate for bortezomib retreatment was 50% (9% complete responses). The median length of retreatment was 5.1 months in responding patients and 2.4 months in nonresponding patients. Therapy was terminated due to unmanageable toxicity in 2 patients during retreatment, compared with 6 patients during initial treatment. During retreatment, no patients required dose reduction due to peripheral neuropathy, compared to 4 patients during their initial treatment. Thus, bortezomib retreatment appears to be safe and effective. Favorable observed response rates with bortezomib retreatment suggest that it may be a viable option for relapsed or refractory multiple myeloma, even in patients previously exposed to bortezomib [78].

An important aspect of all these studies is the toxicity profile of bortezomib, particularly when used in combinations with other agents. The most common side effects of bortezomib were gastrointestinal symptoms, fatigue, and anorexia, although these were mostly grade 1-2 [79]. Thrombocytopenia grade 3-4, due to a reversible blockage in platelet release, was found in 30% of cases, while anemia and neutropenia are uncommon (<10%). The major dose-limiting adverse effect is painful peripheral neuropathy (37% with only 9% grade 3 and more) [80]. Unusual toxicities such as tumor lysis syndrome, severe pulmonary failure, toxic hepatitis or rhabdomyolysis have been also reported [79, 81, 82]. Thus, the toxicity profile of bortezomib is well defined and most complications are predictable and manageable.

Combinations of Bortezomib with Conventional Anti-Multiple Myeloma Agents

Bortezomib was combined in a phase 1 trial with liposomal doxorubicin in advanced MM patients [83]. The response rate among 22 evaluable patients was 73%, including 36% of complete response. An updated analysis [84] after extended follow-up showed the time to progression 9.3 months, the median time from start of therapy to start of subsequent therapy 24.2 months and median overall survival 38.3 months. The phase 3 international study compared the efficacy and safety of a combination of pegylated liposomal doxorubicin (PLD) plus bortezomib with bortezomib monotherapy in patients with relapsed or refractory multiple myeloma [85]. 646 patients were randomly assigned to receive either intravenous bortezomib 1.3 mg/m(2) on days 1, 4, 8, and 11 of an every 21-days cycle, or the same bortezomib regimen with PLD 30 mg/m(2) on day 4. Median time to progression was increased from 6.5 months for bortezomib to 9.3 months with the PLD + bortezomib combination. The 15-month survival rate for PLD + bortezomib was 76% compared with 65% for bortezomib alone. The complete plus partial response rate was 41% for bortezomib and 44% for PLD + bortezomib, a difference that was not statistically significant. Median duration of response was increased from 7.0 to 10.2 months with PLD + bortezomib. Grade 3/4 adverse events were more frequent in the combination group (80% vs 64%), with safety profiles consistent with the known toxicities of the two agents. An increased incidence in the combination group was seen of grade 3/4 neutropenia, thrombocytopenia, asthenia, fatigue, diarrhea, and hand-foot syndrome. PLD with bortezomib is superior to bortezomib monotherapy for the treatment of patients with relapsed or refractory multiple myeloma. The combination therapy is associated with a higher incidence of grade 3/4 myelosuppression, constitutional symptoms, gastrointestinal symptoms, and dermatologic toxicities.

Following the remarkably positive results of a large phase 3 trial comparing bortezomib and PLD with bortezomib monotherapy, the FDA approved the use of this combination in May 2007 for patients who have not previously received bortezomib and who have received at least one prior therapy. Bortezomib can sensitize MM cells to conventional chemotherapeutics to which a patient has previously become resistant [59, 86].

Bortezomib has shown activity in relapsed and or refractory MM, even in patients refractory to thalidomide or lenalidomide (immunomodulatory drug [IMiD]) treatment [87]. Combination therapies with bortezomib - thalidomide - dexamethasone [88], bortezomib-melphalan-prednisone-thalidomide [89] or with bortezomib - lenalidomide - dexamethasone [90] were highly effective in advanced and refractory MM. These treatment strategies will hopefully further prolong the survival of patients with myeloma.

The Second-Generation Proteasome Inhibitors with More Potency and Fewer Side-Effects Studied in Multiple Myeloma

The good clinical results obtained with bortezomib have validated the proteasome as a therapeutic target in MM. Two second-generation proteasome inhibitors have entered phase 1 and phase 2 trials: NPI-0052 (salinosporamide A) and carfilzomib (formerly PR-171) (see Figure 3). Salinosporamide A related to lactacystin is a natural product derived from the fermentation of the marine gram-positive actinomycete *Salinospora tropica* [91-97]. Preclinical studies in MM models showed that NPI-0052induces apoptosis of MM cells, including cells resistant to conventional anti-MMtherapies as well as cells isolated from patients who had developed resistance to bortezomib-based therapies [93]. NPI-0052 is distinct from bortezomib in terms of chemical structure (Figure 3) and effects on individual proteolytic activities of the proteasome activities. While bortezomib inhibits exclusively the chymotrypsin-like activity of the 20S proteasome, NPI-0052 inhibits all three protease activities in the proteasome (Figure 8): the chymotrypsin-like, trypsin-like, and caspase-like activities [93]. Another important difference is that NPI-0052 is orally bioavailable, while bortezomib is not amenable to oral administration. Schematic representation of the mechanism of action of salinosporamide A is shown in Figure 8. Inhibition of all three proteolytic activities of the 20S proteasome in leukemia cells by NPI-0052 results in activation of caspase-8. This leads to proapoptotic protein Bid cleavage and to the considerable decrease of mitochondrial transmembrane potential [97]. Mitochondrial membrane permeabilization, release of cytochrome c and activation of caspase-9 follow. Apoptosis proceeds then by activation of effector caspase-3 and consequent DNA fragmentation and increased levels of intracellular reactive oxygen species were detected [97].

Combination of NPI-0052 and bortezomib induces synergistic anti-MM activity (Figure 9) [96]. These studies therefore provide the rationale for clinical protocols evaluating NPI-0052, alone and together with bortezomib, to improve patient outcome in MM.

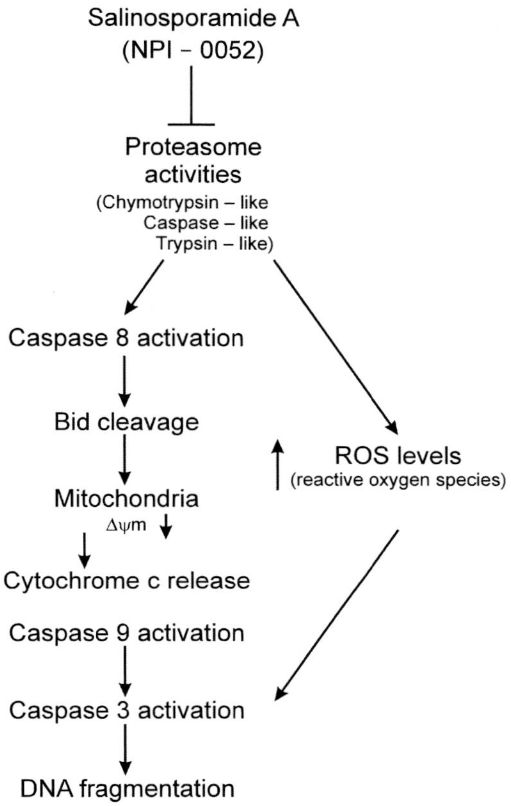

Figure 8. Schema of the mechanism of inhibition of all three proteasome proteolytic activities (the chymotrypsin-like, caspase-like, and trypsin-like activities) by salinosporamide A (NPI-0052). NPI-0052 induces caspase-8, which initiates Bid cleavage and drops of mitochondrial membrane potential (Δψm). Mitochondrial perturbations lead to the release of cytochrome c from the mitochondria, which then activates the mitochondrial – mediated proapoptotic pathway (activation of caspases-9 and -3 and consequent DNA fragmentation). Parallel pathway of cell death induction by NPI-0052 is connected with reactive oxygen species generation.

Another new proteasome inhibitor of next generation is PR-171 (carfilzomib) (Figure 3). PR-171 is epoxyketone-based irreversible proteasome inhibitor that exhibits a high level of selectivity for a single active site in the proteasome, as well as minimal cross reactivity to other protease classes [98-101]. In models of MM, carfilzomib potently bound and specifically inhibited the chymotrypsin-like proteasome and immunoproteasome activities, resulting in accumulation of ubiquitinated substrates. Carfilzomib induced a dose- and time-dependent inhibition of proliferation, ultimately leading to apoptosis. Programmed cell death was associated with activation JNK, mitochondrial membrane depolarization, release of cytochrome c, and activation of both intrinsic and extrinsic caspase pathways.

This agent also inhibited proliferation and activated apoptosis in patient-derived MM cells, as well as neoplastic cells from patients with other hematologic malignancies. Importantly, carfilzomib showed increased efficacy compared to bortezomib (Figure 10), and was active against bortezomib-resistant MM cell lines, and samples from patients with clinical bortezomib resistance.

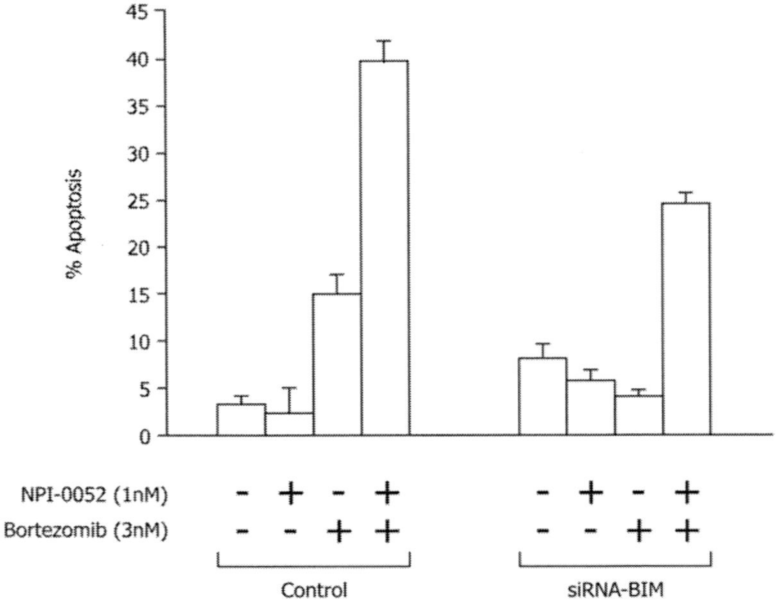

Figure 9. The role of Bim, a proapoptotic relative of Bcl-2, in apoptosis induced by the second generation proteasome inhibitor NPI-0052 in comparison with bortezomib. MM.1S dexamethasone sensitive cells were transfected with Bim siRNA for 48 hours, followed by 12-hour of treatment with indicated proteasome inhibitor/s abd analysis for apoptosis by annexinV/propidium iodide staining. Experimental data from [96] were used.

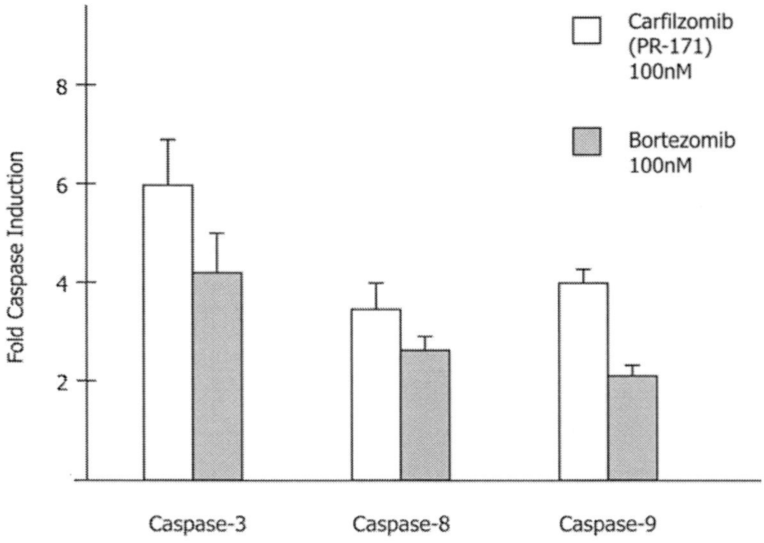

Figure 10. Caspase induction by the second generation proteasome inhibitor carfilzomib (PR-171) in compatison with bortezomib in ANBL-6 MM cells. Cells were exposed to a 1-hour pulse of 100 nM carfilzomib or bortezomib and allowed to recover for 8 hours. Cellular lysates (30μg per reaction) were then incubated with 40μM fluorogenic substrate specific for caspase-3, caspase-8, and caspase-9 activity. Experimental data from [100] were used.

Carfilzomib also overcame resistance to other conventional agents, and acted synergistically with dexamethasone to enhance cell death. In addition to the Phase II trial in solid tumors, carfilzomib is currently being evaluated in two Phase II single-agent trials in multiple myeloma and a Phase I study in lymphoma. Phase I clinical studies have shown that patients with hematologic malignancies (MM and Waldenström´s macroglobulinemia) who have relapsed or progressed following multiple therapies can achieve durable anti-tumor responses with carfilzomib [100, 101].

The third novel orally active proteasome inhibitor CEP-18770 / [(1R)-1-[[(2 S,3 R)-3-hydroxy-2-[(6-phenylpyridine-2-carbonyl)amino]-1-oxobutyl]amino]-3-methylbutyl]boronic acid 20 / was also studied in preclinical trials [102, 103]. CEP-18770 potently induces apoptotic cell death in MM cell lines and in primary purified CD138-positive cultures from untreated and bortezomib-treated MM patients [103]. In vitro, CEP-18770 has a strong antiangiogenic activity and potently represses RANKL-induced osteoclastogenesis. CEP-18770 exhibits a favorable cytotoxicity profile toward normal human epithelial cells, bone marrow progenitors, and bone marrow-derived stromal cells. Thus, CEP-18770 has a favorable tumor selectivity profile for the treatment of MM and other malignancies responsive to proteasome inhibition.

Conclusion and Perspectives

The heterogeneity of MM biology and prognosis has become apparent over the last decade. The prognosis and treatment of an individual with MM depends on many patient-specific factors, including age, overall state of health, and comorbidities. A more personalized approach to treatment is likely to become standardas increasingly robust molecularly based prognostic information becomes available. Insights into the role of the tumor microenvironment have provided new targets for for the novel therapies. Pharmacogenomic analysis promises a new era of therapy tailored to the individual MM patient.

The first clinical trials evaluating the therapeutic potential of proteasome inhibition began before about 10 years. Since then, remarkable progress has been made. The role of bortezomib in the treatment of MM has evolved since the drug was introduced to the market. Bortezomib-based combinations in newly diagnosed patients have resulted in high overall and complete response rates. Additionally, there does not seem to be a negative impact on stem cell harvest or engraftment in patients who received bortezomib as part of their induction regime [104].

A new next generation proteasome inhibitors (NPI-0052 and PR-171) are currently being evaluated in phase 1 and phase 2 trials of patients with relapsed and or refractory MM. As with bortezomib, next generation proteasome inhibitors trigger apoptosis in MM cells but are distinct from bortezomib in their chemical structure, effects on proteasome activities, and mechanism of action. The cellular response to next generation proteasome inhibitors occurs much earlier than that of bortezomib. Orally administered next generation proteasome inhibitors are cytotoxic to myeloma cells, with reduced toxicity against normal cells, compared with bortezomib. Because of the different kinetics and cellular responses, bortezomib and next generation proteasome inhibitors can be used in combination with synergistic apoptotic activity.

Acknowledgments

This work was supported by the research intention VZ 00023736 from the Ministry of Health of the Czech Republic (MZO UHKT 2005), and grant LC 06044 from Ministry of Education, Youth and Sport of the Czech Republic.

References

[1] Cook, R. Economic and clinical impact of multiple myeloma to managed care. *J. Manag. Care Pharm*. 2008, 14, Suppl. S, S19-S25.

[2] Kyle, R.; Rajkumar, SV. Multiple myeloma. *N. Engl. J. Med*. 2004, 351, 1860-1873.

[3] Chng, WJ.; Glebov, O.; Bergsagel, PL.; Kuehl, WM. Genetic events in the pathogenesis of multiple myeloma. *Best Pract. Res. Clin. Haematol*. 2007, 20, 571-596.

[4] Tonon, G. Molecular pathogenesis of multiple myeloma. *Hematol. Oncol. Clin. N. Am*. 2007, 21, 985-1006.

[5] Podar, K.; Richardson, PG.; Hideshima, T.; Chauhan, D.; Anderson, KC. The malignant clone and the bone marrow environment. *Best Pract. Res. Clin. Haematol*. 2007, 20, 597-612.

[6] Mitsiades, CS.; McMillin, DV.; Klippel, S.; Hideshima, T.; Chauhan, D.; Richardson, PG. et al. The role of the bone marrow microenvironment in the pathophysiology of myeloma and its significance in the development of more effective therapies. *Hematol. Oncol. Clin. N. Am*. 2007, 21, 1007-1034.

[7] Richardson, PG.; Barlogie, B.; Berenson, J.; Singhal, S.; Jagannath, S.; Irwin, D. et al. Clinical factors predictive of outcome with bortezomib in patients with relapsed, refractory multiple myeloma. *Blood* 2008, 106, 2977-2981.

[8] Barlogie, B.; Shaughnessy, J.; Tricot, G.; Jacobson, J.; Zangari, M.; Anaissie, E. et al. Treatment of multiple myeloma. *Blood 2*004, 103, 20-32.

[9] Mitsiades, CS.; Hayden, PJ.; Anderson, KC.; Richardson, PG. From the bench to the bedside: emerging new treatments in multiple myeloma. *Best Pract. Res. Clin. Haematol*. 2007, 20, 797-816.

[10] Kastritis, E.; Mitsiades, CS.; Dimopoulos, MA.; Richardson, PG. Management of relapsed and relapsed refractory myeloma. *Hematol. Oncol. Clin. N. Am*. 2007, 21, 1007-1034.

[11] Schwartz, RN. Current and emerging treatments for multiple myeloma. *J. Manag. Care Pharm*. 2008, 14, Suppl. S, S12-S18.

[12] Hershko, A.; Ciechanover, A. The ubiquitin system. *Annu. Rev. Biochem*. 1998, 67, 425-479.

[13] Pickart, C.M. Mechanisms underlying ubiquitination. *Annu. Rev. Biochem*. 2001, 70, 503-533.

[14] Glickman, M.H.; Ciechanover, A. The ubiquitin-proteasome proteolytic pathway: destruction for the sake of construction. *Physiol. Rev.* 2002, 82, 373-428.

[15] Pickart, C.M.; Cohen R.E. Proteasomes and their kin: proteases in the machine age. *Nat. Rev. Mol. Cell. Biol.* 2004, 5, 177-187.

[16] Hershko, A. Review: Nobel Lecture. The ubiquitin system for protein degradation and some of its roles in the control of the cell division cycle. *Cell Death Differ.* 2005, 12, 1191-1197.

[17] Ciechanover, A. Intracellular protein degradation from a vague idea through the lysosome and the ubiquitin-proteasome system and on to human diseases and drug targeting: Nobel Lecture, December 8, 2004. *Ann.. N.Y. Acad. Sci.* 2007, 1116, 1-28.

[18] Rose, I. Review: Nobel Lecture. Ubiquitin at Fox Chase. *Cell Death Differ.* 2005, 12, 1162-1166.

[19] Wilkinson, KD. Ubiquitin: A Nobel protein. *Cell* 2004, 119, 741-745.

[20] Koegl, M; Hoppe, T.; Schlenker, S.; Ulrich, HD.; Mayer, TU.; Jentsch, S. A novel ubiquitination factor, E4, is involved in multiubiquitin chain assembly. *Cell* 1999, 96, 635-644.

[21] Staub, O.; Rotin, D. Role of ubiquitylation in cellular membrane transport. *Physiol. Rev.* 2006, 86, 669-707.

[22] Savory, PJ.; Rivett, AJ. Leupeptin-binding site(s) in the mammalian multicatalytic proteinase complex. *Biochem. J.*1993, 289, 45-48.

[23] Vinitsky, A.; Cardozo, C.; Sepp-Lorenzino, L.; Michaud, C.; Orlowski, M. Inhibition of the proteolytic activity of the multicatalytic proteinase complex (proteasome) by substrate-related peptidyl aldehydes. *J. Biol. Chem.* 1994, 269, 29860-29866.

[24] Delic, J.; Masdehors, P.; Omura, S.; Cosset, JM.; Dumont, J.; Binet, JL. et al. The proteasome inhibitor lactacystin induces apoptosis and sensitizes chemo- and radioresistant human chronic lymphocytic leukemia lymphocytes to TNF-alpha-initiated apoptosis. *Br. J. Cancer* 1998, 77, 1103-1107.

[25] Masdehors, P.; Omura, S.; Merle-Beral, H.; Mentz, F.; Cosset, JM.; Dumont, J. et al. Increased sensitivity of CLL-derived lymphocytes to apoptotic death activation by the proteasome-specific inhibitor lactacystin. *Br. J. Haematol.* 1999, 105, 752-757.

[26] Orlowski, RZ.; Eswara, JR.; Lafond-Walker, A.; Grever, MR.; Orlowski, M.; Dang, CV. Tumor growth inhibition induced in a murine model of human Burkitt´s lymphoma by a proteasome inhibitor. *Cancer Res.* 1998, 58, 4342-4348.

[27] Hideshima, T.; Richardson, PG.; Chauhan, D.; Palombella, VI.; Elliott, PJ.; Adams, J. et al. The proteasome inhibitor PS-341 inhibits growth, induces apoptosis and overcomes drug resistance in human multiple myeloma cells. *Cancer Res.* 2001, 61, 3071-3076.

[28] Kisselev, AF.; Goldberg, AL. Proteasome inhibitors: from research tools to drug candidates. *Chem. Biol.* 2001, 8, 739-758.

[29] Voorhees, PM.; Dees, EC.; O´Neil, B.; Orlowski, RZ. The proteasome as a target for cancer therapy. *Clin. Cancer Res.* 2003, 9, 6316-6325.

[30] Almond, JB.; Cohen, GM. The proteasome: a novel target for cancer chemotherapy. *Leukemia* 2002, 16, 433-443.

[31] Vinitsky, A.; Michaud, C.; Powers, J.C.; Orlowski, M. Inhibition of the chymotrypsin – like activity of the pituitary multicatalytic proteinase complex. *Biochemistry* 1992, 31, 9421-9428.

[32] Palombella, V.J., Rando, O.J., Goldberg, A.L., Maniatis, T. The ubiquitin-proteasome pathway is required for processing the NF-kappa B1 precursor protein and the activation of NF-kappa B. *Cell* 1994, 78, 773-785.

[33] Rock KL.; Gramm, C.; Rothstein, L.; Clark, K.; Stein, R.; Dick, L. et al. Inhibitors of the proteasome block the degradation of most cell proteins and the generation of peptides presented on MHC class I molecules. *Cell* 1994, 78, 761-771.

[34] Adams, J.; Behnke, M.; Chen, S.; Cruickshank, AA.; Dick, LR.; Grenier, L. et al. otent and selective inhibitors of the proteasome: dipeptidyl boronic acids. *Bioorg. Med.Chem.Lett.* 1998, 8, 333-338.

[35] Adams, J.; Kauffman, M. Development of the proteasome inhibitor Velcade (Bortezomib). *Cancer Invest.* 2004, 22, 304-311.

[36] Adams, J. The proteasome: a suitable antineoplastic target. *Nat. Rev. Cancer* 2004, 4, 349-360.

[37] Kane, RC.; Bross, PF.; Farrell, AT.; Pazdur, R. Velcade: U.S. FDA approval for the treatment of multiple myeloma progressing on prior therapy. *Oncologist* 2003, 8, 508-513.

[38] Kane, RC.; Farrell, AT.; Sridhara, R.; Pazdur, R. United States Food and Drug Administration approval summary: bortezomib for the treatment of progressive multiple myeloma after one prior therapy. *Clin.. Cancer Res.* 2006, 12, 2955-2960.

[39] Richardson, PG.; Sonneveld, P.; Schuster, MW.; Irwin, D.; Stadtmauer, EA., Facon, T. et al. Safety and efficacy of bortezomib in high-risk and elderly patients with relapsed multiple myeloma. *Br. J. Haematol.* 2007, 137, 429-435.

[40] Chauhan, D.; Hideshima, T.; Anderson, KC. Targeting proteasomes as therapy in multiple myeloma. *Adv. Exp. Med. Biol.* 2008, 615, 251-260.

[41] Goy, A.; Younes, A.; McLaughlin, P.; Pro, B.; Romaguera, JE.; Hagemeister, F. et al. Phase II study of proteasome inhibitor bortezomib in relapsed or refractory B-cell non-Hodgkin's lymphoma. *J. Clin. Oncol.* 2005, 23, 667-675.

[42] O'Connor, OA.; Wright, J.; Moskowitz, C.; Muzzy, J.; MacGregor-Cortelli, B.; Stubblefield, M. Phase II clinical experience with the novel proteasome inhibitor bortezomib in patients with indolent non-Hodgkin's lymphoma and mantle cell lymphoma. *J. Clin.. Oncol.* 2005, 23, 676-684.

[43] Suh, KS.; Gay, A. Bortezomib in mantle cell lymphoma. *Future Oncol.* 2008, 4, 149-168.

[44] Hideshima, T.; Chauhan, D.; Richardson, P.; Mitsiades, C.; Mitsiades, N.; Hayashi, T. et al. NF-kappa B as a therapeutic target in multiple myeloma. *J. Biol. Chem.* 2002, 277, 16639-16647.

[45] Roccaro, AM.; Vacca, A.; Ribatti, D. Bortezomib in the treatment of cancer. *Recent Patents Anticancer Drug Discov.* 2006, 1, 397-403.

[46] Roccaro, AM.; Hideshima, T.; Raje, N.; Kumar, S.; Ishitsuka, K.; Yasui, H. et al. Bortezomib mediates antiangiogenesis in multiple myeloma via direct and indirect effects on endothelial cells. *Cancer Res.* 2006, 66,184-191.

[47] Hideshima, T.; Bradner, J.E.; Wong, J.; Chauhan, D.; Richardson, P.; Schreiber, S.L.; Anderson, K.C. Small-molecule inhibition of proteasome and aggresome function induces synergistic antitumor activity in multiple myeloma. *Proc. Natl. Acad. Sci. USA* 2005, 102, 8567-8572.

[48] Nawrocki, ST.; Carew, JS.; Dunner, K. Jr.; Boise, LH.; Chiao, PJ.; Huang, P. et al. Bortezomib inhibits PKR-like endoplasmic reticulum (ER) kinase and induces apoptosis via ER stress in human pancreatic cancer cells. *Cancer Res.* 2005, 65, 11510-11519.

[49] Nawrocki, ST.; Carew, JS.; Pino, MS.; Highshaw, RA.; Dunner, K. Jr.; Huang, P. et al. Bortezomib sensitizes pancreatic cancer cells to endoplasmic reticulum stress-mediated apoptosis. *Cancer Res.* 2005, 65, 11658-11666.

[50] Lee, AH.; Iwakoshi, NN.; Anderson, KC.; Glimcher, LH. Proteasome inhibitors disrupt the unfolded protein response in myeloma cells. *Proc. Natl. Acad. Sci. USA* 2003, 100, 9946-9951.

[51] Obeng, EA.; Carlson, LM.; Gutman, DM.; Harrington, WJ. Jr.; Lee, KP.; Boise, H. Proteasome inhibitors induce a terminal unfolded protein response in multiple myeloma cells. *Blood* 2006, 107, 4907-4916.

[52] Gupta, D.; Treon, SP.; Shima, Y.; Hideshima, T.; Podar, K.; Tai, YT. et al. Adherence of multiple myeloma cells to bone marrow stromal cells upregulates vascular endothelial growth factor secretion: therapeutic applications. *Leukemia* 2001, 15, 1950-1961.

[53] Chauhan, D.; Uchiyama, H.; Akbarali, Y.; Urashima, M.; Yamamoto, K.; Libermann, TA. et al. Multiple myeloma cell adhesion – induced interleukin-6 expression in bone marrow stromal cells involves activation of NF-kappa B. *Blood* 1996, 87, 1104-1112.

[54] Chauhan, D.; Pandey, P.; Hideshima, T.; Treon, S.; Raje, N.; Davies, FE. et al. SHP2 mediates the protective effect of interleukin-6 against dexamethasone – induced apoptosis in multiple myeloma cells. *J. Biol. Chem.* 2000, 275, 27845-27850.

[55] Dankbar, B.; Padro, T.; Leo, R.; Feldmann, B.; Kropff, M.; Mesters, RM. et al. Vascular endothelial growth factor and interleukin-6 in paracrine tumor-stromal cell interactions in multiple myeloma. *Blood* 2000, 95, 2630-2636.

[56] Ogata, A.; Chauhan, D; Teoh, G; Treon, SP; Urashima, M; Schlossman RL.; Anderson KC. IL-6 triggers cell growth via the Ras-dependent mitogen-activated protein kinase cascade. *J. Immunol.* 1997, 159, 2212-2221.

[57] Lichtenstein, A.; Tu, Y.; Fady, C.; Vescio, R.; Berenson, J. Interleukin-6 inhibits apoptosis of malignant plasma cells. *Cell Immunol.* 1995, 162, 248-255.

[58] Hideshima, T.; Chauhan, D.; Richardson, P.; Anderson, KC. Identification and validation of novel therapeutic targets for multiple myeloma. J. *Clin. Oncol.* 2005, 23, 6345-6350.

[59] Mitsiades, N.; Mitsiades, CS.; Richardson, PG.; Poulaki, V.; Tai, YT.; Chauhan, D. et al. The proteasome inhibitor PS-341 markedly enhances sensitivity of multiple myeloma cells to conventional chemotherapeutic agents: therapeutic applications. *Blood* 2003, 101, 2377-2380.

[60] Hideshima, T.; Chauhan, D.; Schlassman, R.; Richardson, P.; Anderson, RC. The role of tumor necrosis factor alpha in the pathophysiology of human multiple myeloma: therapeutic applications. *Oncogene* 2001, 20, 4519-4527.

[61] Mitsiades, N.; Mitsiades, CS.; Poulaki, V.; Chauhan, D.; Fanourakis, G.; Gu X. et al. Molecular sequelae of proteasome inhibition in human multiple myeloma cells. *Proc. Natl.Acad. Sci. USA* 2002, 99, 14374-14379.

[62] Gomez-Bougie, P.; Wuilléme-Toumi, S.; Ménoret, E.; Trichet, V.; Robillard, N.; Philippe, M. et al. Noxa up-regulation and Mcl-1 cleavage are associated to apoptosis induction by bortezomib in multiple myeloma. *Cancer Res.* 2007, 67, 5418-5424.

[63] Hideshima, T.; Mitsiades, CS.; Akiyama, M.; Hayashi, T.; Chauhan, D.; Richardson, P. et al. Molecular mechanisms mediating antimyeloma activity of proteasome inhibitor PS-341. *Blood* 2003, 101, 1530-1534.

[64] Zangari, M.; Esseltine, D.; Lee, CK.; Barlogie, B.; Elice, F.; Burns, MJ. et al. Response to bortezomib is associated to osteoblastic activation in patients with multiple myeloma. *Br. J. Haematol.* 2005, 131, 71-73.

[65] Oyajobi, BO.; Garrett, IR.; Gupta, A.; Flores, A.; Esparza, J.; Muñoz, S. et al. Stimulation of new bone formation by the proteasome inhibitor, bortezomib: implications for myeloma bone disease. *Br. J. Haematol.* 2007, 139, 434-438.

[66] Giuliani, N,; Morandi, F.; Tagliaferri, S.; Lazzaretti, M.; Bonomini, S.; Crugnola, M. et al. The proteasome inhibitor bortezomib affects osteoblast differentiation in vitro and in vivo in multiple myeloma patients. *Blood* 2007, 110, 334-338.

[67] Mukherjee, S.; Raje, N.; Schoonmaker, JA,; Liu JC.; Hideshima, T.; Wein, MN. et al. Pharmacologic targeting of a stem/progenitor population in vivo is associated with enhanced bone regeneration in mice. *J. Clin. Invest.* 2008, 118, 491-504.

[68] Yaccoby, S.; Wezeman, MJ.; Zangari, M.; Walker, R.; Cottler-Fox, M.; Gaddy, D. et al. Inhibitory effects of osteoblasts and increased bone formation on myeloma in novel culture systems and a myelomatous mouse model. *Haematologica* 2006, 91, 192-199.

[69] Terpos, E.; Heath, DJ.; Rahemtulla, A.; Zervas, K.; Chantry, A.; Anagnostopoulos, A. et al. Bortezomib reduces serum dickkopf-1 and receptor activator of nuclear factor-kappaB ligand concentrations and normalises indices of bone remodelling in patients with relapsed multiple myeloma. *Br. J. Haematol.* 2006, 135, 688-692.

[70] Uy, GL.; Trivedi, R.; Peles, S.; Fisher, NM.; Zhang, QJ.; Tomasson, MH.; Dipersio, JF.; Vij, R. Bortezomib inhibits osteoclast activity in patients with multiple myeloma. *Clin. Lymphoma Myeloma* 2007, 7, 587-589.

[71] Boissy, P.; Andersen, TL.; Lund, T.; Kupisiewicz, K.; Plesner, T.; Delaissé, JM. Pulse treatment with the proteasome inhibitor bortezomib inhibits osteoclast resorptive activity in clinically relevant conditions. *Leuk. Res.* 2008, 32, 1661-1668.

[72] Westendorf, JJ.; Kahler, RA.; Schroeder, TM. Wnt signaling in osteoblasts and bone diseases. *Gene* 2004, 341, 19-39.

[73] Richardson, PG.; Barlogie, B.; Berenson, J.; Singhal, S.; Jagannath, S.; Irwin, D. et al. A phase 2 study of bortezomib in relapsed, refractory myeloma. *N. Engl. J. Med.* 2003, 348, 2609-2617.

[74] Jagannath, S.; Barlogie, B.; Berenson, J.; Siegel, D.; Irwin, D.; Richardson, PG. et al. A phase 2 study of two doses of bortezomib in relapsed or refractory myeloma. *Br. J. Haematol.* 2004, 127, 165-172.

[75] Jagannath, S.; Richardson, PG.; Barlogie, B.; Berenson, J.; Singhal, S.; Irwin, D. et al. Bortezomib in combination with dexamethasone for the treatment of patients with relapsed and or refractory multiple myeloma with less than optimal response to bortezomib alone. *Haematologica* 2006, 91, 929-934.

[76] Richardson, PG.; Barlogie, B.; Berenson, J.; Singhal, S.; Jagannath, S.; Irwin, D. et al. Clinical factors predictive of outcome with bortezomib in patients with relapsed refractory multiple myeloma. The SUMMIT Investigators. *Blood* 2005, 106, 2977-2981.

[77] Richardson, PG.; Sonneveld, P.; Schuster, M.; Irwin, D.; Stadtmauer, E.; Facon T. et al. Extended follow-up of a phase 3 trial in relapsed multiple myeloma: final time-to-event results of the APEX trial. *Blood* 2007, 110, 3557-3560.

[78] Wolf, J.; Richardson, PG.; Schuster, M.; LeBlanc, A.; Walters, IB.; Battleman DS. Utility of bortezomib retreatment in relapsed or refractory multiple myeloma patients: a multicenter case series. *Clin. Adv. Hematol. Oncol.* 2008, 6, 755-760.

[79] San Miguel, J.; Bladé, J.; Boccadoro, M.; Cavenagh, J.; Glasmacher, A.; Jagannath, S. et al. A practical update on the use of bortezomib in the management of multiple myeloma. *Oncologist* 2006, 11, 51-61.

[80] Richardson, PG.; Briemberg, H.; Jagannath, S.; Wen, PY.; Barlogie, B.; Berenson, J. et al. Frequency, characteristics, and reversibility of peripheral neuropathy during treatment of advanced multiple myeloma with bortezomib. *J. Clin. Oncol.* 2006, 24, 3113-3120.

[81] Rosiñol, L.; Montoto, S.; Cibeira, MT.; Bladé, J. Bortezomib-induced severe hepatitis in multiple myeloma: a case report. *Arch. Intern. Me*d. 2005, 165, 464-465.

[82] Cibeira, MT.; Mercadal, S.; Arenillas, L.; Muntañola, A.; Salamero, O.; Bladé J. Bortezomib-induced rhabdomyolysis in multiple myeloma. *Acta Haematol.* 2006, 116, 203-206.

[83] Orlowski, RZ.; Voorhees, PM.; Garcia, RA.; Hall, MD.; Kudrik, FJ.; Allred, T. et al. Phase 1 trial of the proteasome inhibitor bortezomib and pegylated liposomal doxorubicin in patients with advanced hematologic malignancies. *Blood* 2005, 105, 3058-3065.

[84] Biehn, SE.; Moore, DT.; Voorhees, PM.; Garcia, RA.; Lehman, MJ.; Dees, EC.; Orlowski RZ. Extended follow-up of outcome measures in multiple myeloma patients treated on a phase I study with bortezomib and pegylated liposomal doxorubicin. *Ann. Hematol.* 2007, 86, 211-216.

[85] Orlowski, RZ.; Nagler, A.; Sonneveld, P.; Bladé, J.; Hajek, R.; Spencer, A. et al. Randomized phase III study of pegylated liposomal doxorubicin plus bortezomib compared with bortezomib alone in relapsed or refractory multiple myeloma: combination therapy improves time to progression. *J. Clin. Oncol.* 2007, 25, 3892-3901.

[86] Ma, MH.; Yang, HH.; Parker, K.; Manyak, S.; Friedman, JM.; Altamirano C. et al. The proteasome inhibitor PS-341 markedly enhances sensitivity of multiple myeloma tumor cells to chemotherapeutic agents. *Clin. Cancer Res.* 2003, 9, 1136-1144.

[87] Sonneveld, P.; Hajek, R.; Nagler, A.; Spencer, A.; Bladé, J.; Robak, T. et al. Combined pegylated liposomal doxorubicin and bortezomib is highly effective in patients with recurrent or refractory multiple myeloma who received prior thalidomide/lenalidomide therapy. *Cancer* 2008, 112, 1529-1537.

[88] Pineda-Roman M, Zangari M, van Rhee F, Anaissie E, Szymonifka J, Hoering A. et al. VTD combination therapy with bortezomib-thalidomide-dexamethasone is highly effective in advanced and refractory multiple myeloma. *Leukemia* 2008, 22, 1419-1427.

[89] Palumbo, A.; Ambrosini, MT.; Benevolo, G.; Pregno, P.; Pescosta, N.; Callea, V. et al. Bortezomib, melphalan, prednisone, and thalidomide for relapsed multiple myeloma. *Blood* 2007, 109, 2767-2772.

[90] Fonseca, R.; Rajkumar, SV. Consolidation therapy with bortezomib/lenalidomide/ dexamethasone versus bortezomib/dexamethasone after a dexamethasone-based induction regimen in patients with multiple myeloma: a randomized phase III trial. *Clin. Lymphoma Myeloma* 2008, 8, 315-317.

[91] Feling, RH.; Buchanan, GO.; Mincer, TJ.; Kauffman, CA.; Jensen, PR.; Fenical, W. Salinosporamide A: a highly cytotoxic proteasome inhibitor from a novel microbial source, a marine bacterium of the new genus salinospora. *Angew. Chem. Int. Ed. Engl.* 2003, 42, 355-357.

[92] Macherla, VR.; Mitchell, SS.; Manam, RR.; Reed, KA.; Chao, TH.; Nicholson, B. et al. Structure-activity relationship studies of salinosporamide A (NPI-0052), a novel marine derived proteasome inhibitor. *J. Med.. Chem.* 2005, 48, 3684-3687.

[93] Chauhan, D.; Catley, L.; Li, G.; Podar, K.; Hideshima, T.; Velankar, M. et al. A novel orally active proteasome inhibitor induces apoptosis in multiple myeloma cells with mechanisms distinct from Bortezomib. *Cancer Cell* 2005, 8, 407-419.

[94] Chauhan, D.; Hideshima, T.; Anderson, KC. A novel proteasome inhibitor NPI-0052 as an anticancer therapy. *Br. J. Cancer* 2006, 95, 961-965.

[95] Williamson, MJ.; Blank, JL.; Bruzzese, FJ.; Cao, Y.; Daniels, JS.; Dick, LR. et al. Comparison of biochemical and biological effects of ML858 (salinosporamide A) and bortezomib. *Mol. Cancer Ther.* 2006, 5, 3052-3061.

[96] Chauhan, D.; Singh, A.; Brahmandam, M.; Podar, K.; Hideshima, T.; Richardson, P. et al. Combination of proteasome inhibitors bortezomib and NPI-0052 trigger in vivo synergistic cytotoxicity in multiple myeloma. *Blood* 2008, 111, 1654-1664.

[97] Miller, CP.; Ban, K.; Dujka, ME.; McConkey, DJ.; Munsell, M.; Palladino, M.; Chandra, J. NPI-0052, a novel proteasome inhibitor, induces caspase-8 and ROS-dependent apoptosis alone and in combination with HDAC inhibitors in leukemia cells. *Blood* 2007, 110, 267-277.

[98] Demo, SD., Kirk, CJ.; Aujay, MA.; Buchholz, TJ.; Dajee, M.; Ho, MN. et al. Antitumor activity of PR-171, a novel irreversible inhibitor of the proteasome. *Cancer Res.* 2007, 67, 6383-6391.

[99] Stapnes, C.; Døskeland, AP.; Hatfield, K.; Ersvaer, E.; Ryningen, A.; Lorens JB. et al. The proteasome inhibitors bortezomib and PR-171 have antiproliferative and

proapoptotic effects on primary human acute myeloid leukaemia cells. *Br. J. Haematol.* 2007, 136, 814-828.

[100] Kuhn, DJ.; Chen, Q.; Voorhees, PM.; Strader, JS.; Shenk, KD.; Sun, CM. et al. Potent activity of carfilzomib, a novel, irreversible inhibitor of the ubiquitin-proteasome pathway, against preclinical models of multiple myeloma. *Blood* 2007, 110, 3281-3290.

[101] Orlowski, RZ.; Kuhn, DJ. Proteasome inhibitors in cancer therapy: lessons from the first decade. *Clin. Cancer Res.* 2008, 14, 1649-1657.

[102] Dorsey, BD.; Iqbal, M.; Chatterjee, S.; Menta, E.; Bernardini, R.; Bernareggi, A. et al. Discovery of a potent, selective, and orally active proteasome inhibitor for the treatment of cancer. *J. Med. Chem.* 2008, 51, 1068-1072.

[103] Piva, R.; Ruggeri, B.; Williams, M.; Costa, G.; Tamagno, I.; Ferrero, D. et al. CEP-18770: A novel, orally active proteasome inhibitor with a tumor-selective pharmacologic profile competitive with bortezomib. *Blood* 2008, 111, 2765-2775.

[104] Manochakian, R.; Miller, KC.; Chanan-Khan AA. Clinical impact of bortezomib in frontline regimens for patients with multiple myeloma. *Oncologist* 2007, 12, 978-990.

In: Multiple Myeloma: Symptoms, Diagnosis and Treatment ISBN 978-1-60876-108-1
Editors: M. Georgiev and Ev. Bachev

Chapter 5

Plasma Cell Dyscrasias

Cherie H. Dunphy
Professor of Pathology and Laboratory Medicine,
Director of Hematopathology and Hematopathology Fellowship
University of North Carolina at Chapel Hill, Chapel Hill, NC, USA

Introduction

Plasma cell dyscrasias (PCDs) include plasmacytomas and various forms of plasma cell myeloma (multiple myeloma-MM). Diagnosis of plasmacytoma requires demonstration of a monoclonal/aberrant plasma cell (PC) population in a tissue biopsy; whereas, diagnosis of a PCD involving the bone marrow (BM) (i.e., various forms of MM) requires quantitation of the PCs in the BM in addition to the demonstration of monoclonality/aberrancy. This chapter will describe the definitions of the various forms of PCD (including the International Staging System-ISS), the morphological variants and immunophenotypic features of neoplastic PCs, the diagnostic laboratory techniques useful in establishing a diagnosis (including immunophenotypic techniques), and the ancillary studies that may aid in diagnosis, prognostication, and therapeutic decision-making (i.e., immunophenotypic features, as well as cytogenetic and molecular findings).

Definitions of Various Forms of Plasma Cell Dyscrasia (See Table 1)

Plasmacytoma

Solitary plasmacytoma of bone and extramedullary plasmacytoma and multiple solitary plasmacytomas are defined as distinct entities. If a solitary lytic lesion of PCs is found on skeletal survey in an otherwise asymptomatic patient, and a BM examination from an uninvolved site contains less than 5% to 10% PCs, the patient has an isolated plasmacytoma of bone. Likewise, patients with isolated PC tumors of soft tissues, most commonly occurring in the tonsils, nasopharynx, or paranasal sinuses, should have skeletal x-rays and a BM biopsy [1-3]. If these tests are negative, the patient has extramedullary plasmacytoma.

Table 1. Definitions in Multiple Myeloma

Solitary Plasmacytoma All four criteria must be met: Biopsy-proven solitary lesion of bone or soft tissue with evidence of clonal plasma cells Normal bone marrow with no evidence of clonal plasma cells Normal skeletal survey and MRI of spine and pelvis (except for the primary solitary lesion) Absence of end-organ damage such as CRAB (see below)
Clinical features of end-organ damage: hypercalcemia, renal insufficiency, anemia, or bone lesions (CRAB) Calcium levels increased: 0.5 mg/dL above the upper limit of normal or 10.5 mg/dL Renal insufficiency: creatinine >2 mg/dL Anemia: hemoglobin 2 g/dL below the lower limit of normal or hemoglobin <10 g/dL Bone lesions: lytic lesions or osteoporosis with compression fractures (MRI or CT may clarify) Other: symptomatic hyperviscosity, amyloidosis, recurrent bacterial infections (>2 episodes in 12 months)
Monoclonal gammopathy of undetermined significance (MGUS) All three criteria must be met: Serum monoclonal protein <3g/dl Clonal BM plasma cells <10% and Absence of end-organ damage such as hyper*c*alcemia, *r*enal insufficiency, *a*nemia and bone lesions (CRAB) that can be attributed to the plasma cell proliferative disorder No evidence of other B-cell lymphoproliferative disorder AL amyloid and the IgM paraprotien-related neurological syndromes would be instance of "MG associated with..."
Asymptomatic myeloma (smoldering myeloma) Both criteria must be met: M protein in serum >3 g/dL and/or bone marrow clonal plasma cells >10% No CRAB
Symptomatic multiple myeloma All three criteria must be met except as noted: Clonal bone marrow plasma cells ≥ 10% or plasmacytoma Presence of serum and/or urinary monoclonal protein (except in patients with true non-secretory multiple myeloma) and Evidence of end-organ damage that can be attributed to the underlying plasma cell proliferative disorder, specifically Hypercalcemia: serum calcium ≥ 11.5 mg/100 ml or Renal insufficiency: serum creatinine >1.73 mmol/l) Anemia: normochromic, normocytic with a hemoglobin value of >2 g/100 ml below the lower limit of normal or a hemoglobin value <10 g/100 ml Bone lesions: lytic lesions, severe osteopenia, or pathologic fractures +CRAB (Some patients may have no symptoms, but have CRAB.)
Plasma Cell Leukemia Circulating plasma cells exceed 2,000/ul or 20% of the peripheral white blood cells

MRI=magnetic resonance imaging.

Monoclonal Gammopathy of Undetermined Significance (MGUS)

Monoclonal gammopathy of undetermined significance (MGUS) is characterized by a serum monoclonal protein <30g/l, <10% PCs in the BM, and the absence of end-organ damage (i.e., CRAB–hypercalcemia, renal insufficiency, anemia, or bone lesions).

Smoldering Multiple Myeloma

Smoldering (asymptomatic) MM is characterized by having a serum IgG or IgA monoclonal protein of 30g/l or higher and/or 10% or more PCs in the BM but no evidence of end-organ damage.

Symptomatic Multiple Myeloma

Symptomatic MM requires evidence of related organ or tissue impairment (ROTI). The diagnostic criteria for symptomatic MM include the following:

- Monoclonal PCs in the BM (≥ 10%)
- Monoclonal protein in serum and/or urine by electrophoresis
- One or more of the CRAB features of organ damage (elevated calcium (> 10.5 mg/dl); renal dysfunction (creatinine > 2 mg/dl); anemia (Hgb < 10 g/dl or 2 g below normal); and bone disease (lytic lesions or osteoporosis).

Non-Secretory Multiple Myeloma

Non-secretory multiple myeloma is characterized by the absence of an M-protein in the serum and urine, but with BM plasmacytosis and ROTI.

Plasma Cell Leukemia

Plasma cell leukemia is defined as circulating PCs exceeding 2,000/ul or exceeding 20% of the peripheral white blood cells.

Multiple Myeloma International Staging System

The MM ISS consists of the following stages: stage I, serum β_2 microglobulin ($S\beta_2M$) less than 3.5 mg/L plus serum albumin ≥3.5 g/dL (median survival, 62 months); stage II, neither stage I nor III (median survival, 44 months); and stage III, $S\beta_2M$ ≥5.5 mg/L (median survival, 29 months).[5]

Morphologic Variants of Neoplastic Plasma Cells (See Table 2)

Neoplastic PCs may be so well-differentiated cytologically as to be indistinguishable from normal/reactive PCs.

This mature appearance is known as the Marshalko type morphology. Russell bodies (large intracytoplasmic globules of proteins) and Dutcher bodies (pale intranuclear inclusions) are relatively common findings in neoplastic PCs. However, in addition, various unusual cytological appearances of neoplastic PCs seen have been well described in the literature [6]. These include the following:

- "Flame cells" (deep magenta to pink staining in the peripheral part of the cytoplasm)
- "Mott, morular, or grape cells" (cells with multiple small globular cytoplasmic inclusions similar to multiple small Russell bodies)
- "Thesaurocytes" (plasma cells with abundant reticulated cytoplasm and/or cytoplasm trabeculated by eosinophilic bands): The appearance of flame cells and thesaurocytes is due to the accumulation of flocculent or granular material in the endoplasmic reticulum, as observed ultrastructurally.
- Cells intermediate in appearance between flame cells and thesaurocytes may be seen, possibly representing stages in the development of a shared subcellular composition
- Plasma cells with the presence of cytoplasmic spindle-shaped crystalline deposits (single or multiple)
- Cleaved, Multilobated, and Monocytoid Cells/Polymorphous Variant: These cytological variants may be confused with poorly differentiated carcinoma, lymphoma, and myeloid or monocytic leukemia. The multilobated cells may resemble neutrophils or histiocytes.
- Histiocytic variant: Neoplastic PCs may have abundant homogeneous eosinophilic cytoplasm and dense nuclei, mimicking epithelioid histiocytes or histiocytes of a storage disorder. The neoplastic PCs in such cases contain paranuclear cytoplasmic inclusions, representing clonal light chain.
- Plasma cell dyscrasia mimicking erythrophagocytosis: Recently Pillai et al. [7] have documented a case of plasmacytoma in which the neoplastic PCs mimicked erythrocyte-laden macrophages. This was the result of accumulation of waxy, pale eosinophilic material in the cytoplasm. Rarely, true erythrophagocytosis may be seen in myelomas.
- Clear cell variant: The cells contain abundant clear cytoplasm. Signet-ring cells (see next variant description) may also be present in this variant. Occasionally multiple clear vacuoles are present within the cytoplasm and may mimic a germ cell tumor or clear cell carcinoma.
- Signet-ring cell variant: Signet-ring cell MM is an extremely rare neoplasm. This variant may be easily confused with metastatic carcinoma. Signet-ring cell morphology has also been described in lymphomas. The cells in this variant contain peripheral crescentic nuclei and empty cytoplasmic vacuoles. Immunostains for light and heavy chains show a delicate ring of positivity around the vacuoles.
- Pleomorphic variant: Rarely, neoplastic PCs exhibit marked cellular pleomorphism and multinuclearity. These neoplasms simulate an anaplastic carcinoma or anaplastic large cell lymphoma.
- Blastic variant: This variant is composed of either plasmablasts (large PCs with hyperchromatic nuclei and prominent nucleoli) or cells closely resembling large-cell non-Hodgkin lymphoma. The cells in the latter type contain centrally placed large hyperchromatic or vesicular nuclei with one or more prominent nucleoli and scanty cytoplasm. Pleomorphic cells may also be seen in the blastic variant.
- Small cell (lymphoid) variant: The small-cell type of MM in the marrow may mimic a small cell lymphocytic leukemia/lymphoma or an acute leukemic infiltrate. This is a particular problem since acute leukemia may coexist with MM in the marrow. It

may also be confused with other types of small-cell malignancies. The small cells in these neoplasms contain dense, round, angulated or notched nuclei and scanty cytoplasm.

- Spindle cell variant: The neoplastic PCs may assume a spindle cell morphology or may be associated with a fibroblastic stromal response, closely resembling a spindle cell mesenchymal tumor.
- Oncocytic variant: This is an extremely rare variant of non-secretory MM.

Table 2. Morphologic Features of Neoplastic Cells

Morphologic Variants of Neoplastic Cells	Inclusions Within or Structures Associated With Neoplastic Plasma Cells
Marshalko (Mature plasma cell morphology)	Russell Bodies
Flame	Dutcher Bodies
Mott	Intracytoplasmic Crystals
Thesaurocyte	
Histiocytic variant	
Mimicking erythrophagocytosis	
Clear cell variant	
Signet-ring cell variant	
Pleomorphic variant	
Blastic variant	
Small cell (lymphoid) variant	
Spindle cell variant	
Oncocytic variant	

Thus, neoplastic PCs may histologically mimic carcinomas of various types (including anaplastic carcinoma), lymphomas (including anaplastic lymphoma), leukemias, germ-cell tumours, and very rarely sarcomas and histiocytic lesions. The clue to the correct diagnosis is finding PCs with typical morphology. However, such typical PCs may not always be readily identified, and thus recognition of these variants of neoplastic cells ultimately relies on their immunophenotypic features, described in the next section.

Immunophenotypic Features of Neoplastic Plasma Cells

The single best marker for identifying neoplastic PCs is syndecan-1 (i.e., CD138) combined with demonstration of monoclonal cytoplasmic light chain expression. Neoplastic PCs may display a heterogeneous phenotype consistent with the fact that the neoplastic clone is able to undergo a certain degree of differentiation. Although neoplastic PCs usually lack surface expression of B-cell associated antigens (i.e., CD19 and CD20), weak expression of CD20 may be seen in less than 1/3 of cases, and strong expression of CD20 may be seen in the majority of cells in <10% of cases. Likewise, CD19 may be expressed by neoplastic PCs.

CD79a is typically, though not invariably, positive. Although normal PCs and most neoplastic PCs lack surface light chain expression, they do demonstrate cytoplasmic light chain expression (restricted in neoplastic PCs). In addition, restricted surface light chain expression may be demonstrated in some neoplastic PCs. Likewise, although leukocyte common antigen (CD45) is not expressed by normal PCs and most neoplastic PCs, it may be expressed in some neoplastic PCs. Of note, neoplastic PCs also frequently display reactivity for markers which are not restricted to the B-cell lineage, such as the neural cell adhesion molecule-CD56, CD31, [8] CD43, UCHL1 (CD45RO), [9] CD10, [10] and myelomonocytic markers (i.e., CD13 and CD33), [11] as well as cyclin D1, [12] cytokeratin, [11] and epithelial membrane antigen (EMA). Thus, cytokeratin and EMA positivity, with LCA negativity, could lead to an erroneous diagnosis of carcinoma.

Likewise, the small cell, 'lymphocyte-like' variant of MM may be a particular diagnostic challenge, being confused morphologically and immunophenotypically with other CD20+ mature B-cells neoplasms. Furthermore, this variant frequently demonstrates over-expression of cyclin D1, as seen in mantle cell lymphoma (MCL). Immunophenotyping using a panel of antibodies, including CD3, CD5, CD20, CD23, CD103, CD11c, surface and cytoplasmic light chain expression, and CD138 aid in distinguishing the small cell variant of MM from MCL, chronic lymphocytic leukemia, lymphoplasmacytic lymphoma, and marginal zone lymphoma.

Of the immunophenotypic markers described above, some have prognostic and/or clinicopathologic significance. The presence of CD56 expression by plasma cells has been shown to indicate clonality, since they have been identified in plasma cell myeloma and lymphoplasmacytic lymphoma, but not in any cases of reactive plasmacytosis [13]. CD56 has also been associated with the presence of lytic bone lesions. In addition, it has been demonstrated that CD56 expression is inversely and significantly linked to the degree of BM involvement as well as peripheral blood and central nervous system involvement [14-16]. As mentioned previously, cyclin D1 expression has been associated with the small cell variant of MM. The prognostic significance of cyclin D1 expression in MM is controversial. Cyclin D1 protein expression has been associated with a significantly unfavorable overall and progression-free survival [17]. However, other studies using conventional chemotherapy or high dose chemotherapy with autologous stem cell transplantation have generally shown either no effect or a slightly favorable effect on prognosis [18-20]

Expression of CD10 and/or myelomonocytic markers (i.e., CD13 and CD33) by neoplastic PCs has likewise been associated with a worst prognosis.

Not only are CD138 and the demonstration of monoclonal cytoplasmic light chain expression important in recognizing neoplastic PCs, particularly in the morphologic variant cases, but the evaluation of the percentage and clonality of PCs in BM specimens is essential in establishing a diagnosis of a MM. Unfortunately, PCs tend to strip in BMA smear preparations. Based on this stripping artifact, as well as the occurrence of atypical morphological forms, PCs may be difficult to recognize and thus, tend to be underestimated in BMA differential counts. However, immunohistochemical (IHC) analysis of CD138 has been shown to be useful in quantitating PCs in paraffin sections of BM clots and cores and is superior to BMA differential counts in evaluating an accurate percentage of PCs in the BM, and preferentially in the BM core biopsy sections than in the BM clot sections [13].

Immunophenotypic Techniques in Diagnosing Plasma Cell Dyscrasias

The following markers may be detected by both flow cytometric (FC) and IHC or in-situ hybridization (ISH) techniques: CD138, CD56, cytoplasmic and surface light chains, CD45, CD10, CD13, CD33, CD19, CD20, CD3, CD5, CD23, CD103, CD11c, and CD43. the ISH technique is much superior to IHC technique in evaluating light chain expression, since it better detects surface light chain expression and has much less background staining. The following markers are detected by IHC techniques, but not by FC techniques: CD31, UCHL-1, cytokeratin, EMA, and cyclin D1. Immunohistochemistry is the preferred technique in quantifying PCs, since the cellular processing involved in performing flow cytometry appears to reduce PC percentages in many cases [21]. In addition, CD56 may be particularly helpful in determining the presence of neoplastic PCs, particularly in cases of PCD with "biclonal" populations and in the non-secretory variant.

Clinically Significant Molecular Abnormalities in Plasma Cell Myeloma (See Table 3)

Chromosome 13 Abnormalities

Monosomy of chromosome 13 or deletions of chromosome 13q represent one of the most frequent abnormalities in MM, being detectable by FISH in approximately 50% of cases [19,22,23]. In cases with interstitial 13q deletions, the deleted segment appears to be centered about 13q14. However, in the great majority of cases, chromosome 13 abnormalities consist of monosomy 13. [24]. In cases with chromosome 13 abnormalities detected by FISH, the percent of PC nuclei carrying the deletion varies from approximately 25% to >95%, suggesting this abnormality represents a secondary change in the pathogenesis of MM.

Table 3. Correlation of Cytogenetic and Molecular Abnormalities with Prognosis in Multiple Myeloma

Cytogenetic/Molecular Abnormality	Prognostic Impact/**Stage of Disease**
Chromosome 13 abnormalities	Adverse
17p13 deletion/p53 mutation	Adverse
t(11;14)	No effect or slightly favorable
t(4;14)	Adverse
t(14:16)	Adverse
MYC translocation	Advanced Disease
Chromosome 1p21 deletion	Adverse
Hypodiploidy	Adverse
K-ras mutation	Adverse

However, chromosome 13 abnormalities are also detectable in 25-50% of cases of MGUS, indicating this abnormality appears to occur relatively early in the evolution of plasma cell neoplasms [19,22].

In patients treated with either standard chemotherapy or high dose chemotherapy and autologous bone marrow transplantation (BMT), the presence of a chromosome 13 abnormality is associated with an adverse prognosis [25-29]. Chromosome 13 abnormalities are also highly associated with other molecular abnormalities with an adverse prognosis, such as t(4;14), discussed later. Of interest, the prognostic impact of chromosome 13 abnormalities is greater when the abnormality is detected by metaphase cytogenetics rather than by FISH, likely reflecting the combined influence of chromosome 13 abnormalities and the PC proliferative rate. [30,31].

Del(17p) and P53 Abnormalities

Somatic point mutations or hemizygous deletions of the tumor suppressor gene p53, located at locus 17p13, are observed in many malignant neoplasms [32]. As detected by FISH, deletions of the 17p13 locus are found in 5-10% of cases of MM. 17p deletions have been shown to be more common in patients with advanced MM and in more than 60% of human myeloma cell lines, suggesting that p53 mutations and deletions develop as secondary abnormalities during the course of disease progression [19,22]. In patients treated with conventional chemotherapy or high dose chemotherapy with autologous BMT, the FISH detection of 17p13 deletions is associated with short survival [20,33-35].

Although most of the data in the literature regarding the clinical and prognostic significance of p53 abnormalities comes from studies employing FISH, other techniques, such as metaphase cytogenetics, may also be of clinical utility. Furthermore, deletions of the 17p13 locus may represent a marker for functional abnormalities of the p53 tumor suppressor pathway, rather than being of intrinsic biologic significance.

In general, the hemizygous loss of one p53 locus is thought to be associated with acquired mutations in the remaining locus that lead to abnormal function. Sequencing based studies have suggested that point mutations in p53 are less common than 17p deletions [36]. Furthermore, because p53 mutations lead to an abnormally long half-life of the protein, the presence of p53 mutations is associated with increased nuclear p53 expression as detected by IHC techniques.

The presence of nuclear p53 staining by IHC techniques has been shown to be associated with deletions of 17p13 by FISH, and with poor survival [37]. IHC studies, which are much more widely available in routine pathology practice than FISH studies, may be useful to examine for p53 abnormalities in MM.

It is currently unclear which of these methodologies (FISH, sequencing, or IHC) provides the most clinically relevant assessment of the p53 pathway in MM.

Immunoglobulin Heavy Chain (14q32) Translocations

General

Translocations involving the immunoglobulin heavy chain locus (*IGH*) at chromosome 14q32 are identified in approximately 50-60% of cases of MM, and are associated with non-hyperdiploid karyotypes [19]. The incidence of *IGH* translocations has also been shown to be inversely correlated with patient age [38]. Unlike several B-cell non-Hodgkin lymphomas that are associated with specific translocations involving the *IGH* locus and one partner gene (e.g. *IGH/BCL2* in follicular lymphoma), numerous *IGH* translocation partner genes have been described in myeloma. The major recurring partner genes include *CCND1* (11q13), *MMSET* (4p16), and *CMAF* (14q62). These recurring translocations can be detected in cases of MGUS and are therefore thought to arise early in the pathogenesis of MM.[19,39] Other *IGH* translocations, however, such as the *IGH/CMYC* translocation, are thought to represent secondary abnormalities acquired during disease progression [40]. The major recurring translocations, discussed below, are associated with specific pathologic and clinical features.

t(11;14)(q13;q32) *IGH/CCND1*

The t(11;14)(q13;q32) is found in approximately 15-20% of cases of MM using FISH techniques.[19,22,41] This translocation is also found in essentially all cases of mantle cell lymphoma. The precise translocation breakpoints, however, differ between MM and MCL, consistent with differing molecular pathogenesis (i.e. translocations arising during VDJ recombination for mantle cell lymphoma versus during class switching for MM) [19,42,43]

Cases of MM containing the *IGH/CCND1* translocation are associated with distinct clinicopathologic features including a small cell (i.e., lymphoid) morphology and CD20 expression, as previously discussed. Oligosecretory/non-secretory myeloma and IgM myeloma are also associated with the presence of the *IGH/CCND1*.[18,44,45]. The influence of *IGH/CCND1* on prognosis has been controversial. As discussed previously, studies using conventional chemotherapy or high dose chemotherapy with autologous stem cell transplantation have generally shown either no effect or a slightly favorable effect on prognosis [18-20]

Several techniques have been used for the detection of *IGH/CCND1* in routine practice. When informative karyotypes are available, the translocation is typically readily identified by metaphase cytogenetics. Many *IGH/CCND1* positive cases, however, may yield non-informative results by standard karyotyping. Using modern, sensitive antibodies to Cyclin D1 protein, the vast majority of cases containing the *IGH/CCND1* show strong, uniform positivity for Cyclin D1 protein by IHC analysis (as discussed previously). One should keep in mind that approximately 30% of MM also show weak, partial expression of Cyclin D1 in the absence of the t(11;14) through other mechanisms of dysregulation of the *CCND1* locus [46]. The detection of Cyclin D1 mRNA by RT-PCR has also been shown to be of prognostic significance; however, this technique did not discriminate between *IGH/CCND1* and other forms of *CCND1* dysregulation [47]. FISH studies offer the most sensitive and specific method for detection of this translocation, especially when using simultaneous phenotyping (such as cIg-FISH or CD138 gating) or purification of plasma cells prior to FISH analysis.

t(4;14)(p16;q32) *MMSET/IGH*

The t(4;14)(p16;q32) is found by FISH studies in approximately 15-20% of cases of MM.[18,48-50]. The translocation leads to the production of an *IGH/MMSET* fusion gene. The normal function of the *MMSET* gene and the role of the dysregulated *IGH/MMSET* fusion gene in MM pathogenesis are largely unknown. In addition, the t(4;14) also leads to dysregulation of the *FGFR3* gene at chromosome 4p16 in about 80% of cases containing this translocation. Dysregulation of the FGFR3 protein is also thought to contribute to the molecular pathogenesis of t(4;14) positive MM. [19,22,48]

In MM treated with either conventional chemotherapy or high dose chemotherapy with autologous BMT, the presence of the t(4;14) has been associated with an adverse prognosis.[18,33,48] The prognosis appears to be poor in cases with the t(4;14), regardless of whether or not *FGFR3* expression is detectable [51]. This latter observation suggests that the *IGH/MMSET* fusion gene contributes directly to the adverse prognosis in these patients. Cases with the t(4;14) also show a strong association with chromosome 13q abnormalities that may also contribute to the adverse prognosis [19,22,50]. MM cases containing the t(4;14) are also associated with specific clinicopathologic features, including a blastoid morphology, IgA paraproteins, and preferential restriction of lambda light chains.[19,22,52] Novel small molecule inhibitors targeting the function of FGFR3 and cytotoxic anti-FGFR3 antibodies are currently in development for treatment of t(4;14) positive MM [53-55].

The t(4;14)(p16;q32) is cryptic by routine banded karyotyping. The *IGH-MMSET* fusion transcript may be detected by RT-PCR or interphase FISH studies [19,22]. More recently, studies have shown that IHC detection of FGFR3 protein may also be used to screen for the presence of t(4;14).[56,57]. However, since FGFR3 protein expression is found in only 75-80% of cases containing the t(4;14), FISH studies remain the gold standard for detection of this abnormality.

t(14;16)(q32;q23) *IGH/CMAF*

A t(14;16)(q32;q23) involving the *IGH* locus and the *CMAF* oncogene is identified in 2-10% of MM cases by FISH [19,22]. Due to the rarity of this translocation, there is limited data regarding the prognosis of cases carrying this abnormality. However, the available findings suggest the abnormality is associated with an adverse prognosis [33]. The *IGH/CMAF* translocation is generally cryptic by metaphase cytogenetics, and is best detected by interphase FISH (dual fusion FISH probes specific for this abnormality are commercially available). Rare MM cases contain a variant t(14;20)(q32;q12) involving *IGH* and another member of the maf family, *MAFB*. [58]. Although only a small number of cases with this abnormality have been described, it also appears to be associated with short survival.

Other *IGH* Translocations

Several other *IGH* translocation partner genes have also been identified in MM. Translocations involving *MYC* are frequent in MM cell lines, but are found in only a small percentage of MM patient samples [59,60]. The *IGH/CMYC* translocations are generally found in patients with advanced disease and are thought to generally represent secondary, acquired abnormalities. A t(6;14)(p21;q32) involving *IGH* and the Cyclin D3 gene (*CCND3*) is found in <5% of cases. A t(6;14)(p25;q32) involving the *MUM1/IRF4* locus has also been described in several patients [19,22,61,62]. The clinical significance of CCND3 and MUM1/IRF4 translocations are not presently well characterized.

Other Chromosomal Abnormalities

Abnormalities of chromosome 1 are frequently found in MM. Duplication or amplification of the *CKS1B* gene on chromosome 1q21 is found in approximately 30% of cases of MM using FISH [63,64]. The *CKS1B* protein regulates the degradation of p27, thereby promoting cell cycle progression. Amplification of the CKS1B locus is associated with the presence of other prognostically significant abnormalities, including 17p13 deletions and chromosome 13 abnormalities, and the presence of CKS1B amplification conveys poor survival. Another chromosome 1 abnormality, deletion of chromosome 1p21, has been reported in 20% of MM cases [65]. The deleted locus contains the cyclin dependant kinase phosphatase, *CDC14A*. Deletion of 1p21 is also associated with other chromosomal abnormalities, including chromosome 13 abnormalities and the t(4;14)(p16;q32). Cases with the 1p21 deletion display an adverse prognosis in cases treated with high dose chemotherapy and autologous BMT.

In addition, the presence of hypodiploidy predicts a significantly reduced survival [66].

Other Genetic Abnormalities

Activating *Ras* mutations have been noted in 35–50% of MM patients. The prevalence of the mutations may increase somewhat with advancing stages of the disease. Most mutations involve K- and N-*ras* at codons 12, 13, and 61. MM cases with t(4;14)(p16.3;q32) can have activating mutations of *FGFR3* or *Ras*, but these events appear to be mutually exclusive, suggesting that activating mutations of *Ras* or *FGFR3* have a similar effect. *Ras* mutations appear to be rare in MGUS, suggesting that this is a molecular marker if not causative in the progression from MGUS to MM for some tumors. Mutations of K-*ras*, but not of N-*ras*, have been associated with shorter survival. Treatment strategies addressing the constitutive activation of *ras* are being explored [19].

A Practical Approach to Molecular Evaluation of MM

To allow for identification of these abnormalities in routine practice, metaphase cytogenetic studies and FISH studies for IGH translocations, chromosome 13 abnormalities, and p53 are suggested in all cases at initial diagnosis. The p53 pathway may also be assessed by IHC methods. Although other recurring abnormalities may also be of prognostic significance, it is currently unclear how such information should be incorporated into routine practice.

Current Therapeutic Guidelines for MM [66]

In the past decade, there have been major advances in the treatment of myeloma. Thalidomide,67 bortezomib, [68,69] and lenalidomide [70,71] have emerged as highly active agents in the treatment of myeloma. There is no evidence that early treatment of patients with smoldering MM prolongs survival. However, clinical trials are ongoing to determine whether newer agents can delay progression.

The treatment of symptomatic MM depends on eligibility for stem-cell transplantation and risk assessment. Current therapy for MM relies on the ISS as well as important prognostic factors that stratify patients into high risk and standard risk, including deletion 13 or hypodiploidy on conventional karyotyping, deletion 17p– or immunoglobulin heavy chain translocations [t(4;14) or t(14;16)] on molecular genetic studies, and plasma cell labeling index of 3% or higher [72] The presence of any one or more of these high-risk factors classifies a patient as having high-risk myeloma. The median survival of patients with high-risk features is only 2 to 3 years, even with tandem stem-cell transplantation, compared with 5 or more years in patients with standard-risk disease. Figure 1 outlines the current approach to the treatment of newly diagnosed MM.

Initial Therapy in Patients Eligible for Transplantation

The most common induction regimens used today are *thalidomide–dexamethasone (Thal/Dex), bortezomib-based regimens, and lenalidomide–dexamethasone (Rev/Dex).*

Initial Therapy in Patients Not Eligible for Transplantation

Patients who are not transplant candidates are treated with standard alkylating agent therapy. The 3 most commonly used regimens are *Melphalan, prednisone, thalidomide (MPT); Melphalan, prednisone, bortezomib (MPV; and Melphalan, prednisone, lenalidomide (MPR).*

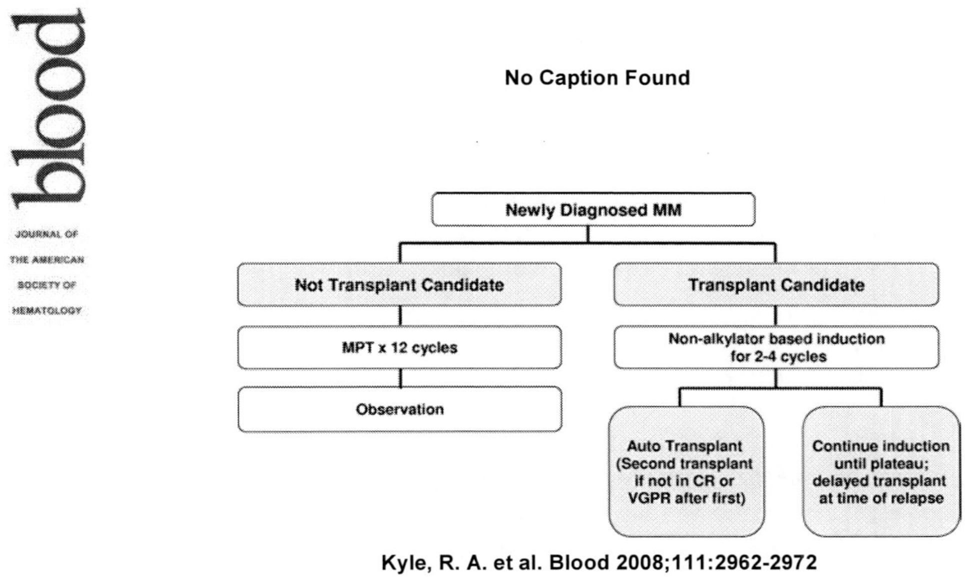

Figure 1. Algorithm outlining the current approach to the treatment of newly diagnosed myeloma. CR indicates complete response; MPT, melphalan, prednisone, thalidomide; and VGPR, very good partial response. Reprinted with permission.

Hematopoietic Stem-Cell Transplantation

Autologous Stem Cell Transplant (ASCT) Although not curative, *ASCT* improves complete response rates and prolongs median overall survival in MM by approximately 12 months [73,74]. The mortality rate is 1% to 2%. Melphalan, 200 mg/m^2, is the most widely used conditioning regimen. Randomized trials have shown similar survival rates in patients in which *ASCT* is done early (immediately after 4 cycles of induction therapy) or later (at the time of relapse as salvage therapy) [75,76]. It has also been shown that patients responding to induction therapy had similar overall and progression-free survival with either *ASCT* or 8 additional courses of chemotherapy, questioning the benefit of *ASCT* in patients responding to induction chemotherapy [77]. The need for early *ASCT* in this era of new promising drugs is the present real therapeutic question in MM.

Tandem Transplantation

With tandem (double) *ASCT*, patients receive a second planned *ASCT* after recovery from the first *ASCT*. This approach has been restricted to patients failing to achieve a complete response or significant partial response with the first *ASCT*. [78,79]

Allogeneic Transplantation

Only a limited number of MM patients are candidates for allogeneic transplantation due to age, availability of an HLA-matched sibling donor, and adequate performance status. The high treatment-related mortality, mainly related to graft-versus-host disease, has made conventional allogeneic transplants unacceptable for most MM patients. Initial trials employing an approach of an *ASCT* followed by a planned reduced intensity (RIC) allogeneic *SCT* have shown promise [80]. However, additional confirmation is needed.

Maintenance Therapy

Observation is still the standard following initial therapy as described (Figure 1). Interferon does not appear to provide significant clinical Benedit [76]. A recent trial (IFM 99-02) randomized 597 patients (age < 65 years) after tandem ASCT to no maintenance, pamidronate, or pamidronate plus thalidomide [81]. The 4-year overall survival rate was superior with thalidomide (77%, 74%, and 87%, respectively, $P < .04$), but these results need further confirmation. Clinical trials are currently evaluating thalidomide, lenalidomide, bortezomib, and other novel approaches as maintenance therapy.

Treatment of High-Risk Myeloma

As mentioned previously, patients with high-risk MM tend to do poorly with median overall survival of approximately 2 years even with tandem *ASCT* [82] Incorporation of new agents early in the disease course is a major option for treatment [72]. *ASCT* followed by RIC-allogeneic SCT may also be an option in selected patients. A third option is to incorporate routine maintenance therapy after treatment as outlined earlier for patients with standard-risk disease.

Supportive Care

Numerous improvements in supportive care have greatly improved the outcome of MM patients. Some of the most important advances are the advent of bisphosphonates to treat hypercalcemia and to prevent MM bone disease, the use of vertebroplasty and kyphoplasty to treat vertebral fractures, and judicious use of prophylactic antibiotics in selected patients.

References

[1] Tournier-Rangeard L, Lapeyre M, Graff-Caillaud P, et al.: Radiotherapy for solitary extramedullary plasmacytoma in the head-and-neck region: A dose greater than 45 Gy

to the target volume improves the local control. *Int. J. Radiat. Oncol. Biol. Phys.* 64 (4): 1013-7, 2006.

[2] Michalaki VJ, Hall J, Henk JM, et al.: Definitive radiotherapy for extramedullary plasmacytomas of the head and neck. *Br. J. Radiol.* 76 (910): 738-41, 2003.

[3] Alexiou C, Kau RJ, Dietzfelbinger H, et al.: Extramedullary plasmacytoma: tumor occurrence and therapeutic concepts. *Cancer* 85 (11): 2305-14, 1999.

[4] The International Myeloma Working Group. Criteria for the classification of monoclonal gammopathies, multiple myeloma, and related disorders: a report of the International Myeloma Working Group. *Br. J. Haematol.* 121:749-757,2003.

[5] Kyle RA, Rajkumar SV. Criteria for diagnosis, staging, risk stratification and response assessment of multiple myeloma. Leukemia. Online publication: doi:10.1038/leu.2008.291.

[6] Banerjee SS, Verma S, Shanks JH. Morphological variants of plasma cell tumours. *Histopathology* 44:2-8, 2004.

[7] Pillai G, Lwin K, Pezzella F, Gatter K. Malignant plasmacytosis mimicking erythrophagocytosis. *Histopathology* 41; 468–470, 2002.

[8] Govender D, Harilal P, Dada M, Chetty R. CD31 (JC70) expression in plasma cells: an immunohistochemical analysis of reactive and neoplastic plasma cells. *J. Clin. Pathol* 50; 490–493, 1997.

[9] Menke DM, Horny HP, Griesser H, Atkinson EJ, Kaiserling E, Kyle RA. Immunophenotyping and genotyping of multiple myelomas with adverse prognosis characterised by immunohistological expression of the T cell related antigen CD45R0 (UCHL-1). *J. Clin. Pathol* 51:432–437, 1998.

[10] San Miguel JF, Gonzalez M, Gascon A et al. Immunophenotypic heterogeneity of multiple myeloma: influence on the biology and clinical course of the disease. Castellano-Leones (Spain) co-operative group for the study of monoclonal gammopathies. *Br. J. Haematol* 77; 185–190, 1991.

[11] Shin JS, Stopyra GA, Warhol MJ, Multhaupt HAB. Plasmacytoma with aberrant expression of myeloid markers, T-cell markers, and cytokeratin. *J. Histochem. Cytochem*. 49:791-792, 2001.

[12] Vasef MA, Medeiros LJ, Yospur LS, Sun NC, McCourty A, Brynes RK. Cyclin D1 protein in multiple myeloma and plasmacytoma: an immunohistochemical study using fixed, paraffin-embedded tissue sections. *Mod. Pathol* 1997; 10; 927–932, 1997.

[13] Dunphy CH, Nies MK, Gabriel DA. Correlation of plasma cell percentages by CD138 immunohistochemistry, cyclin D1 status, and CD56 expression with clinical parameters and overall survival in plasma cell myeloma. *Appl. Immunohistochem Mol. Morphol.* 15:248-254, 2007.

[14] Pellat-Deceunynck C, Barille S, Jego G, et al. The absence of CD56(NCAM) on malignant plasma cells is a hallmark of plasma cell leukemia and of a special subset of multiple myeloma. *Leukemia* 12:1977-1982, 1998.

[15] Rawstron A, Barrans S, Blythe D, et al. Distribution of myeloma plasma cells in peripheral blood and bone marrow correlates with CD56 expression. *Br. J. Haematol* 104:138-143, 1999.

[16] Chang H, Bartlett E, Patterson B, Chen CI, Yi QL. The absence of CD56 on malignant plasma cells in the cerebrospinal fluid is the hallmark of multiple myeloma involving central nervous system. *Br. J. Haematol* 129:539-541, 2005.

[17] Hoechtlen-Vollmar W, Menzel G, Bartl R, et al. Amplification of cyclin D1 gene in multiple myeloma: clinical and prognostic relevance. *Br. J. Haematol.* 109(1): 30-38, 2000.

[18] Moreau, P., et al., Recurrent 14q32 translocations determine the prognosis of multiple myeloma, especially in patients receiving intensive chemotherapy. *Blood* 100(5):1579-83, 2002.

[19] Fonseca, R., et al., The recurrent IgH translocations are highly associated with nonhyperdiploid variant multiple myeloma. *Blood* 102(7): p. 2562-7, 2003.

[20] Gertz, M.A., et al., Clinical implications of t(11;14)(q13;q32), t(4;14)(p16.3;q32), and -17p13 in myeloma patients treated with high-dose therapy. *Blood* 106(8):2837-40, 2005.

[21] Smock KJ, Perkins SL, Bahler DW. Quantitation of plasma cells in bone marrow aspirates by flow cytometric analysis compared with morphologic assessment. *Arch. Pathol. Lab. Med.* 131:951-955, 2007.

[22] Liebisch, P. and H. Dohner, Cytogenetics and molecular cytogenetics in multiple myeloma. *Eur. J. Cancer* 42(11):1520-9, 2006.

[23] Fonseca, R. and J. San Miguel, Prognostic factors and staging in multiple myeloma. *Hematol. Oncol. Clin. North Am.* 21(6):1115-40, ix, 2007.

[24] Avet-Louseau, H., et al., Chromosome 13 abnormalities in multiple myeloma are mostly monosomy 13. *Br. J. Haematol.* 111(4):1116-7, 2000.

[25] Shaughnessy, J., Jr., et al., Prognostic impact of cytogenetic and interphase fluorescence in situ hybridization-defined chromosome 13 deletion in multiple myeloma: early results of total therapy II. *Br. J. Haematol.* 120(1):44-52, 2003.

[26] Zojer, N., et al., Deletion of 13q14 remains an independent adverse prognostic variable in multiple myeloma despite its frequent detection by interphase fluorescence in situ hybridization. *Blood* 95(6):1925-30, 2000.

[27] Facon, T., et al., Chromosome 13 abnormalities identified by FISH analysis and serum beta2-microglobulin produce a powerful myeloma staging system for patients receiving high-dose therapy. *Blood* 97(6):1566-71, 2001.

[28] Desikan, R., et al., Results of high-dose therapy for 1000 patients with multiple myeloma: durable complete remissions and superior survival in the absence of chromosome 13 abnormalities. *Blood* 95(12):4008-10, 2000.

[29] Fonseca, R., et al., Biological and prognostic significance of interphase fluorescence in situ hybridization detection of chromosome 13 abnormalities (delta13) in multiple myeloma: an eastern cooperative oncology group study. *Cancer Res* 62(3):715-20, 2002.

[30] Chiecchio, L., et al., Deletion of chromosome 13 detected by conventional cytogenetics is a critical prognostic factor in myeloma. *Leukemia* 20(9):1610-7, 2006.

[31] Dewald, G.W., et al., Relationship of patient survival and chromosome anomalies detected in metaphase and/or interphase cells at diagnosis of myeloma. *Blood* 106(10):3553-8, 2005.

[32] Soussi, T. and K.G. Wiman, Shaping genetic alterations in human cancer: the p53 mutation paradigm. *Cancer Cell* 12(4):303-12, 2007.

[33] Fonseca, R., et al., Clinical and biologic implications of recurrent genomic aberrations in myeloma. *Blood* 101(11):4569-75, 2003.

[34] Drach, J., et al., Presence of a p53 gene deletion in patients with multiple myeloma predicts for short survival after conventional-dose chemotherapy. *Blood* 92(3):802-9, 1998.

[35] Chang, H., et al., p53 gene deletion detected by fluorescence in situ hybridization is an adverse prognostic factor for patients with multiple myeloma following autologous stem cell transplantation. *Blood* 105(1):358-60, 2005.

[36] Chng, W.J., et al., Clinical significance of TP53 mutation in myeloma. *Leukemia* 21(3):582-4, 2007.

[37] Chang, H., et al., Aberrant nuclear p53 protein expression detected by immunohistochemistry is associated with hemizygous P53 deletion and poor survival for multiple myeloma. *Br. J. Haematol.* 138(3):324-9, 2007.

[38] Ross, F.M., et al., Age has a profound effect on the incidence and significance of chromosome abnormalities in myeloma. *Leukemia* 19(9):1634-42, 2005.

[39] Kaufmann, H., et al., Both IGH translocations and chromosome 13q deletions are early events in monoclonal gammopathy of undetermined significance and do not evolve during transition to multiple myeloma. *Leukemia* 18(11):1879-82, 2004.

[40] Shou, Y., et al., Diverse karyotypic abnormalities of the c-myc locus associated with c-myc dysregulation and tumor progression in multiple myeloma. Proc. Natl. Acad. Sci. *USA* 97(1):228-33, 2000.

[41] Stewart, A.K. and R. Fonseca, Prognostic and therapeutic significance of myeloma genetics and gene expression profiling. *J. Clin. Oncol.* 23(26):6339-44, 2005.

[42] Bergsagel, P.L. and W.M. Kuehl, Chromosome translocations in multiple myeloma. *Oncogene* 20(40):5611-22, 2001.

[43] Bergsagel, P.L. and W.M. Kuehl, Critical roles for immunoglobulin translocations and cyclin D dysregulation in multiple myeloma. *Immunol Rev* 194:96-104, 2003.

[44] Fonseca, R., et al., Myeloma and the t(11;14)(q13;q32); evidence for a biologically defined unique subset of patients. Blood 99(10):3735-41, 2002.

[45] Feyler, S., et al., IgM myeloma: a rare entity characterized by a CD20-CD56-CD117-immunophenotype and the t(11;14). *Br. J. Haematol.* 140(5):547-51, 2008.

[46] Cook, J.R., et al., Immunohistochemistry Identifies Two Cyclin D1 Positive Subsets of Plasma Cell Myeloma, Each Associated With Favorable Survival. *Am. J. Clin. Pathol.* 125:615-24, 2006.

[47] Soverini, S., et al., Cyclin D1 overexpression is a favorable prognostic variable for newly diagnosed multiple myeloma patients treated with high-dose chemotherapy and single or double autologous transplantation. *Blood* 102(5):1588-94, 2003.

[48] Keats, J.J., et al., Ten years and counting: so what do we know about t(4;14)(p16;q32) multiple myeloma. *Leuk Lymphoma* 47(11):2289-300, 2006.

[49] Chesi, M., et al., Frequent translocation t(4;14)(p16.3;q32.3) in multiple myeloma is associated with increased expression and activating mutations of fibroblast growth factor receptor 3. *Nat. Genet.* 16(3):260-4, 1997.

[50] Fonseca, R., M.M. Oken, and P.R. Greipp, The t(4;14)(p16.3;q32) is strongly associated with chromosome 13 abnormalities in both multiple myeloma and monoclonal gammopathy of undetermined significance. *Blood* 98(4):1271-2, 2001.

[51] Keats, J.J., et al., In multiple myeloma, t(4;14)(p16;q32) is an adverse prognostic factor irrespective of FGFR3 expression. *Blood* 101(4):1520-9, 2003.

[52] Garand, R., et al., t(11;14) and t(4;14) translocations correlated with mature lymphoplasmacytoid and immature morphology, respectively, in multiple myeloma. *Leukemia* 17(10):2032-5, 2003.

[53] Xin, X., et al., CHIR-258 is efficacious in a newly developed fibroblast growth factor receptor 3-expressing orthotopic multiple myeloma model in mice. *Clin. Cancer Res.* 12(16):4908-15, 2006.

[54] Trudel, S., et al., CHIR-258, a novel, multitargeted tyrosine kinase inhibitor for the potential treatment of t(4;14) multiple myeloma. *Blood* 105(7):2941-8, 2005.

[55] Trudel, S., et al., The inhibitory anti-FGFR3 antibody, PRO-001, is cytotoxic to t(4;14) multiple myeloma cells. *Blood* 107(10):4039-46, 2006.

[56] Chang, H., et al., Immunohistochemistry accurately predicts FGFR3 aberrant expression and t(4;14) in multiple myeloma. *Blood* 106(1):353-5, 2005.

[57] Larson, A. and J.R. Cook, Fibroblast Growth Factor Receptor 3 (FGFR3) Expression in Malignant Lymphoma. *Appl. Imm. Mol. Morph*. In press.

[58] Boersma-Vreugdenhil, G.R., et al., The recurrent translocation t(14;20)(q32;q12) in multiple myeloma results in aberrant expression of MAFB: a molecular and genetic analysis of the chromosomal breakpoint. *Br. J. Haematol.* 126(3):355-63, 2004.

[59] Fabris, S., et al., Heterogeneous pattern of chromosomal breakpoints involving the MYC locus in multiple myeloma. *Genes Chromosomes Cancer* 37(3):261-9, 2003.

[60] Gabrea, A., P.L. Bergsagel, and W.M. Kuehl, Distinguishing primary and secondary translocations in multiple myeloma. *DNA Repair* 5:1225-1233, 2006.

[61] Yoshida, S., et al., Detection of MUM1/IRF4-IgH fusion in multiple myeloma. *Leukemia* 13(11):1812-6, 1999.

[62] Iida, S., et al., Deregulation of MUM1/IRF4 by chromosomal translocation in multiple myeloma. *Nat. Genet* 17(2):226-30, 1997.

[63] Chang, H., et al., Multiple myeloma patients with CKS1B gene amplification have a shorter progression-free survival post-autologous stem cell transplantation. *Br. J. Haematol.* 135(4):486-91, 2006.

[64] Fonseca, R., et al., Prognostic value of chromosome 1q21 gain by fluorescent in situ hybridization and increase CKS1B expression in myeloma. *Leukemia* 20(11):2034-40, 2006.

[65] Chang, H., et al., Chromosome 1p21 deletion is a novel prognostic marker in patients with multiple myeloma. *Br. J. Haematol.* 139(1):51-4, 2007.

[66] Smadja NV, Bastard C, Brigaudeau C, Leroux D, Fruchart C, Groupe Francais de Cytogenetique H. Hypodiploidy is a major prognostic factor in multiple myeloma. *Blood* 98:2229–2238, 2001.

[67] Singhal S, Mehta J, Desikan R, et al. Antitumor activity of thalidomide in refractory multiple myeloma [see comments]. *N. Engl. J. Med.* 341:1565–1571, 1999.

[68] Richardson PG, Barlogie B, Berenson J, et al. A phase 2 study of bortezomib in relapsed, refractory myeloma. *N. Engl. J. Med.* 348:2609–2617, 2003.

[69] Richardson PG, Sonneveld P, Schuster MW, et al. Bortezomib or high-dose dexamethasone for relapsed multiple myeloma [see Comment]. *N. Engl. J. Med.* 352:2487–2498, 2005.

[70] Rajkumar SV, Hayman SR, Lacy MQ, et al. Combination therapy with lenalidomide plus dexamethasone (Rev/Dex) for newly diagnosed myeloma. *Blood* 106:4050–4053, 2005.

[71] Richardson PG, Blood E, Mitsiades CS, et al. A randomized phase 2 study of lenalidomide therapy for patients with relapsed or relapsed and refractory multiple myeloma. *Blood* 108:3458–3464, 2006.

[72] Dispenzieri A, Rajkumar SV, Gertz MA, et al. Treatment of newly diagnosed multiple myeloma based on Mayo stratification of myeloma and risk-adapted therapy (mSMART): Consensus Statement. *Mayo Clin. Proc.* 82:323–341, 2007.

[73] Attal M, Harousseau JL, Stoppa AM, et al. A prospective, randomized trial of autologous bone marrow transplantation and chemotherapy in multiple myeloma: Intergroupe Francais du Myelome. *N. Engl. J. Med.* 335:91–97, 1996.

[74] Child JA, Morgan GJ, Davies FE, et al. High-dose chemotherapy with hematopoietic stem-cell rescue for multiple myeloma. *N. Engl. J. Med.* 348:1875–1883, 2003.

[75] Fermand JP, Ravaud P, Chevret S, et al. High-dose therapy and autologous peripheral blood stem cell transplantation in multiple myeloma: up-front or rescue treatment? Results of a multicenter sequential randomized clinical trial. *Blood* 92:3131–3136, 1998.

[76] Barlogie B, Kyle RA, Anderson KC, et al. Standard chemotherapy compared with high-dose chemoradiotherapy for multiple myeloma: final results of phase III US Intergroup Trial S9321. *J. Clin. Oncol.* 24:929–936, 2006.

[77] Blade J, Rosinol L, Sureda A, et al. High-dose therapy intensification compared with continued standard chemotherapy in multiple myeloma patients responding to the initial chemotherapy: long-term results from a prospective randomized trial from the Spanish cooperative group PETHEMA. *Blood* 106:3755–3759, 2005.

[78] Attal M, Harousseau JL, Facon T, et al. Single vs double autologous stem-cell transplantation for multiple myeloma [see comment]. *N. Engl. J. Med.* 349:2495–2502, 2003.

[79] Cavo M, Tosi P, Zamagni E, et al. Prospective, randomized study of single compared with double autologous stem-cell transplantation for multiple myeloma: Bologna 96 Clinical Study. *J. Clin. Oncol.* 25:2434–2441, 2007.

[80] Maloney DG, Molina AJ, Sahebi F, et al. Allografting with nonmyeloablative conditioning following cytoreductive autografts for the treatment of patients with multiple myeloma. *Blood* 102:3447–3454, 2003.

[81] Attal M, Harousseau J-L, Leyvraz S, et al. Maintenance therapy with thalidomide improves survival in patients with multiple myeloma. *Blood* 108:3289–3294, 2006.

[82] Stewart AK, Bergsagel PL, Greipp PR, et al. A practical guide to defining high-risk myeloma for clinical trials, patient counseling and choice of therapy. *Leukemia* 21:529–534, 2007.

In: Multiple Myeloma: Symptoms, Diagnosis and Treatment ISBN 978-1-60876-108-1
Editors: M. Georgiev and Ev. Bachev

Chapter 6

Bisphosphonates in Multiple Myeloma Patients

Jasmina Redzepovic, Ronald Gust and Heinz Pertz
Institute of Pharmacy, Free University of Berlin, Berlin, Germany

Abstract

Treatment of multiple myeloma, a B-cell cancer, is usually palliative. Bone disease affects 70% of multiple myeloma patients and causes complications such as pathologic fractures, severe bone pain, impaired mobility, spinal cord compression and hypercalcaemia, resulting in greater morbidity and poorer quality of life (QoL) for patients. Management of these complications can include treatment with bisphosphonates. The therapy choice for a multiple myeloma patient depends optimally on evidence that the selected treatment leads to better QoL and/or a lower risk of side effects. Therefore, a steady updating of the current knowledge of efficacy and safety of the therapy of choice is necessary. This chapter aims at a risk-benefit re-evaluation of bisphosphonates. This is achieved firstly by looking at new clinical studies examining the role of bisphosphonates on skeletal-related effect reduction and mortality, and secondly by analysing observational studies and case reports that constitute the only source of evidence for osteonecrosis of jaw (ONJ), a side effect that has been associated with intravenous bisphosphonates only in recent years, leading to a change in labelling.

1. Introduction

Like all tumor cells, which to a great extent maintain the characteristics of the healthy cells from which they originate, multiple myeloma cancer cells that originate from plasma cells also migrate mainly to the bone marrow (multiple myeloma is a bone marrow cancer) where they produce abnormal antibodies, called M (monoclonal) proteins or paraproteins [Janeway 2002]. When myeloma cell growth occurs inside the marrow-producing bones, healthy cells (e.g. red blood cells, white blood cells, platelets) are crowded out by cancer cells, causing immune system impairment, with an increased susceptibility to infections, as well as tiredness, and weakness. Furthermore, bone-remodeling cells, called osteoclasts are stimulated, whereas bone builders, called osteoblasts, are simultaneously suppressed. The pathogenesis of the oseoclast bone resorption is understood to be reslut of abnormal cytokine signaling between malignant plasma cells, osteoclasts, and osteoblasts. Increased levels of RANK-ligand produced by myeloma cells and marrow stromal cells coupled with a suppression of soluble osteoprotegerin (OPG) favors osteoclast bone resorption [Oxford Handbook of Oncology 2006]. Other cytokines such as interleukin 6 further support an excess of osteoclast activity [Oxford Handbook of Oncology 2006].

In addition, slow and steady bone damage (osteolytic lesions) caused by myeloma may lead to fractures of the long bones or compression fractures in the spine. Bone pain is often a symptom of this disease, especially in the form of a severe back pain.

Considering bisphosphonates as potent osteoclast inhibitors that suppress both natural and pathological bone resorption [Rogers 2000, Berenson 1998, Fleisch 1997], a therapeutic utilisation in multiple myeloma is indicated. Additionally, this is supported by their mechanism of action. Alendronate, risedronate, ibandronate, pamidronate, zoledronate (called aminobisphosphonates, Figure 1) are bisphosphonates containing nitrogen in one of the side chains. Clodronate, etidronate and tiludronate (called non-aminobisphosphonates, Figure 1) do not contain nitrogen.

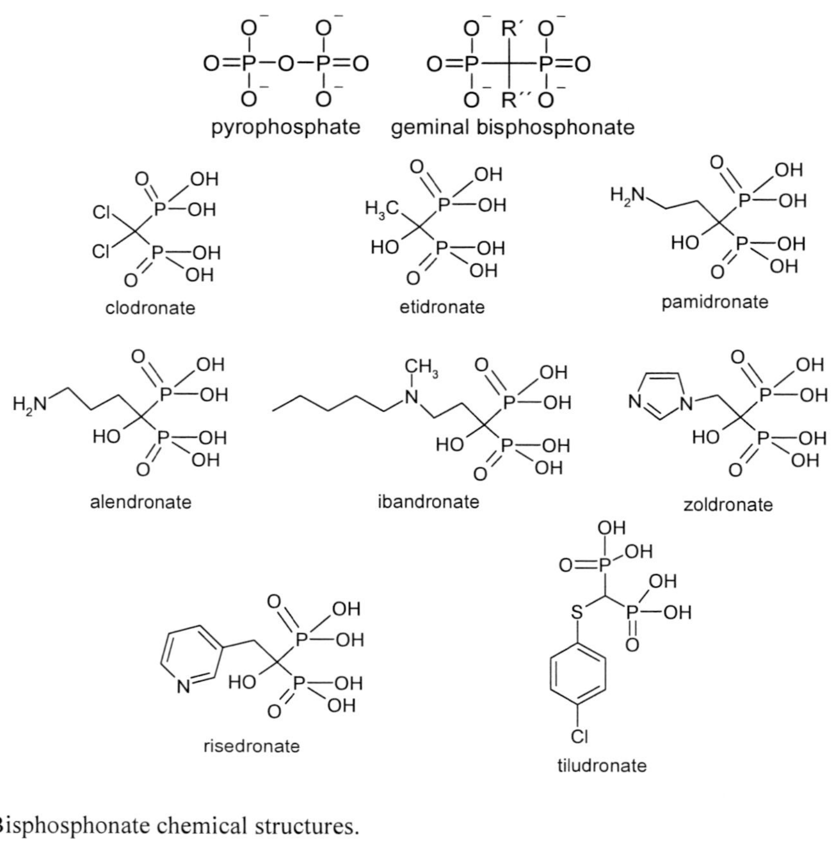

Figure 1. Bisphosphonate chemical structures.

While nitrogen-containing bisphosphonates inhibit the mevalonate pathway (the main target being farnesyl diphosphate synthase), nonnitrogen-containing bisphosphonates are incorporated into hydrolytically stable analogues of adenosine triphosphate. Both events cause impairment of osteoclast cell function and, ultimately, lead to osteoclast apoptosis [Brawn 2004]. Their role in mortality reduction and improvement of QoL of multiple myeloma patients has been examinded in numerous clinical studies. Consequently, their supportive application for bone complications in symptomatic patients is recommended by current multiple myeloma guidelines [Harrouseau 2008, Kyle 2007, Smith 2005, Barosi 2004, Durie 2003, NCCN 2008].

This chapter develops a systematic review of therapy evidence on bisphosphonate effects in multiple myeloma patients. In addition, data from observational studies and case reports on osteonecrosis of jaw (ONJ), a side-effect only associated with bisphosphonates in recent years, was analyzed in order to gain a new evidence for a risk-benefit re-evaluation of bisphosphonate therapy.

2. Method

Systematic Review and Meta-Analysis

A systematic review as a method for reviewing research evidence was used because it involves the careful and systematic collection of data from clinical trials, an assessment of each study, an unbiased synthesis and measurement of the findings from individual studies mostly by means of a statistical tool called meta-analysis, and it includes due consideration of any flaws in the evidence. The aim was to arrive at conclusions that are stronger and more reliable for clinical practice than the results of the individual trials.

A methodologically effective approach for conducting a systematic review requires a constant updating of the analysis through the integration of data coming from new studies, and an attentive reviewing process.

Search Strategy

As is generally accepted, randomized controlled trials (RCT) are considered the best source of evidence for reviews that attempt to evaluate effectiveness [Hayward 1995, Girling 2003, Altman 2001].

Searched for in this chapter, were RCTs for bisphosphonates that evaluate treatment benefits. However, because RCTs generally assess safety data less rigorously in respect to efficacy data [Lassere 2005] (bisphosphonate RCTs also report almost exclusively gastro-intestinal (GI) side-effects), it was necessary to obtain evidence on bisphosphonate side-effects from either descriptive studies such as case reports or case series, or observational studies without any control group.

The review of published ONJ case reports and observational studies was undertaken to investigate the quantity of evidence on this particular side-effect. It was examined whether, a critical quantity of evidence exists that shows that ONJ frequency is not rare, which would lead to the conclusion that authorities require that the manufacturers conduct an in-depth investigation into this issue. An analogous analysis for other bisphosphonate side-effects would go beyond the aim and scope of this work.

In this chapter, two searching strategies were applied, according to expected findings of different methodological quality, which had to be analyzed separately.

1) Search Strategy Aimed At Identifying Randomized Multiple Myeloma Trials

MEDLINE (1966 until Januar 2008), EMBASE (1974 until Januar 2008) and the Cochrane Controlled Trials Register (all years until October 2007) were searched to identify all randomized trials in multiple myeloma. The searched MeSH (Medical Subject Heading) and EMTREE terms for clodronate, pamidronate, etidronate, ibandronate, alendronate, risedronate, tiludronate and zoledronate were each cross-referenced with MeSH/EMTREE terms for multiple myeloma. The identified MeSH/EMTREE key words are listed in Table 12. The searches were limited to reports of clinical trials in humans. The relevant references in the articles published in peer-reviewed journals were also checked.

Broad searches of the Cochrane Controlled Trials Register, and of the meeting proceedings of the American Society of Clinical Oncology from 2005 to 2006, were performed using the following key words: bisphosphonates / disphosphonates, clodronate / clodronic acid, pamidronate / amidronate, ibadronate / ibadronic acid, alendronate, etidronate / etidronic acid, risedronate / risedronic acid, tiludronate / tiludronic acid, zoledronate / zoledronic acid, multiple, myeloma / plasma cell.

Finally, after the search was completed, the sensitivity and specificity of the search strategy were tested on the findings resulting from the search conducted by Cochrane Collaboration for their last bisphosphonate therapy review in 2002 [Djulbegovic 2002].

2) Search Strategy Aimed at Identifying either Observational Studies or Case Reports Examining Osteonecrosis of the Jaw (ONJ)

Daily search of Medline and PubMed MEDLINE (January 2003 until October 2007) with the MeSH/EMTREE key-words for clodronate, pamidronate, etidronate, ibandronate alendronate, risedronate, tiludronate, zoledronate were each cross-referenced with MeSH/EMTREE identified key-words for multiple myeloma, ostenecrosis and jaw diseases (Table 12, Table 13). A broad search of the meeting proceedings of the American Society of Clinical Oncology from 2005 to 2006 was performed using the following key words: bisphosphonates / disphosphonates, clodronate / clodronic acid, pamidronate / amidronate, ibadronate / ibadronic acid, alendronate, etidronate / etidronic acid, risedronate / risedronic acid, tiludronate / tiludronic acid, zoledronate / zoledronic acid, multiple, myeloma/plasma cell, jaw, diseases, mandible, maxilla, osteonecrosis, necrosis. Important references in ONJ reviews published in peer-reviewed journals were also taken into account.

3. Results

1. Efficacy

Numerous clinical trials (Table 1) examining benefits of the bisphosphonate therapy. Measured outcomes include: reduction of mortality, skeletal-related effects (SREs), hypercalcemia, pain, and improvement of QoL.

The evaluation of efficacy in this chapter is based on mortality and SRE data. Hypercalcemia, being only a preliminary end point of clinical trials, has not been taken into account.

In the identified clinical trials, pain reduction has not been adequately measured against an opiat therapy. For this reason, such data have also not been evaluated in this chapter. QoL data have been insufficiently reported, meaning that an extraction could not be performed. Clinical studies examining bisphosphonate therapy in asymptomatic patients [Musto 2003, Musto 2008, Barlogie 2008] were excluded, because it's the benefit of this therapy in this population is highly controversial and is not recommended by current clinical guidelines [Harrouseau 2008, Kyle 2007, Smith 2005, Barosi 2004, Durie 2003, NCCN 2008]. Other excluded publications are listed in Table 2.

Meta-Analysis of Mortality Reduction Data

Data extracted from 9 out of 13 randomized trials took in 1826 patients. There were 499 deaths among 927 patients treated with bisphosphonates, and 509 deaths among 899 control patients. There was a significant heterogeneity among the trials (Chi^2=18.11; degrees of freedom (df)=8; p=0.02). The corresponding odds ratio of 0.89 (95% CI: 0.72-1.10; p=0.27) indicates an advantage regarding mortality of the patients treated with bisphosphonates (Figure 2).

Meta-Analysis of SRE Reduction Data

Data from seven trials were included in the meta-analysis of skeletal related effects reduction. Among 880 patients treated with bisphosphonates, 298 experienced skeletal related events in comparison with 301 skeletal related events experienced by patients among 973 controls. The Chi^2 test (Chi^2 =8.55; degrees of freedom (df)=6; p=0.20) shows that there was no significant heterogeneity among trials. The odds ratio of 0.89 (95% CI: 0.72-1.09; p=0.27) indicates no beneficial effect of bisphosphonates on the number of patients experiencing general skeletal events (Figure 3).

Table 1. Summary of included multiple myeloma trial

First author, year	Study type	Treatment groups	No. of BP pts E (enrolled) /R (randomized)	No. of control pts E (enrolled) / R (randomized)	Route, dose, frequency	Treatmen t duration	Outcomes
Clodronate							
Delmas 982	Double-blind	Clodronate vs placebo	E=R= 7	E=R=7	1600 mg/d po.	18 mo	SRE (total) total fractures(%) vertebral fractures non-vertebral fractures total mortality pain calcium adverse events
Heim 1995	Not double blind, not placebo controlled	Clodronate vs observation	R= 39	R=32	1600 mg/d po	12 mo	SRE (total), total fractures, pain, calcium, adverse events
Lahtinen 1992	Double blind	Clodronate vs placebo	E=R=168	E=R=168	400 mg capsules po tid	24 mo	Mortality, non-vertebral fractures, pain, calcium
McCloskey 2001	Double blind	Clodronate vs placebo	E=R=264	E=R=272	400 mg capsules po tid	24 mo	SRE (total), total fractures, vertebral fractures, non-vertebral fractures, total mortality, pain, calcium
Pamidronate							
Attal 2006	Not double blind, not placebo controlled	Pamidronate vs pamidronate and thalidomide vs placebo	R (pamidronate)= 196 R (pamidronate and thalidomide)=201	R=200	Pamidronate 90 mg IV, every 4 weeks and 400 mg pamidronate and	30 mo	SRE (total), response rates, event-free, relapse-free, overall survival

First author, year	Study type	Treatment groups	No. of BP pts E (enrolled) /R (randomized)	No. of control pts E (enrolled) / R (randomized)	Route, dose, frequency	Treatment duration	Outcomes
					thalidomide, po a minimum dose reduction of 50 mg for treatment related toxicity.		
Berenson 1998	Double blind	Pamidronate vs placebo	E=205 R=198	E=187 R= 173	90 mg in 500 ml of 5% dextrose in water every 4 weeks.	21 mo	SRE (total), vertebral fractures, non-vertebral fractures, total mortality, pain, calcium, adverse events
Brincker 1998	Double blind	Pamidronate vs placebo	R=152	R=148	75 mg capsules po bid	24 mo	SRE (total), pain, calcium, adverse events
Kraja 2000	Not double blind, not placebo controlled	Pamidronate vs placebo	E=R=23	E=R=23	60 mg IV, every 4 weeks		Total mortality, vertebral fractures
Terpos 2000	Not double blind, not placebo controlled	Pamidronate vs placebo	E=R=32	E=R=30	90 mg iv, every 4 weeks	14 mo	Total mortality, total fractures, vertebral fractures, non-vertebral fracture, pain, hypercalcemia, abdominal pain.
Etidronate							
Belch 1991	Double blind	Etidronate vs placebo	E=98 R=92	E=78 R=74	5 mg/kg/d	Until death or discontinuation	SRE (total), pain, calcium, survival

Table 1. (Continued)

First author, year	Study type	Treatment groups	No. of BP pts E (enrolled) /R (randomized)	No. of control pts E (enrolled) / R (randomized)	Route, dose, frequency	Treatment duration	Outcomes
Daragon 1993	Double-blind	Etidronate vs placebo	E=49 R=39	E=45 R=39	10 mg/kg po qd	4 mo	SRE (total) total fractures vertebral fractures non-vertebral fractures total mortality pain calcium adverse events
Ibandronate							
Menssen 2002	Double blind	Ibandronate vs placebo	E=107 R=99	E=107R=99	2 mg IV every mo.	24 mo	SRE/year, vertebral fractures, non-vertebral fractures, total mortality, pain, hypercalcemia
Zoldronate							
Rosen 2004	Double-blind Phase III comparison study	Zoledronate 4 mg vs zoledronate 8 mg vs pamidronate	Breast and myeloma patients: E=1090 R=1087	Breast and myeloma patients: E=558 R=556	IV Zoledronate (4 mg or 8 mg) OR amidronate 90 mg iv every 3-4 weeks	12 mo	SRE (incidence at 13 months) pain morbidity time to event bone pain.

Table 2. Summary of the excluded multiple myeloma RCTs trials

First author, year	Reason for exclusion
Clodronate	
Adam 1996	Not randomized
Clemens 1993	More up-to-date data published in 1995 (Heim 1995)
Merlini 1990	Pseudorandomized study (treatment allocation was performed on alternate days, and not according to randomized allocation sequence)
McCloskey 1998	More up-to-date data published in 2001 (McCloskey 2001)
Pamidronate	
Abildgaard 1998	Subgroup analysis of a larger trial (Brinker 1998)
Ali 2001	Not randomized (see also zoldronate)
Berenson 1996	More up-to-date data published in 1998 (Berenson 1998)
Musto 2003	Asymptomatid patients
Caparrotti 2003	Not randomized. A combination therapy
Ciepłuch 2002	Not randomized. A combination therapy
Martin 2002	Asymptomatic patients
Morris 2001	Not randomized. A combination therapy
Barlogie 2008	Asymptomatic patients
Kraj 2000b	Duplicate publication (Kraj 2000)
Terpos 2003	No published outcomes of interest
Ibandronate	
Bergner 2007	Not randomized
Coleman 1999	Not extractable data for MM patients
Fontana 1998	More up-to-date published in 2002 (Menssen 2002)
Terpos 2003	No published outcomes of interest
Zoldronate	
Ali 2001	Not randomized (see also pamidronate)
Musto 2008	Asymptomatic patients
Spencer 2008	Not randomized. A combination therapy
Tassinari 2007	An observational study
Tosi 2006 a	A combination therapy
Vogel 2004	Not randomized

Study or Subgroup	Bisphosphonates Events	Bisphosphonates Total	Control Events	Control Total	Weight	Odds Ratio M-H, Fixed, 95% CI
1.1.1 Etidronate						
Belch 2001	65	92	37	74	6.7%	2.41 [1.27, 4.56]
Daragon 1993	20	39	19	39	5.1%	1.11 [0.46, 2.69]
Subtotal (95% CI)		**131**		**113**	**11.8%**	**1.84 [1.10, 3.08]**
Total events	85		56			
Heterogeneity: $Chi^2 = 1.93$, df = 1 (P = 0.16); $I^2 = 48\%$						
Test for overall effect: Z = 2.33 (P = 0.02)						
1.1.2 Clodronate						
Delmas 1982	4	7	1	6	0.3%	6.67 [0.49, 91.33]
Lahtinen 1992	54	168	68	168	25.6%	0.70 [0.45, 1.09]
McCloskey 2001	234	264	253	271	15.7%	0.55 [0.30, 1.02]
Subtotal (95% CI)		**439**		**445**	**41.5%**	**0.68 [0.48, 0.97]**
Total events	292		322			
Heterogeneity: $Chi^2 = 3.36$, df = 2 (P = 0.19); $I^2 = 40\%$						
Test for overall effect: Z = 2.14 (P = 0.03)						
1.1.3 Pamidronate						
Berenson 1998	67	203	77	189	29.6%	0.72 [0.47, 1.08]
Kraj 2003	13	23	12	23	2.9%	1.19 [0.37, 3.81]
Terpos 2000	0	32	2	30	1.4%	0.18 [0.01, 3.81]
Subtotal (95% CI)		**258**		**242**	**33.9%**	**0.73 [0.50, 1.08]**
Total events	80		91			
Heterogeneity: $Chi^2 = 1.51$, df = 2 (P = 0.47); $I^2 = 0\%$						
Test for overall effect: Z = 1.58 (P = 0.11)						
1.1.4 Ibandronate						
Menssen 2001	42	99	40	99	12.8%	1.09 [0.62, 1.91]
Subtotal (95% CI)		**99**		**99**	**12.8%**	**1.09 [0.62, 1.91]**
Total events	42		40			
Heterogeneity: Not applicable						
Test for overall effect: Z = 0.29 (P = 0.77)						
Total (95% CI)		**927**		**899**	**100.0%**	**0.89 [0.72, 1.10]**
Total events	499		509			
Heterogeneity: $Chi^2 = 18.11$, df = 8 (P = 0.02); $I^2 = 56\%$						
Test for overall effect: Z = 1.10 (P = 0.27)						
Test for subgroup differences: Not applicable						

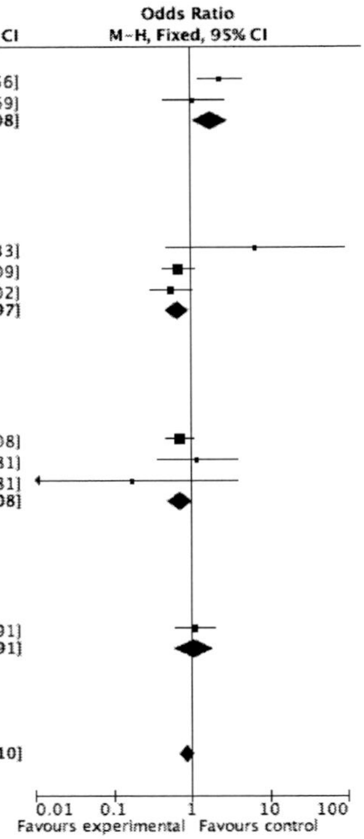

Figure 2. Mortality reduction.

Study or Subgroup	Bisphosphonates Events	Bisphosphonates Total	Control Events	Control Total	Weight	Odds Ratio M-H, Fixed, 95% CI
1.2.1 Etidronate						
Belch 2001	20	92	21	74	9.6%	0.70 [0.35, 1.42]
Subtotal (95% CI)		**92**		**74**	**9.6%**	**0.70 [0.35, 1.42]**
Total events	20		21			
Heterogeneity: Not applicable						
Test for overall effect: Z = 0.98 (P = 0.33)						
1.2.2 Clodronate						
Heim 1995	19	39	21	32	6.2%	0.50 [0.19, 1.30]
Lahtinen 1992	23	96	13	108	4.9%	2.30 [1.09, 4.85]
Subtotal (95% CI)		**135**		**140**	**11.1%**	**1.29 [0.73, 2.28]**
Total events	42		34			
Heterogeneity: $Chi^2 = 6.08$, df = 1 (P = 0.01); $I^2 = 84\%$						
Test for overall effect: Z = 0.89 (P = 0.38)						
1.2.3 Pamidronate						
Attal 2006	41	196	48	200	19.8%	0.84 [0.52, 1.34]
Berenson 1998	62	198	66	179	25.0%	0.78 [0.51, 1.20]
Brincker 1998	79	152	80	148	20.5%	0.92 [0.58, 1.45]
Subtotal (95% CI)		**546**		**527**	**65.2%**	**0.84 [0.65, 1.09]**
Total events	182		194			
Heterogeneity: $Chi^2 = 0.27$, df = 2 (P = 0.87); $I^2 = 0\%$						
Test for overall effect: Z = 1.30 (P = 0.19)						
1.2.4 Ibandronate						
Menssen 2001	54	107	52	99	14.1%	0.92 [0.53, 1.59]
Subtotal (95% CI)		**107**		**99**	**14.1%**	**0.92 [0.53, 1.59]**
Total events	54		52			
Heterogeneity: Not applicable						
Test for overall effect: Z = 0.30 (P = 0.77)						
Total (95% CI)		**880**		**840**	**100.0%**	**0.89 [0.72, 1.09]**
Total events	298		301			
Heterogeneity: $Chi^2 = 8.55$, df = 6 (P = 0.20); $I^2 = 30\%$						
Test for overall effect: Z = 1.11 (P = 0.27)						
Test for subgroup differences: Not applicable						

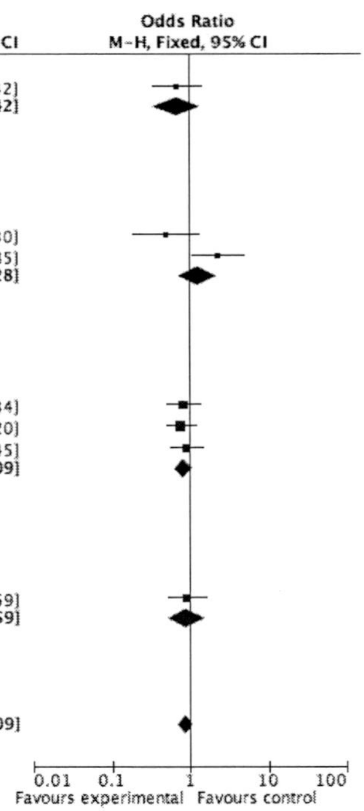

Figure 3. Reduction of skeletal related events.

2. Safety

As mentioned earlier, the identified bisphosphonate RCTs report almost only gastro-intestinal (GI) side-effects (Table 4). Other bisphosphonate side-effect evidence can be found in either descriptive studies such as case reports or in case series, or in observational studies without a control group. Here, credibility depends on the number of cases reported. The reason behind this difference in assessment in clinical trials is that the regulatory agencies (US Food and Drug Administration or FDA, the European Medicines Agency or EMEA) give drug market authorizations based primarily on the determination of efficacy and not of safety. Furthermore, because a rare side effect may come to light when the drug is approved, and used in the larger population, the post-marketing surveillance is a very important issue. However, safety report submissions to the agencies are made on a voluntary basis.

Even though only one randomized trial reports on osteonecrosis of jaw ONJ [Attal 2006], a growing number of ONJ case reports and observational studies evaluating ONJ have been published in recent years (Tables 5, 6, 7). Typical symptoms for ONJ are pain, soft-tissue swelling and infection, loose teeth and exposed bone. Since 2003, when the first reports were published, several groups and organizations have developed or issued recommendations, position papers, or statements regarding bisphosphonate-associated ONJ. In order to gain evidence of ONJ frequency for medical decisions, case reports or case series in either descriptive studies or observational studies are the only source of evidence. Since no comparison is made with any controls, contributory causes cannot be provided. Descriptive studies are subjective and are at risk of being abused or misinterpreted. At best they can suggest future directions for research into the treatment, or for the test being reported, using more stringent study design.

Moreover, their credibility depends on the number of reported cases. This means, for example, that if ONJ is a rare side-effect ($p<0.001$) and is very unlikely to occur on a regular basis, then descriptive studies may be be regarded as evidence.

Seven identified observational trials with 1068 examined patients regarding ONJ were analyzed. The highest frequencies were demonstrated by a combination of Pamidrnonate and Zoldronate (4.55%, 9.1%, 23.3%, 24.71% and 51.51%). Zoldronate demonstrated frequencies ranging from 2.7% to 10.9%. Pamidronate showed frequencies ranging from 0% to 17.65%. If this 0% regarded as an outlier, then the lowest frequency for pamidronate is 1.28%. These frequencies show that ONJ is not a rare side-effect, in patients using Pamidronate, Zoldronate, or a combination thereof. This means that regulatory agencies should require from manufacturers that the true incidence be investigated using more stringent study design.

Inadequate evidence exists for conclusions to be drawn for other bisphosphonates. There are also other bisphosphonate side-effects that are not visible in RCTs, but should be regarded as important by physicians and policy makers. All bisphosphonates can cause hypocalcemia, regardless of the method of administration, although this is found to be a clinically symptomatic problem only infrequently. The most common side-effects with oral bisphosphonates (depending on whether an aminobisphosphonate or a non-aminobisphosphonate is being applied) are upper gastrointestinal trouble, such as gastritis [Van Holten-Verzantvoort 1993] and diarrhea [Atula 2003]. IV infusions can be associated with injection site reaction and acute systematic inflammatory reactions [Tanvetyanon 2006].

Renal dysfunction is a particularly problematic adverse event that can also occur after infusion of IV bisphosphonates. However, the incidence may vary between agents, depending on renal uptake and elimination. The US Food and Drug Administration (FDA) reported that 72 patients suffered renal failure following zoledronate therapy [Chang 2003]. As a result, the product labels for Pamidronate and Zoledronate were amended to include additional nephrotoxicity warnings.

Table 4. Commonest side-effects reported in the multiple myeloma studies

Reference	Route, dose and frequency	Commonest toxicity	Comments
Clodronate			
Delmas 1982	1600 mg/d po	Not reported	
Heim 1995	1600 mg/d po	Leukopenia, nausea, loss of appetite, vomiting, dyspnoea	
Lahtinen 1992	400 mg capsules po tid	Nausea, diarrhoea, constipation, abdominal pain, alergic reations. No difference between clodronate and placebo group	
McCloskey 2001	400 mg capsules po tid	Not reported	
Pamidronate			
Attal 2006	Pamidronate 90 mg IV, every 4 weeks, and 400 mg pamidronate plus thalidomide po. a minimum dose reduction of 50 mg	Peripheral neuropathy, fatigue, constipation, neutropenia, thrombocytopenia, anemia, infection, osteonecrosis, nausea	
Berenson 1998	90 mg po. every 4 weeks	Anemia, fever, nausea, upper respiratory tract infection, fatigue, constipation, diarrhea, coughing	Two withdrawals due toxicities: an apparently allergic reaction and hypocalcemia (7.5 mg per deciliter)
Brincker 1998	75 mg capsules po. bid	Nausea, dysphagia/ dyspepsia and gastrointestinal ulcerations (56 vs. 43)	Only gastrointestinal events were reported
Kraj 2000	60 mg IV, every 4 weeks	Not reported	
Terpos 2000	90 mg IV, every 4 weeks	Not reported	
Etidronate			
Belch 1991	5 mg/kg/d	Not reported.	
Reference	Route, dose and frequency	Commonest toxicity	Comments

Ibandronate			
Daragon 1993	10 mg/kg po qd	Not adequately reported. No GIT	Two withdrawals due to toxicities: skin allergy was experienced by a patient in the pamidronate group and pancreatitis by a patient in placebo group
Menssen 2002	2 mg IV every month	Not spezified	40 placebo and 42 ibandronate patients dropped out because of severe adverse advents
Zoldronate			
Rosen 2004	Zoledronate 4/8 mg iv or Pamidronate 90 mg iv, every 3-4 weeks	Bone pain, nausea, fatigue, pyrexia, emesis, anemia, diarrhea, dyspnea, myalgia, constipation (1077 with Zoldronate and 556 with Pamidronate)	Data are not stratified by multiple myeloma or breast cancer

Table 5. Included ONJ studies

First author, year	Study type
Badros 2006	Retrospective study
Calvo-Villas 2006	Not clear
Corso 2007	Retrospective study
Dimopouloulos 2006	Retrospective study from 1997; Prospective from 2003 to 2005
Garcia-Gara 2006	Retrospective study
Tosi 2006 b	Retrospective study
Zervas 2006	Retrospective study from 1991, prospective from 2001 to 2006

Table 6. Summary of excluded ONJ studies

1st author, year	Reason for exclusion
Bujanda 2007	No multiple myeloma pts with ONJ
Hoff 2006	Not extractable data for MM pts (abstract)
Kut 2004	ASH 2004 (abstract No-4933): Approximately 600 MM pts. The reported frequency: 7 pts. Exclusion due to not imprecise reporting (e.g. “approximately 600 MM pts”)

Table 7. Summary of ONJ case reports

1st author, year		Purcell and Boyd 2005
Abu-Id 2006		Ruggiero 2004
Agrillo 2006		Pastor-Zuazaga 2006
Bagan 2006		Phal 2007
Battley 2006		Polizzotto 2006
Braun 2006		Salesi 2006
Broglia 2006		Senel 2007
Capalbo 2006		Sitters 2005
Carneiro 2006		Treister 2006
Carter 2005		Vannucchi 2005
Clarke 2007		Walter 2007
Curi 2007		Wutzl 2006
Dannemann 2007		Yeo 2005
Diego 2007		Zarychanski 2006
Dimitrakopoulos 2006		
Elad 2006		
Estilo 2004		
Ficarra 2005		
Gibbs 2005		
Hansen 2006		
Hay 2006		
Herbozo 2007		
Kademani 2006		
Katz 2005		
Khamaisi 2006		
Kumar 2007		
Lenz 2005		
Lugassy 2004		
Magopoulos 2007		
Marunick 2005		
Marx 2005		
Mavrokokki 2007		
Melo 2005		
Merigo 2006		
Migliorati 2005		
Montazeri 2007		
Mortensen 2007		
Murad 2007		
Pires 2005		
Pozzi 2007		

Conclusion

The current meta-analysis, as well as all identified clinical trials, demonstrates that there is no practical survival advantage. Therefore future studies should investigate bisphosphonate treatments as a palliative treatment by measuring its influence on true QOL end points. The QOL assessment using solely surrogate end points such as SRE reduction is inappropriate from a methodological point of view, and can in fact be misleading because such QOL outcomes are only surrogate responses [Tassinari 2003].

Although it is recommended by current guidelines [Harrouseau 2008, Kyle 2007, Smith 2005, Barosi 2004, Durie 2003, NCCN 2008], this meta-analysis does not show significant benefits in the use of bisphosphonates for reduction of skeletal-related events. These results are consistent with those of a majority of studies [Attal 2006, Menssen 2002, Brincker 1998, Berenson 1998, Lahtinen 1992, Heim 1995, Belch 1991, Daragon 1993]. These results also contradict the findings of Cochrane Collaboration that indicate benefits of bisphosphonates regarding osteolytic fraction. This discrepancy may be due to the different measures included in the meta-analysis. In this chapter, we meta-analysed the total number of SREs, whereas the Cochrone group meta-analysed vertebral and non-vertebral fraction reduction [Djulbegovic 2002].

In this chapter, a critical analysis of ONJ conducted by means of a thorough review of all descriptive studies, showed that ONJ is not a rare side-effect of Zoldronate, Pamidronate, or their combination, and that these results should call attention to existing concerns regarding current standards for clinical studies. Other bisphosphonate side-effects were not investigated, as this would go beyond the scope of this work, but a general requirement for higher examination standards for other relevant side-effects should be also considered legitimate.

Physicians' choices regarding which bisphosphonates to apply must be ideally based on evidence from comparative trials. Unfortunately, there is only a comparative Rosen 2004 study [Rosen 2001, 2003, 2004, Berenson 2001], the data from which were not adequately reported. Comparative investigations should be urgently carried out in the future to enable appropriate health care decisions to be made.

References

Abildgaard N, Rungby J, Glerup H, et al. (1998). Long-term oral pamidronate treatment inhibits osteoclastic bone resorption and bone turnover without affecting osteoblastic function in multiple myeloma. *Eur. J. Hematol.* 61:128–134.

Abu-Id MH, Açil Y, Gottschalk J, Kreusch T. (2006). Bisphosphonate-associated osteonecrosis of the jaw. *Mund Kiefer Gesichtschir.* 10(2):73-81.

Adam Z, Prokes B, Znojil V, et al. (1996). Effect of clodronate on bone density of patients in multiple myeloma-2 year study [Vliv clodronatu na kostin denzitu pacientu s mnohocenym myelomem-dvoulete sledeovani lecebneho ucinku]. *Vnitr Lek.* 42:379–385.

Agrillo A, Petrucci MT, Tedaldi M, et al. (2006). New therapeutic protocol in the treatment of avascular necrosis of the jaws. J 3. 3. 3. *Craniofac Surg.* 17(6):1080-1083.

Ali SM, Esteva FJ, Hortobagyi G, et al. (2001). Safety and efficacy of bisphosphonates beyond 24 months in cancer patients. *J. Clin. Oncol.* 19(14):3434-3437.

Altman DG, Schulz KF, Moher D et al. (2001). The revised CONSORT statement for reporting randomized trials: explanation and elaboration. *Ann. Intern. Med.* 134:63–694.

Atula S, Powles T, Paterson A, et al. (2003). Extended safety profile of oral clodronate after long term nuse in primary breast cancer patients. *Drug Safety*. 26: 661 – 671.

Attal M, Harousseau JL, Leyvraz S, et al. (2006). Maintenance therapy with thalidomide improves survival in multiple myeloma patients. *Blood.* 108(10):3289-3294.

Badros A, Weikel D, Salama A, et al. (2006). Osteonecrosis of the Jaw in Multiple Myeloma Patients: Clinical Features and Risk Factors. *J. Clin. Oncol.* 24(6):945-952.

Bagan JV, Jimenez Y, Murillo J, et al. (2006). Jaw osteonecrosis associated with bisphosphonates: multiple exposed areas and its relationship to teeth extractions. Study of 20 cases [Letter]. *Oral Oncol.* 42:327-329.

Barlogie B, van Rhee F, Shaughnessy JD Jr, et al. (2008). Seven-year median time to progression with thalidomide for smoldering myeloma: partial response identifies subset requiring earlier salvage therapy for symptomatic disease. *Blood.* 112(8):3122-3125.

Barosi G, Boccadoro M, Cavo M, et al. (2004). Management of multiple myeloma and related-disorders: guidelines from the Italian Society of Hematology (SIE), Italian Society of Experimental Hematology (SIES) and Italian Group for Bone Marrow Transplantation (GITMO). *Haematologica*. 89:717 – 741.

Battley J, Jayathissa S, Seneviratne E. (2006). Jaw osteonecrosis associated with bisphosphonates. *N Z Med. J.* 119(1246):U2341.

Belch AR, Bergsagel DE, Wilson K. (1991). Effect of daily etidronate on the osteolysis of multiple myeloma. *J. Clin. Oncol.* 9:1397-1402.

Berenson JR, Lichtenstein A, Porter L, et al. (1996). Efficacy of pamidronate in reducing skeletal events in patients with advanced multiple myeloma. Myeloma Aredia Study Group. *N. Engl. J. Med.* 334:488–493.

Berenson JR, Lichtenstein A, Porter L. (1998). Long-term pamidronate treatment of advanced multiple myeloma patients reduces skeletal events. *J. Clin. Oncol.* 16:593–602.

Berenson JR, Rosen LS, Howell A, et al. (2001). Zoledronic acid reduces skeletal-related events in patients with osteolytic metastases. *Cancer.* 91(7):1191-1200.

Bergner R, Henrich DM, Hoffmann M, et al. (2007). Renal safety and pharmacokinetics of ibandronate in multiple myeloma patients with or without impaired renal func-tion. *J. Clin. Pharmacol.* 47(8):942-950.

Braun E, Iacono VJ. (2006). Bisphosphonates: case report of nonsurgical periodontal therapy and osteochemonecrosis. *Int. J. Periodontics Restorative Dent.*2006; 26(4):315-319.

Brincker JW, Abildgaard N. (1998). Failure of oral pamidronate to reduce skeletal morbidity in multiple myeloma : a double-blind placebo-controlled trial. *Br. J. Haematol.*101:280-286.

Broglia C, Merlati G, Valentino F, et al. (2006). Avascular jaw osteonecrosis associated with bisphophonate therapy. *Recenti Prog Med.* 97(3):140-144.

Brown JE, Neville-Webbe H, Coleman RE. (2004). The role of bisphosphonates in breast and prostate cancers. *Endocr. Relat. Cancer.* 11:207 – 224.

Bujanda AD, Sarmiento BU, Suárez CMA, Morales AJ. (2007). Assessment of renal toxicity and osteonecrosis of the jaws in patients receiving zoledronic acid for bone metastasis. *Ann. Oncol.* 18(3):556-560.

Calvo-Villas JM, Tapia Torres M, Govantes Rodriguez J, et al. (2006). Osteonecrosis of the jaw in patients with multiple myeloma during and after treatment with zoledronic acid. *Med. Clin.* (Barc). 127(15):576-579.

Capalbo S, Delia M, Diomede D, et al. (2006). Jaw osteonecrosis associated with use of bisphosphonates and chemotherapy: paradoxical complication of treatment of bone lesions in multiple myeloma patients. *Int. J. Hematol.* 83(5):439-442.

Caparrotti G, Catalano L, Feo C, et al. (2003). Perspective study on pamidronate in stage I multiple myeloma. *Hematol. J.* 4(6):459-460.

Carneiro E, Vibhute P, Montazem A, Som PM. (2006). Bisphosphonate-associated mandibular osteonecrosis. *AJNR Am. J. Neuroradiol.* 27(5):1096-1097.

Carter G, Goss AN, Doecke C. (2005). Bisphosphonates and avascular necrosis of the jaw: a possible association. *Med. J. Aust.* 182:413-415.

Chang JT, Green L, Beitz J. (2003). Renal failure with the use of zoledronic acid. *N. Engl. J. Med.* 349:1676 – 1679.

Ciepłuch H, Baran W, Hellmann A. (2002). Combination of pamidronate and thalidomide in the therapy of treatment-resistant multiple myeloma. *Med. Sci. Monit.* 8(4):PI31-PI36.

Clarke BM, Boyette J, Vural E, et al. (2007). Bisphosphonates and jaw osteonecrosis: the UAMS experience. *Otolaryngol Head Neck Surg.* 136(3):396-400.

Clemens MR, Fessele K, Heim ME. (1993). Multiple myeloma: effect of daily dichloromethylene bisphosphonate on skeletal complications. *Ann. Hematol.* 66:141–146.

Coleman RE, Purohit OP, Black C, et al. (1999). Double-blind, randomised, placebo-controlled, dose-finding study of oral ibandronate in patients with metastatic bone disease. *Ann. Oncol.* 10(3):311-316.

Corso A, Varettoni M, Zappasodi P, et al. (2007). A different schedule of zoledronic acid can reduce the risk of the osteonecrosis of the jaw in patients with multiple myeloma. *Leukemia.* 21(7):1545-1548.

Curi MM, Cossolin GS, Koga DH, et al. (2007). Treatment of avascular osteonecrosis of the mandible in cancer patients with a history of bisphosphonate therapy by combining bone resection and autologous platelet-rich plasma: Report of 3 cases. *J. Oral Maxillofac Surg.* 65(2):349-355.

Dannemann C, Grätz KW, Riener MO, Zwahlen RA. (2007). Jaw osteonecrosis related to bisphosphonate therapy: a severe secondary disorder. *Bone.* 40(4):828-834.

Daragon A, Humez C, Michot CXLL. (1993). Treatment of multiple myeloma with etidronate results of a multicentre double-blind study. *Eur. J. Med.* 2:449-452.

Delmas PD, Charhon S, Chapuy MC, et al. (1982). Long-term effects of dichloromethylene diphosphonate (CI2MDP) on skeletal lesions in multiple myeloma. *Metab. Bone Dis. Relat. Res.* 4(3):163-168.

Diego R, D'Orto O, Pagani D, et al. (2007). Bisphosphonate-associated osteonecrosis of the jaws: a therapeutic dilemma. *Oral. Surg. Oral. Med. Oral Pathol. Oral. Radiol. Endod.* 103(3):e1-5.

Dimopoulos MA, Kastritis E, Bamias A, et al. (2006). Osteonecrosis of the jaw in patients with multiple myeloma treated with bisphosphonates: evidence of increased risk after treatment with zoledronic acid. *Haematologica.* 91:968-971.

Dimitrakopoulos I, Magopoulos C, Karakasis D. (2006). Bisphosphonate-induced avascular osteonecrosis of the jaws: a clinical report of 11 cases. *Int. J. Oral Maxillofac Surg.* 35(7):588-593.

Djulbegovic B, Wheatley K, Ross J, et al. (2002). Bisphosphonates in multiple myeloma. *The Cochrane Database of Systematic Reviews.* 4. John Wiley and Sons, Ltd Chichester, UK.

Durie BG, Kyle RA, Belch A, et al. (2003). Myeloma management guidelines: a consensus report from the Scientific Advisors of the International Myeloma Foundation. *Hematology J.* 4:379 – 398.

Elad S, Yarom N, Hamed W, et al. (2006). Osteomylelitis and necrosis of the jaw in patients treated with bisphosphonates: a comparative study focused on multiple myeloma. *Clin. Lab. Haematol.* 28(6):393-398.

Estilo CS, Van Poznak CH, Williams T, et al. (2004). Osteonecrosis of the maxilla and mandible in patients treated with bisphosphonates: a retrospective study [Abstract]. *Proc. Am. Soc. Clin. Oncol.* 22:750.

Ficarra G, Beninati F, Rubino I, et al. (2005). Osteonecrosis of the jaws in periodontal patients with a history of bisphosphonates treatment. *J. Clin. Periodontol.* 32:1123-1128.

Fleisch H. (1997). Bisphosphonates in Bone Disease-From the Labratory to the Patient (ed 3). New York, NY, The Pathenon Publishing Group.

Fontana A, Herrmann Z, Menssen HD, et al. (1998). Effects of intravenous ibandronate therapy on skeletal related events (SRE) and survival in patients with advanced multiple myeloma. *Blood.* 92(1):106a.

Garcia-Gara C, Gonzalez-Garcia C, Juliana Majado M, et al. (2006). Osteonecrosis of the Jaw in Multiple Myeloma Patients. Experience of Two Hospitals. *Blood.* 108 (11):5086.

Gibbs SD, O'Grady J, Seymour JF, Prince HM. (2005). Bisphosphonate-induced osteonecrosis of the jaw requires early detection and intervention [Letter]. *Med. J. Aust.* 183:549-550.

Girling DJ. (2003). *Clinical Trials in Cancer: Principles and Practice.* New York: Oxford University Press.

Hansen T, Kunkel M, Weber A, Kirkpatrick CJ. (2006). Osteonecrosis of the jaws in patients treated with bisphosphonates - histomorphologic analysis in comparison with infected osteoradionecrosis. *J. Oral Pathol. Med.* 35(3):155-160.

Harrouseau JL, Dreyling M. (2008). Multiple myeloma: ESMO Clinical Recommendations for diagnosis, treatment and follow-up. *Ann. Oncol.* 19(2): ii55-ii57.

Hay KD, Bishop PA. (2006) Association of osteonecrosis of the jaws and bisphosphonate pharmacotherapy: dental implications. *N Z Dent. J.* 102(1):4-9.

Hayward RS, Wilson MC, Tunis SR et al. (1995). Users' guides to the medical literature VIII. How to use clinical practice guidelines. A. Are the recommendations valid? The Evidence-Based Medicine Working Group. *J. Am. Med. Assoc.* 274:570–574.

Heim ME, Clemens MR, Queißer W, et al. (1995). Prospective randomized trial of dichloromethilene bisphosphonate (clodronate) in patients with multiple myeloma. *Onkologie.* 18: 439-448.

Herbozo PJ, Briones DL, Ferres AJ, Torrealba RL. (2007). Severe spontaneous cases of bisphosphonate-related osteonecrosis of the jaws. *J. Oral Maxillofac Surg*. 65(8):1650-1654.

Hoff AO, Toth BB, Altunday K et al. (2006). Osteonecrosis of the jaw in patients receiving intravenous bisphosphonate therapy. *J. Clin. Oncol*. 24:8528a.

Imrie K, Stevens A, Makarski J, et al. (2007). The role of bisphosphonates in the management of skeletal complications for patients with multiple myeloma: A clinical practice guideline. Published online: http://www.cancercare.on.ca/pdf/pebc6-4f.pdf

Janeway C. (2002). Immunologie. 5 Aufl.- Heidelberg; Berlin: Spektrum, *Akad. Verl*. 304.

Kademani D, Koka S, Lacy MQ, Rajkumar SV. (2006). Primary surgical therapy for osteonecrosis of the jaw secondary to bisphosphonate therapy. *Mayo Clin. Proc*. 81(8):1100-1103.

Katz H. (2005). Endodontic implications of bisphosphonate-associated osteonecrosis of the jaws: a report of three cases. *J. Endod*. 31:831-834.

Khamaisi M, Regev E, Yarom N, et al. (2007). Possible association between diabetes and bisphosphonate-related jaw osteonecrosis. *J. Clin. Endocrinol. Metab*. 92(3):1172-1175.

Kraj M, Poglód R, Pawlikowsky J, Maj S. (2000 a). The effect of long-term pamidronate treatment on skeletal morbidity in advanced multiple myeloma. *Acta Haematologica Polonica*. 31:379-389.

Kraj M, Póglod R, Pawlikowski J, Maj S, Nasiloska B. (2000 b). Effect of pamidronate on skeletal morbidity in myelomatosis. Part 1: The results of the 12 months of pamidronate therapy. *Acta Poloniae Pharmaceutica*. 57 (1):113–116.

Kumar V, Pass B, Guttenberg SA, Ludlow J, et al. (2007). Bisphosphonate-related osteonecrosis of the jaws: a report of three cases demonstrating variability in outcomes and morbidity. *J. Am. Dent. Assoc*. 138(5):602-609.

Kut V, Mehta J, Tariman J, et al. (2004). Osteonecrosis of the Jaw in Myeloma Patients Receiving Pamidronate or Zoledronate. *Blood*. 104: 4933.

Kyle RA, Yee GC, Somerfield MR, et al. (2007). American Society of Clinical Oncology 2007 clinical practice guideline update on the role of bisphosphonates in multiple myeloma. *J. Clin. Oncol*. 25(17):2464-2472.

Lahtinen R, Laakso M, Palva I, et al. (1992). Randomized, placebo-controlled multicentre trial of clodronate in multiple myeloma. *Lancet*. 340:1049-1052.

Lassere MND, Johnson KR, Woodworth TG, et al. (2005). Challenges and progress in adverse event ascertainment and reporting in clinical trials. *Journal of Rheumatology*. 32(10): 2030-2032.

Lenz JH, Steiner-Krammer B, Schmidt W, et al. (2005). Does avascular necrosis of the jaws in cancer patients only occur following treatment with bisphosphonates? *J. Craniomaxillofac Surg*. 33:395-403.

Lugassy G, Shaham R , Nemets A , Ben-Dor D, Nahlieli O. (2004). Severe osteomyelitis of the jaw in long-term survivors of multiple myeloma: a new clinical entity, *Am. J. Med*. 117:440–441.

Magopoulos C, Karakinaris G, Telioudis Z, et al. (2007). Osteonecrosis of the jaws due to bisphosphonate use. A review of 60 cases and treatment proposals. *Am. J. Otolaryngol*. 28(3):158-163.

Martin A, Garcia-Sanz R, Hernandez J, et al. (2002). Pamidronate induces bone formation in patients with smoldering or indolent myeloma, with no significant anti-tumor effect. *Br. J. Haematol.* 118:239–242.

Marunick M, Miller R, Gordon S. (2005). Adverse oral sequelae to bisphosphonate administration. *J. Mich. Dent. Assoc.* 87:44-49.

Marx RE, Sawatari Y, Fortin M, Broumand V. (2005). Bisphosphonate-induced exposed bone (osteonecrosis/osteopetrosis) of the jaws: risk factors, recognition, prevention, and treatment. *J. Oral Maxillofac Surg.* 63:1567-1575.

Mavrokokki T, Cheng A, Stein B, Goss A. (2007). Nature and frequency of bisphosphonate-associated osteonecrosis of the jaws in Australia. *J. Oral Maxillofac Surg.* 65(3):415-423.

McCloskey EV, MacLennan IC, Drayson MT, et al. (1998). A randomized trial of the effect of clodronate on skeletal morbidity in multiple myeloma. MRC Working Party on Leukaemia in Adults. *Br. J. Hematol.* 100:317–325.

McCloskey EV, Dunn JA, Kanis JA, et al. (2001). Long-term follow-up of a prospective, double-blind, placebocontrolled randomised trial of clodronate in multiple myeloma. *Br. J. Haematol.* 113:1035-1043.

Menssen HD, Sakalová A, Fontana A, et al. (2002). Effects of long-term intravenous ibandronate therapy on skeletal-related events, survival, and bone resorption markers in patients with advanced multiple myeloma. *J. Clin. Oncol.* 20(9):2353-2359.

Melo MD, Obeid G. (2005). Osteonecrosis of the jaws in patients with a history of receiving bisphosphonate therapy: strategies for prevention and early recognition. *J. Am. Dent Assoc.* 136(12):1675-1681.

Merigo E, Manfredi M, Meleti M, et al. (2006). Bone necrosis of the jaws associated with bisphosphonate treatment: a report of twenty-nine cases. *Acta Biomed.* 77(2):109-117.

Migliorati CA, Schubert MM, Peterson DE, Seneda LM. (2005). Bisphosphonate-associated osteonecrosis of mandibular and maxillary bone: an emerging oral complication of supportive cancer therapy. *Cancer.*104:83-93.

Merlini G, Parrinello GA, Piccinini L, et al. (1990). Long-term effects of parenteral dichloromethylene bisphosphonate (CL2MBP) on bone disease of myeloma patients treated with chemotherapy. *Hematol. Oncol.* 8:23–30.

Montazeri AH, Erskine JG, McQuaker IG. (2007). Oral sodium clodronate induced osteonecrosis of the jaw in a patient with myeloma. *Eur. J. Haematol.* 79(1):69-71.

Morris TC, Ranaghan L, Morrison J. (2001). Phase II trial of clarithromycin and pamidronate therapy in myeloma. *Med. Oncol.*18(1):79-84.

Mortensen M, Lawson W, Montazem A. (2007). Osteonecrosis of the jaw associated with bisphosphonate use: Presentation of seven cases and literature review. *Laryngoscope.* 117(1):30-34.

Murad OM, Arora S, Farag AF, Guber HA. (2007). Bisphosphonates and osteonecrosis of the jaw: a retrospective study. *Endocr. Pract.* 13(3):232-238.

Musto P, Falcone A, Sanpaolo G, et al. (2003). Pamidronate Reduces Skeletal Events but does not Improve Progression-free Survival in Early-stage Untreated Myeloma: Results of a Randomized Trial.Leukemia and Lymphoma. 44 (9):1545–1548.

Musto P, Petrucci MT, Bringhen S, et al. (2008). A multicenter, randomized clinical trial comparing zoledronic acid versus observation in patients with asymptomatic myeloma. *Cancer.* 113(7):1588-1595.

NCCN. National Comprehensive Cancer Network, Inc. The Multiple Myeloma Clinical Practice Guidelines in Oncology (Version 2.2008). Available at www.nccn.org/professionals/physician_gls/PDF/myeloma.pdf. Accessed November 20, 2008.

Oxford Handbook of Oncology. (2006). *Oxford University press.* New York. 504-505.

Pastor-Zuazaga D, Garatea-Crelgo J, Martino-Gorbea R, et al. (2006). Osteonecrosis of the jaws and bisphosphonates. Report of three cases. *Med. Oral Patol. Oral Cir. Bucal.* 11:76-79.

Phal PM, Myall RW, Assael LA, Weissman JL. (2007). Imaging findings of bisphosphonate-associated osteonecrosis of the jaws. *AJNR Am. J. Neuroradiol.* 28(6):1139-1145.

Pires FR, Miranda A, Cardoso ES, et al. (2005). Oral avascular bone necrosis associated with chemotherapy and biphosphonate therapy. *Oral Dis.* 11:365-369.

Polizzotto MN, Cousins V, Schwarer AP. (2006). Bisphosphonate-associated osteonecrosis of the auditory canal. *Br. J. Haematol.* 132(1):114.

Pozzi S, Marcheselli R, Sacchi S, et al. (2007). Bisphosphonate-associated osteonecrosis of the jaw: a review of 35 cases and an evaluation of its frequency in multiple myeloma patients. *Leuk Lymphoma.* 48(1):56-64.

Purcell PM, Boyd IW. (2005). Bisphosphonates and osteonecrosis of the jaw. *Med. J. Aust.* 2005; 182:417-418.

Rogers MJ, Gordon S, Benford HL, et al. (2000). Cellular and molecular mechanisms of action of bisphosphonates. *Cancer.* 88:2961 – 2978.

Rosen LS, Gordon D, Kaminski M, et al. (2001). Zoledronic acid versus pamidronate in the treatment of skeletal metastases in patients with breast cancer or osteolytic lesions of multiple myeloma: a phase III, double-blind, comparative trial. *Cancer J.* 7(5):377-387.

Rosen L, Gordon D, Kaminski M, et al. (2003). Long term efficacy and safety of zolendronic acid compared with pamidronate disodium in the treatment of skeletal complications in patients with advanced multiple myeloma or breast carcinoma. *Cancer.* 98(8):1735-1744.

Rosen LS, Gordon DH, Dugan W Jr, et al. (2004). Zoledronic acid is superior to pamidronate for the treatment of bone metastases in breast carcinoma patients with at least one osteolytic lesion. *Cancer.* 100:36–43.

Ruggiero SL, Meherotra B, Rosenberg TJ, Engroff SL. (2004). Osteonecrosis of the jaws associated with the use of bisphosphonates: a review of 63 cases, *J. Oral Maxillofac.* Surg. 62:527–534.

Salesi N, Pistilli R, Marcelli V, et al. (2006). Bisphosphonates and oral cavity avascular bone necrosis: a review of twelve cases. *Anticancer Res.* 26(4B):3111-3115.

Senel FC, Saracoglu Tekin U, et al. (2007). Severe osteomyelitis of the mandible associated with the use of non-nitrogen-containing bisphosphonate (disodium clodronate): report of a case. *J. Oral Maxillofac Surg.* 65(3):562-565.

Sitters MA, Caldwell CS. (2005). Bisphosphonates, dental care and osteonecrosis of the jaws. *Tex Dent J.* 122:968-72.

Smith A, Finn W, Samson D. (2005). Guidelines on the diagnosis and management of multiple myeloma. *Br. J. Haematol.* 132:410-451.

Spencer A, Roberts A, Kennedy N, et al. (2008). Renal safety of zoledronic acid with thalidomide in patients with myeloma: a pharmacokinetic and safety sub-study. *BMC Clin. Pharmacol.* 8:2.

Tanvetyanon T, Stiff PJ. (2006). Management of the adverse effects associated with intravenous bisphosphonates. *Ann. Oncol.* 17:897 – 907.

Tassinari D. (2003). Surrogate end points of quality of life assessment: have we really found what we are looking for? *Health Qual Life Outcomes.* 1:71.

Tassinari D, Poggi B, Nicoletti S, et al. (2007). Zoledronic acid treatment at home: safety data from an observational prospective trial. *J. Palliat Med.* 10(2):352-358.

Terpos E, Palermos J, Tsionos K, et al. (2000). Effect of pamidronate administration on markers of bone turnover and disease activity in multiple myeloma. *Eur. J. Haematol.* 65:331-336.

Terpos E, Viniou N, de la Fuente J, et al. (2003). Pamidronate is superior to ibandronate in decreasing bone resorption, interleukin-6 and beta 2-microglobulin in multiple myeloma. *Eur. J. Haematol.* 70(1):34-42.

Tosi P, Zamagni E, Cellini C, et al. (2006 a). First-line therapy with thalidomide, dexamethasone and zoledronic acid decreases bone resorption markers in patients with multiple myeloma. *Eur. J. Haematol.* 76(5):399-404.

Tosi P, Zamagni E, Cangini D, et al. (2006 b). Osteonecrosis of the jaws in newly diagnosed multiple myeloma patients treated with zoledronic acid and thalidomide-dexamethasone. *Blood.* 108(12):3951-3952.

Treister N, Woo SB. (2006). Images in clinical medicine. Bisphosphonate-associated osteonecrosis of the jaw. *N. Engl. J. Med.* 355(22):2348.

Van Holten-Verzantvoort AT, Kroon HM, Bijvoet OL, et al. (1993). Palliative pamidronate treatment in patients with bone metastases from breast cancer. *J. Clin. Oncol.* 11:491–498.

Vannucchi AM, Ficarra G, Antonioli E, Bosi A. (2005). Osteonecrosis of the jaw associated with zoledronate therapy in a patient with multiple myeloma. *Br. J. Haematol.* 28:738.

Walter C, Grötz KA, Kunkel M, Al-Nawas B. (2007). Prevalence of bisphosphonate associated osteonecrosis of the jaw within the field of osteonecrosis. *Support Care Cancer.* 15(2):197-202.

Wutzl A, Eisenmenger G, Hoffmann M, et al. (2006). Osteonecrosis of the jaws and bisphosphonate treatment in cancer patients. *Wien Klin Wochenschr.* 118:15-16:473-478.

Yeo AC, Lye KW, Poon CY. (2005). Bisphosphonate-related osteonecrosis of the jaws. *Singapore Dent J.* 27:36-40.

Zarychanski R, Elphee E, Walton P, Johnston J. (2006). Osteonecrosis of the jaw associated with pamidronate therapy. *Am. J. Hematol.* 81:73-75.

Zervas K, Verrou E, Teleioudis Z, et al. (2006). Incidence, risk factors and management of osteonecrosis of the jaw in patients with multiple myeloma: a single-centre experience in 303 patients. *Br. J. Haematol.* 134(6):620-623.

In: Multiple Myeloma: Symptoms, Diagnosis and Treatment ISBN 978-1-60876-108-1
Editors: M. Georgiev and Ev. Bachev

Chapter 7

Immune Defects in Multiple Myeloma

***Krzysztof Giannopoulos*[*1,2#], *Iwona Hus*[1#] and *Anna Dmoszynska*[1]**
[1]Hematooncology Department and Bone Marrow Transplantation, Medical University of Lublin, Poland
[2]Clinical Immunology Department, Medical University of Lublin, Poland

Abstract

Multiple myeloma (MM) is associated with many immune defects, that are responsible both for impaired anti-tumor responses, as well as frequent and recurrent infections. It was primary found that immune defects in MM patients included abnormalities in number and function of B, T and NK cells. More recent data revealed convincing evidences on an important role of dendritic cells (DC) and T regulatory cells in the impairment of the immune system.

B cell population in MM patients was found to be severely deficient. The suppression of $CD19^+$ B lymphocytes is reversible, correlates inversely with the disease stage, and specifically affects the early and late stages of normal B-cell differentiation. Low number of normal B cells results in reduced levels of polyclonal immunoglobulins (Ig). The inhibition of normal B cell proliferation and Ig secretion might be caused by altered cytokine activities, including decreased peripheral blood IL-4 level, or increased production of TGF-β by bone marrow stroma cells. DC are professional antigen-presenting cells which play a crucial role in initiation and potentiation of immune responses. Impaired DC function was described in a wide range of cancers. There is also a convincing evidence that defect in DC function may be responsible for the impairment of an immune system in MM. The reduced number of circulating myeloid (MDC) and plasmacytoid dendritic cells (PDC) characterized by low HLA-DR, CD40, as well as CD80 expression was found in patients with MM. Although MM is a B-cell malignancy, there are many abnormalities concerning T-cell compartment, such as impaired Th1/Th2

---

[*] Corresponding author: Prof. Anna Dmoszynska, Hematooncology Department and Bone Marrow Transplantation Medical University of Lublin, Poland. ul. Staszica 11. 20-081 Lublin. tel. 0048815346468. annadmosz@wp.pl

[#] Both authors contributed equally.

ratio as well as changes in regulatory T cells frequencies. In this chapter we summarized the current knowledge on the immune defects in MM.

Immunodeficiency is a typical finding in patients suffering from multiple myeloma (MM). Infections, mostly bacterial are frequent and serious complication of the disease, being one of the leading causes of morbidity and mortality. The immune deficit observed in myeloma patients is multifactorial. Impairments of both innate, as well as adapted immune system described in MM patients, not only contribute to susceptibility to infections, but also play an important role in disease pathogenesis and progression. At the diagnosis, mainly humoral arm of the immune system is depressed. Though T cell impairment was also described in MM, fungal and viral infections are relatively uncommon, suggesting that T cell defects are less clinically significant. However T cells were reported to play a crucial role in tumor immunosurveillance therefore their impairment might lead to disease progression.

Innate Immunity

Among innate immunity alterations, defective opsonization [1,2], decreased granulocyte adhesiveness [3], low level of C4 component of complement system [4] and impaired leukocyte migration [3] could be responsible for increased infection incidence. Recently, genetic polymorphisms of the immune system were found to influence the risk of infections in MM patients. Certain variant of the mannose-binding lectin gene (MBL2) was reported as a probable risk factor for sepsis during induction chemotherapy [5] and high dose chemotherapy with autologous stem cell transplantation [6]. MBL is known to be an important component of the innate immune defense system against a broad array of bacterial, viral, fungal, and protozoal pathogens opsonizing them directly or via complement activation for immunophagocytosis [7,8].

Several studies reported a significant decrease of natural-killer (NK) cells in patients with advanced MM when compared to the patients with low tumor burden [9,10]. Dhodapkar et al. [11] found that natural killer T (NKT) cells from both the blood and tumor bed of patients with progressive MM, in contrast to non-progressive cases have a marked deficiency of ligand-dependent interferon-gamma (IFN-γ) production. These data suggest that NK and NKT effector function represents an important host factor maintaining control of tumor growth *in vivo* in patients with MM [10,11].

B Cells

B cell population in MM patients was found to be severely deficient in a number [12-14] as well as in a function [15-16]. Low number of normal B cells results in reduced levels of polyclonal immunoglobulins (Ig) that are responsible for recurrent bacterial infections. The impaired capacity to respond to antigen challenge was also well recognized in MM patients [17]. The risk of infection is significantly higher during active disease and during first two months of therapy. The respiratory and urinary tracts are the main sites of infection and septicemia. The most implicated pathogens are: *Streptococcus aureus* and *Haemophilus influenzae* for a respiratory tract infections, *Escherichia coli*, species of *Pseudomonas*, *Proteus* and *Klebsiella* for the infections of urinary tract [18]. The suppression of $CD19^+$ B lymphocytes is reversible, correlates inversely with the disease stage, and specifically affects the early and late stages of normal B-cell differentiation. In murine plasmocytoma, B-cell suppression was traced to a plasma cell factor that drived monocytes and macrophages to suppress normal B cell proliferation [19]. An alternative mechanism concerns the suppression of normal B cells by immunoglobulin binding factor (IgBF) that may be characteristic to the Ig-Fc receptor shed by the T cells [20]. The inhibition of normal B cell proliferation and Ig secretion might be caused by altered cytokine activities, including decreased peripheral blood IL-4 level or increased production of transforming growth factor-β (TGF-β) by bone marrow stroma cells [21]. Plasmocytoma bearing mice develop a marked impairment of B cell function attributable to up to 30-fold increments in serum levels of TGF-β [21]. In contrast, malignant plasma cells are resistant to inhibitory effects of TGF-β. According to Pilarski et al.[15], terminal differentiation of B cells in myeloma patients is blocked by suppressor T cells. The authors postulate the existence of an autoimmune inhibitory network involving suppressor T cells mediating the arrest in B-cell differentiation and the humoral immune deficiency [15]. The other reasons for Ig synthesis impairment include a low number or a poor function of antigen-binding cells, an inhibition of Ig production by immunoregulatory macrophages, a presence of „chalones" that might block the expansion of B lymphocytes in response to antigen challenge [22]. The absolute count of $CD19^+$ blood cells has been showed to correlate directly and positively with the response to the therapy, as well as with survival throughout the course of MM, suggesting that non-malignant cell population can directly or indirectly control the myeloma disease [23]. Moreover, low blood $CD19^+$ cell levels are strongly associated with patients' propensity for infection and for deaths attributable to infection during first 2 months of treatment [24,25].

T Cells

T cell immunity has been also shown to be affected in MM patients. Several reports described alterations in the proportion, absolute numbers, as well as function of T cell subsets [13,26,27]. Deficient T cell count in MM patients results mostly from reduction in $CD4^+$ cells, particularly $CD4^+/CD45RA^+$ cells that causes also significant reduction in $CD4^+/CD8^+$ ratio[9,23,28]. The depression of $CD4^+/CD8^+$ ratio is even more evident in patients with progressive disease [28,29]. Ogawara et al. [30] found comparable values of $CD4^+/CD8^+$ in patients with monoclonal gammapathy of unknown significance (MGUS, $CD4^+/CD8^+$ ratio of 1.06) as well as in MM patients in the initial diagnosis phase ($CD4^+/CD8^+$ ratio of 1.2) when compared with healthy controls with $CD4^+/CD8^+$ ratio of 1.28. In MM patients, this ratio was further reduced to 0.89 in a plateau phase to achieve the lowest value of 0.58 in a refractory phase of disease. In untreated patients reduced $CD4^+$ cell counts have been shown to be linked to a poor prognosis [24]. The absolute numbers of $CD8^+$ T cells remain normal in MM patients, but according to Pilarski et. al. [26], clonogenic potential of T cells, especially $CD8^+$ lymphocytes is significantly compromised.

T cell immunity alterations in MM include also Th1/Th2 imbalance [30,31]. Th1 polarization is facilitated by IFN-γ and Th2 by IL-4 (Figure 1). Th1/Th2 ratio is high in MM patients due to decrease in the absolute number of Th2 cells.

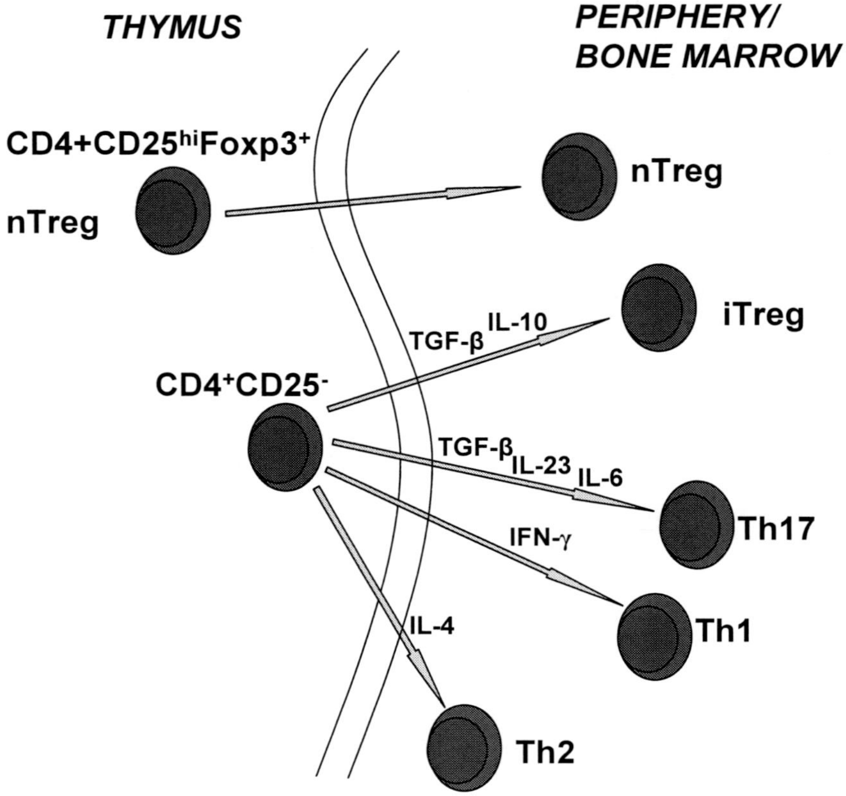

Abbreviations: MM – multiple myeloma, CTL – cytotoxic T lymphocyte, Th - T helper lymphocyte, DC – dendritic cell, Treg – regulatory T cell, TCR – T-cell receptor, MHC – major histocompatibility complex, Th17 – IL-17 producing T helper cells.

Figure 1. Immune interactions in a tumor bed of multiple myeloma patient. Antigens specific for multiple myeloma (MM) cells are located on apoptotic bodies created as a result of immune attack of cytotoxic T cells (CTL) or/and Th17 on MM cells. Myeloma-specific antigens are processed and presented by dendritic cells (DC) to effector CTL and T helper cells (Th). Activated antigen-specific CTL attack MM cell in a processed controlled by a specific peptide-MHC-TCR recognition. In a tumor bed two other important T-cell population are primed by antigen-experienced DC, T regulatory cells able to inhibit CTL reaction as well as Th17 cells able to attack MM cells by IL-17.

Decreased IL-4 levels found in MM might be responsible for this process [32]. Th2 cells are significantly lower at initial diagnosis and in refractory disease. The decrease of Th2 cells is closely related to the tumor burden and might be though one of the causes of the polyclonal Ig depression and impaired B-cell responses [30,31]. Yi et al. [33] observed predominantly Th1 polarized immune response in indolent disease, while in advanced and refractory MM, Th2 arm of immune response was more pronounced.

T-cell incompetence has been partly attributed to abnormalities within T-cell receptor (TCR)/CD3-associated signal transduction as well as co-stimulatory molecules [34].

Mozzafari et al. [34] reported a marked reduction in the proportion of CD4 and CD8 cells expressing CD28, CD152, CD3zeta, p56lck, ZAP-70 and PI3-k in patients with MM. The reduction decreased along with the disease progression, showing the lowest values in stage III MM patients. Moreover these changes were even more pronounced after stimulation with *Staphylococcal enterotoxin B* (SEB) pointing to a functional dysfunction of TCR signaling pathway. Interestingly, CD154 (CD40L) expressed on both $CD4^+$ and $CD8^+$ T cells tended to be higher in MM patients. However upon SEB activation only T cells of healthy controls up-regulated CD154 expression. Further the same group characterized intracellular levels of IFN-γ, IL-2 and IL-4 in T cells. The intracellular IFN-γ and IL-4 levels tended to be higher in stage I MM patients when compared to T cells of age-matched healthy controls as well as advanced MM patients. Notably, upon SEB activation, only T cells of healthy people showed increased cytokine production while T cells of MM patients responded marginally. In contrast, intracellular levels of IL-2, both in controls and MM patients, increased after SEB stimulation. Impaired activation-induced cytokine production might therefore indicate profound and multiple T-cell signaling defects, especially in advanced stages of MM [34]. An impairment of cell mediated immune response in MM patients was found to be associated with an expansion of peripheral $CD3^+$ lymphocytes with the phenotype of activated memory T cells [35,36]. As the results of Frassanito et al.[37] indicated, both the immunosuppressive effect of $CD8^+/CD57^+$ T cells and the enhanced susceptibility to apoptosis of peripheral T lymphocytes could be involved in the pathogenesis of the immunodeficiency observed in MM. Another study of these authors showed increased percentages of $IL\text{-}6^+/CD3^+$ lymphocytes and a defective polarization of Th1 immune responses in parallel with MM clinical stage [38]. Authors suggest that elevated IL-6 production by activated $CD3^+$ lymphocytes may thus be supposed to modulate anti-tumor Th1 polarization contributing to the disease progression [38].

Regulation of the Immune Response

Not only Th1/Th2 polarization modulate the immune response. There is a growing interest in T regulatory cells (Treg) able to suppress T- and B-cell mediated immune responses. Treg were originally defined as $CD4^+CD25^{hi}$ T-cells by Sakaguchi et al.[39]. Two subpopulations of Treg might be distinguished, naïve regulatory T cells and induced Treg. Naïve regulatory T cells (nTreg) are generated in a thymus as T cells with a high affinity to auto-peptides presented in a great groove of MHC class II molecules. These cells prevent auto-immune reactions. In periphery, IL-10 and TGF-β polarize differentiation of CD4+CD25- T cells towards induced Treg (iTreg, Figure 1). This subpopulation was reported to be overrepresented during cancer development [40,41]. Recently the intracellular Forkhead box protein 3 (Foxp3) was identified as a crucial molecule that characterizes both nTreg and iTreg. Foxp3 is required for the suppressive activity and mediates Treg function and differentiation. Foxp3 was found to directly interact with NFAT, NFκβ, as well as AP-1 molecules involved in T-cell mediated cytotoxicity. Treg might act both directly via cell-contact-dependent mechanisms and indirectly via the production of cytokines such as IL-10 or TGF-β[42]. In the first original report on Treg in MM patients, Prabhala et al.[43] found increased percentages of Treg in patients with MGUS as well as MM when Treg cells were characterized as $CD4^{+}CD25^{hi}$ T cells. Strikingly, when expression of *FOXP3* transcription factor was analyzed, reduced frequencies of $CD4^{+}Foxp3^{+}$ T cells were observed, both in MGUS and MM patients. Flow cytometric results were further confirmed by confocal microscopy and Western blot analysis. In proliferation assays, addition of Treg to anti-CD3-stimulated T cells inhibited effectively thymidine incorporation in healthy individuals, but not in patients with MGUS and MM. This study provides the first evidence on reduced frequencies of Treg in patients with hematological malignancies. Authors point also to a significant Treg dysfunction found early in MM development and therefore representing an immunological highlight of the disease. In contrast, Beyer et al.[44] found increased frequencies of Treg when compared with those of healthy controls, both characterized as $CD4^{+}CD25^{hi}$ and $CD4^{+}CD25^{hi}Foxp3^{+}$. These cells were positive for other markers found on Treg, such as CTLA-4, CD62L, GITR, OX40, TGF-β as well as IL-10. In our study, Treg were identified as $CD4^{+}CD25^{hi}Foxp3^{+}$. Similarly to Beyer et al.[44],we found significantly higher percentages of Treg among $CD4^{+}$ T lymphocytes in MM patients when compared to the healthy volunteers (HV), 5.1% vs. 3.7% respectively [45].

The suppressive function was showed in allogeneic mixed lymphocyte reaction, where addition of Treg inhibited both T cell proliferation and IFN-γ production. Treg of MM patients suppressed proliferation of both mitogen and anti-CD3/CD28 induced $CD4^{+}$ T cells, pointing to a preserved functionality. Frequencies of Treg in peripheral blood were comparable with those of bone marrow. Authors did not find changes of Treg frequencies after chemotherapy and allogeneic stem cell transplantation (SCT). Interestingly, auto-SCT significantly reduced the percentage of Treg. Beyer et al.[44] also assessed the phenotype of Treg and found increased frequencies of cells showing central-memory (mainly in bone marrow), effector-memory (overrepresented on periphery) and surprisingly naïve phenotype (expressed in equal proportions in peripheral blood and bone marrow). In further experiments they assessed numbers of T-cell receptor excision circles (TREC) to estimate developmental vicinity of these naive T cells and their division history. Low TREC numbers in naive Treg subpopulation along with no-detectable TREC levels in central-memory and effector-memory suggests that Tregs are generated on the periphery as an immune response to myeloma.

Functionally Treg are also potent inhibitors of antigen presenting cells (APC) including dendritic cells (DC). In mice, Treg significantly suppressed the expression of co-stimulatory molecules CD80 and CD86 on DC. DC are professional APC which play a crucial role in initiation and potentiation of immune response. Impaired DC function was described in a wide range of cancers. There is also a convincing evidence that defect in DC function may be responsible for the impairment of an immune system in MM patients [46]. The reduced number of circulating myeloid (MDC) and plasmacytoid dendritic cells (PDC) characterized by low HLA-DR, CD40 as well as CD80 expression was found in patients with MM [46]. In study performed in our Department, we evaluated the number of peripheral blood DC in newly diagnosed MM patients [45]. The percentage of both MDC and PDC was significantly lower in MM patients as compared to HV (0.13% vs. 0.99% and 0.05% vs. 0.3%, respectively). Ratta et al. [47] found that DC were functionally defective showing impaired capacity to stimulate allogeneic T-cell proliferation. Authors attributed this deficit to IL-6, since IL-6 inhibited the colony growth of CD34(+) DC progenitors and switched the commitment of CD34(+) cells from DCs to monocytic cells showing potent phagocytic activity but no antigen-presentation capacity. In blocking experiments, the effect of IL-6 was reversed. Interestingly, stem cells growing in the culture without IL-6 also suppressed the development and function of DC. The results of this study bring into question the advisability of using DC as antigen carriers for future immunotherapy trials in MM, as well as suggest a novel escape mechanism from the tumor immunosurveillance.

Several studies including ours, demonstrated reduced number of MDC and PDC as well as increased number of Treg in patients with MM [45]. Such defects of the immune system might be responsible for disease progression and might facilitate infection complications during the course of disease. Impaired number and function of APC as well as impairment of effector T cells coexisting with the excess of Treg might designate novel strategies for therapy. Immunotherapy with the use of DC might support the defective antigen presentation in MM patients. Moreover, successful manipulation of the immune system might reduce the number of Treg enabling immune-mediated rejection of tumor cells. On the other hand, Quach et al.[48] reported on decreased numbers of Treg that are normalized after lenalidomide therapy. This striking results might emerge from the analysis method since this group calculated absolute numbers of Treg in contrast to other groups who reported on Treg frequency among $CD4^{+}$ T cells [48].

Shaping the Immune Response in Tumor Bed

In physiological setting, the immune response mounted against different stimuli should be stopped at a certain moment to prevent uncontrolled damages of activated immune system, including autoimmune complications. In myeloma patients, MDC were found to be superior in induction of Treg when compared with other APC including B-cells, PDC as well as monocytes. Especially DC matured with inflammatory cytokines were effective not only in induction of cytotoxic T cells but also Tregs [49]. This phenomenon also points to a role of inflammatory cytokines presented in the tumor bed. Several types of cytokines were indentified in tumor microenvironment including inflammatory molecules with a key role of IL-6 as well as angiogenic factors like VEGF [50]. In a paper recently published by Yang et al.[51] authors presented that effective VEGF blockade might overcome defective antigen presentation of tumor antigens by DC from MM patients. Activation signaling pathways in DC pulsed with tumor lysates showed high levels of phospho-STAT3 and phospho-ERK that correlated with VEGF levels presented in MM lysates. Neutralization of VEGF normalized phosphorylation of STAT3, as well as ERK, and also enhanced IL-12 secretion [51].

TGF-β was reported to induce Foxp3 expression on Tregs. On the other hand, TGF-β is able to activate other transcriptic factor, the orphan nuclear receptor RORγt and therefore orchestrate IL-17 producing T cells (Th17) differentiation [52]. Th17 represent a certain subpopulation of T-helper cells that regulate immunity and inflammation [53]. However in human its role, especially in tumor setting, is not well established. Recently, Kryczek at al. [54] reported on increased frequencies of Th17 that increased along with Tregs frequencies in tumor microenvironment. Th17 cells are rarely expressed in peripheral blood of healthy controls. Its representation does not exceed 1.5% of peripheral blood mononuclear cells.

During cancer development, increase of Th17 numbers in peripheral blood was observed. Especially, Th17 lymphocytes are highly represented in tumor microenvironment. Differentiation of Th17 requires presence of IL-23 that shares common domain with IL-12, cytokine produced in large amounts by DC during immune response [55]. In MM Dhodapkar et al.[56] found that frequency of Th17 in bone marrow was higher than in peripheral blood. Interestingly, this enrichment seems to be specific for MM, since no differences between Th17 levels of bone marrow and corresponding proportions in blood were observed in MGUS or healthy controls [50]. In functional assays, mature DC from MM patients effectively induced Th17. This interaction was regulated by IL-1β, IL-6 and IL-23, as proved in inhibition experiments. Further authors found that antigen uptake of dying cells might contribute to Th17 enrichment in tumor microenvironment (Figure 2). In line, IL-17 levels in MM patients were found to be increased [57]. Recently, the angiogenic effect of IL-17 have been postulated, which is-consistent with previously observed Th17 enrichment in tumor bed where angiogenesis seems to take place [57]. Th17 might also link immune response with bone destruction observed in MM patients as IL-17 represent an active osteoclastogenic factor [58].

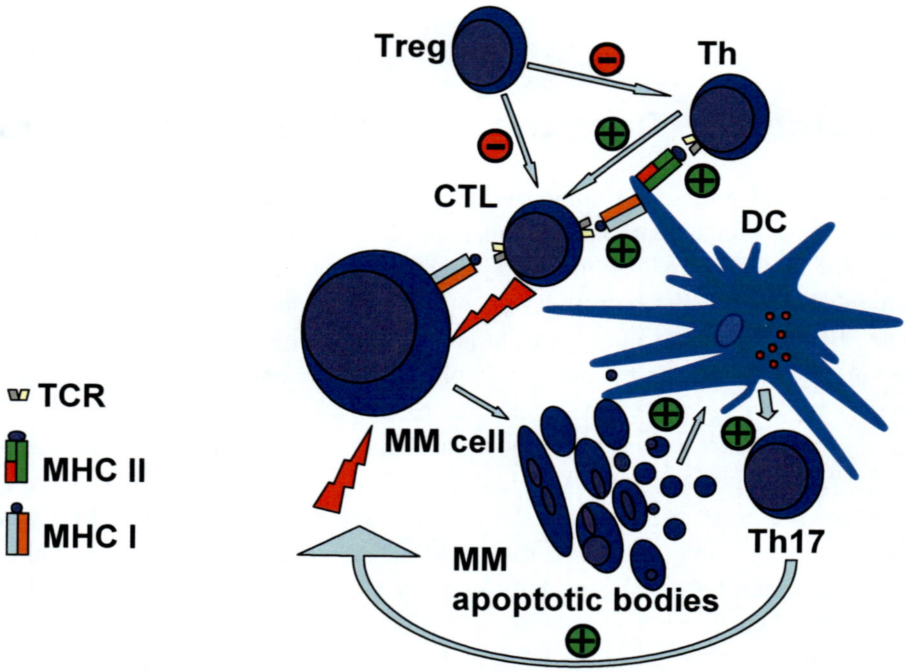

Abbreviations: Th1- type 1T helper lymphocyte, Th2 - type 2 T helper lymphocyte, nTreg – naïve regulatory T cell, iTreg – induced regulatory T cell, Th17 – IL-17 producing T helper cells.

Figure 2. Cytokines shape the T-cell subsets repertoire. Naïve regulatory T cells (nTreg) are generated in a thymus as T cells that recognize auto-peptides presented with a high affinity in MHC-II molecules. In periphery, IL-10 and TGF-β polarize differentiation towards induced Treg (iTreg). High levels of TGF-β, Il-6 and IL-23 might facilitated Th17 lymphocytes induction. Th1 polarization is mediated through IFN-γ and Th2 by IL-4. Decreased IL-4 levels found in multiple myeloma might suppress Th2 subpopulation.

Immune Response during Therapy

The immunodeficient state of myeloma patients, including profound depletion of $CD19^+$ lymphocytes could be aggravated by chemotherapy given at conventional doses, especially during first cycles [25] as well as by high-dose chemotherapy (HD-CTX) [14]. Following HD-CTX, $CD19^+$ cells recover to normal values within 180 days and similar time-course is observed for polyclonal Ig. Interestingly $CD19^+$ lymphocytes were significantly increased in patients within more than 180 days after HD-CPX compared to the values before therapy that might reflect the therapeutic efficacy of HD-CPX and humoral reconstitution in the absence of myeloma disease [14].

Further impairment of cellular immunity with significant reduction of $CD4^+$ and $CD8^+$ cells was observed after conventional chemotherapy [59,60]. The study by Schutt et al.[14] showed that low levels of naïve, and activated $CD4^+$ cell subsets, after both conventional chemotherapy as well as after HD-CTX, correlated with incidence of opportunistic infections, including cytomegalovirus disease, *Pneumocystis carinii* pneumonia and varicella zoster virus (VZV) infections [14]. After HD-CTX, some parameters such as $CD8^+$ lymphocytes recover as early as during 42-60 days, $CD4^+$ lymphocytes remain diminished for a prolonged period of time, from several months even up to 6 years [14,61,62]. Van der Velden et al. [63] showed prolonged impairment of T-cell mediated immunity with suppression of antigen-stimulated IFN-γ production that might contribute to relatively high incidence of viral infections after HD-CPX. Significant increase of VZV reactivation was found to be associated with bortezomib treatment [64]. It has been suggested that bortezomib might suppress the number and function of NK cells and $CD8^+$ T cells [65]. In patients treated with bortezomib or bortezomib-containing regimens the antiviral prophylaxis with acyclovir should be considered. Patients on high doses of glucocorticosteroids are prone to viral and fungal infections, they also should receive a prophylaxis of *Pneumocystis carinii* infection with trimethoprim-sulfamethoxazole. In contrast, immunomodulatory drugs, such as thalidomide and its analogue lenalidomide have been showed to augment cellular immunity. Immunomodulatory effects of thalidomide are mediated at least in part by activation of $CD8^+$ lymphocytes [66], augmentation of the IL-2 production in mononuclear cells [67], induction of Th2 cytokine production [68] and the enhancement of NK cell activity resulting in MM cells lysis [69]. According to Chang et al.[70] lenalidomide greatly enhances ligand-dependent activation, proliferation and cytokine production by human NKT cells ,as well as enhances NKT cells *in vivo*. In the study conducted in our Institution, we found that thalidomide effectively reduced levels of VEGF, HGF, bFGF, TNF as well as IL-6 in MM patients [71]. Since infections might cause serious complications, Robertson et al.72 vaccinated 46 MM patients against *S. pneumonia, Haemophilus influenzae* and influenza. The vaccination mounted a poor humoral responses that were highly disappointing in case of influenza vaccination where only about 1/3 patients achieved protective levels against one of three strains of a vaccine. Concluding, an effective conventional chemotherapy, as well as treatment with novel immunomodulatory drugs including bortezomib, thalidomide and lenalidomide might normalize abnormalities of the certain subpopulations of immune system in MM patients.

In summary, immunodeficiency in patients with MM is polyaethiological and involve both innate and adoptive immunity. Impairment of quantity and function of B, T and NK cells are well defined with established influence on the disease progression and infectious complications (Table 1). More recently, abnormalities in newly identified $CD4^+$ T-cell subsets were found in MM patients, however their role in MM is still to be determined. The definition of defects in the immune system is essential to establish novel therapeutical modalities for patients with MM.

Table 1. Hallmarks of the immune defects in multiple myeloma

B cells	↓
CD4/CD8	↓
CD4	↓
Th1/Th2	↑
Th2	↓
MDC	↓
PDC	↓
Treg	↑

Abbreviations: Th1- type 1 T helper lymphocytes, Th2- type 2 T helper lymphocytes, MDC – myeloid dendritic cells, PDC- plasmacytoid dendritic cells, Treg – regulatory T cells.

References

[1] Kansu E, Akalin E, Civelek C, Tekesin O, Laleli Y, Firat D. Serum bactericidal and opsonic activities in chronic lymphocytic leukemia and multiple myeloma. *Am. J. Hematol.* 1986; 23: 191-6.

[2] Hopen G, Glette J, Halstensen A, Kalager T, Schreiner A, Solberg CO. Granulocyte function in malignant monoclonal gammopathy. *Scand. J. Haematol.* 1983; 31: 133-43.

[3] Hopen G, Glette J, Matre R. Mechanisms of decreased leucocyte adhesiveness and migration in plasma from patients with IgG myelomatosis. *Scand J. Haematol.* 1984; 32: 88-94.

[4] Spitler LE, Spath P, Petz L, Cooper N, Fudenberg HH. Phagocytes and C4 in paraproteinaemia. *Br. J. Haematol.* 1975; 29: 279-92.

[5] Mølle I, Steffensen R, Thiel S, Peterslund NA. Chemotherapy-related infections in patients with multiple myeloma: associations with mannan-binding lectin genotypes. *Eur. J. Haematol.* 2006; 77: 19-26.

[6] Mølle I, Peterslund NA, Thiel S, Steffensen R. MBL2 polymorphism and risk of severe infections in multiple myeloma patients receiving high-dose melphalan and autologous stem cell transplantation. *Bone Marrow Transplant.* 2006; 38: 555-60.

[7] Neth O, Jack DL, Dodds AW, Holzel H, Klein NJ, Turner MW. Mannose-binding lectin binds to a range of clinically relevant microorganisms and promotes complement deposition. *Infect Immun.* 2000; 68: 688-693.

[8] Turner MW. Mannose-binding lectin: the pluripotent molecule of the innate immune system. *Immunol Today*. 1996; 17: 532-540.

[9] Serra HM, Mant MJ, Ruether BA, Ledbetter JA, Pilarski LM Selective loss of CD4+ CD45R+ T cells in peripheral blood of multiple myeloma patients. *J. Clin. Immunol.* 1988; 8: 259-65.

[10] Osterborg A, Nilsson B, Björkholm M, Holm G, Mellstedt H. Natural killer cell activity in monoclonal gammopathies: relation to disease activity. *Eur. J. Haematol.* 1990; 45: 153-7.

[11] Dhodapkar MV, Geller MD, Chang DH, Shimizu K, Fujii S, Dhodapkar KM, Krasovsky J. A reversible defect in natural killer T cell function characterizes the progression of premalignant to malignant multiple myeloma. *J. Exp. Med.* 2003; 197: 1667-76.

[12] Pilarski LM, Mant MJ, Ruether BA, Belch A. Severe deficiency of B lymphocytes in peripheral blood from multiple myeloma patients. *J. Clin. Invest* 1984; 74: 1301-6.

[13] Pilarski LM, Andrews EJ, Serra HM, Ledbetter JA, Ruether BA, Mant MJ. Abnormalities in lymphocyte profile and specificity repertoire of patients with Waldenstrom's macroglobulinemia, multiple myeloma, and IgM monoclonal gammopathy of undetermined significance. *Am. J. Hematol.* 1989; 30: 53-60.

[14] Schütt P, Brandhorst D, Stellberg W, Poser M, Ebeling P, Müller S, Buttkereit U, Opalka B, Lindemann M, Grosse-Wilde H, Seeber S, Moritz T, Nowrousian MR. Immune parameters in multiple myeloma patients: influence of treatment and correlation with opportunistic infections. *Leuk Lymphoma*. 2006; 47: 1570-82.

[15] Pilarski LM, Ruether BA, Mant MJ. Abnormal function of B lymphocytes from peripheral blood of multiple myeloma patients. Lack of correlation between the number of cells potentially able to secrete immunoglobulin M and serum immunoglobulin M levels. *J. Clin. Invest*. 1985; 75: 2024-9.

[16] Pilarski LM, Andrews EJ, Mant MJ, Ruether BA. Humoral immune deficiency in multiple myeloma patients due to compromised B-cell function. J Clin Immunol. 1986; 6: 491-501.

[17] Bladé J, Rosiñol L. Renal, hematologic and infectious complications in multiple myeloma. *Best Pract. Res. Clin. Haematol*. 2005; 18: 635-52.

[18] Hargreaves RM, Lea JR, Griffiths H, Faux JA, Holt JM, Reid C, Bunch C, Lee M, Chapel HM. Immunological factors and risk of infection in plateau phase myeloma. *J. Clin. Pathol*. 1995; 48: 260-6.

[19] Ullrich S, Zolla-Pazner S. Immunoregulatory circuits in myeloma. *Clin. Haematol.* 1982; 11: 87-111.

[20] Preud'Homme JL, Brouet JC, Seligmann M.Membrane-bound IgD on human lymphoid cells, with special reference to immunodeficiency and immunoproliferative diseases. *Immunol Rev.* 1977; 37: 127-51.

[21] Urashima M, Ogata A, Chauhan D, Hatziyanni M, Vidriales MB, Dedera DA, Schlossman RL, Anderson KC. Transforming growth factor-beta1: differential effects on multiple myeloma versus normal B cells. *Blood* 1996; 87: 1928-38.

[22] Paglieroni T, MacKenzie MR. Studies on the pathogenesis of an immune defect in multiple myeloma. *J. Clin.Invest.* 1977; 59: 1120-33.

[23] Kay NE, Leong TL, Bone N, Vesole DH, Greipp PR, Van Ness B, Oken MM, Kyle RA. Blood levels of immune cells predict survival in myeloma patients: results of an Eastern Cooperative Oncology Group phase 3 trial for newly diagnosed multiple myeloma patients. *Blood.* 2001; 98: 23-8.

[24] Kay NE, Leong T, Kyle RA, Greipp P, Billadeau D, Van Ness B, Bone N, Oken MM. Circulating blood B cells in multiple myeloma: analysis and relationship to circulating clonal cells and clinical parameters in a cohort of patients entered on the Eastern Cooperative Oncology Group phase III E9486 clinical trial. *Blood.* 1997; 90: 340-5.

[25] Cesana C, Nosari AM, Klersy C, Miqueleiz S, Rossi V, Ferrando P, Valentini M, Barbarano L, Morra E. Risk factors for the development of bacterial infections in multiple myeloma treated with two different vincristine-adriamycin-dexamethasone schedules. *Haematologica.* 2003; 88: 1022-8.

[26] Pilarski LM, Mant MJ, Ruether BA, Carayanniotis G, Otto D, Krowka JF. Abnormal clonogenic potential of T cells from multiple myeloma patients. *Blood.* 1985; 66: 1266-71.

[27] Kay N, Leong T, Kyle RA, Greipp P, Van Ness B, Bone N, Oken MM. Altered T cell repertoire usage in CD4 and CD8 subsets of multiple myeloma patients, a Study of the Eastern Cooperative Oncology Group (E9487). *Leuk Lymphoma.* 1999; 33: 127-33.

[28] Mellstedt H, Holm G, Pettersson D, Björkholm M, Johansson B, Lindemalm C, Peest D, Ahre A. T cells in monoclonal gammopathies. *Scand. J. Haematol.* 1982; 29: 57-64.

[29] Tienhaara A, Pelliniemi TT. Peripheral blood lymphocyte subsets in multiple myeloma and monoclonal gammopathy of undetermined significance. *Clin. Lab. Haematol.* 1994; 16: 213-23.

[30] Ogawara H, Handa H, Yamazaki T, Toda T, Yoshida K, Nishimoto N, Al-ma'Quol WH, Kaneko Y, Matsushima T, Tsukamoto N, Nojima Y, Matsumoto M, Sawamura M, Murakami H. High Th1/Th2 ratio in patients with multiple myeloma. *Leuk. Res.* 2005; 29: 135-40.

[31] Murakami H, Ogawara H, Hiroshi H.Th1/Th2 cells in patients with multiple myeloma. *Hematology.* 2004; 9: 41-5.

[32] Kyrstsonis MC, Dedoussis G, Baxevanis C, Stamatelou M, Maniatis A. Serum interleukin-6 (IL-6) and interleukin-4 (IL-4) in patients with multiple myeloma (MM). *Br. J. Haematol.* 1996; 92: 420-2.

[33] Yi Q, Osterborg A, Bergenbrant S, Mellstedt H, Holm G, Lefvert AK. Idiotype-reactive T-cell subsets and tumor load in monoclonal gammopathies. *Blood.* 1995; 86: 3043-9.

[34] Mozaffari F, Hansson L, Kiaii S, Ju X, Rossmann ED, Rabbani H, Mellstedt H, Osterborg A. Signalling molecules and cytokine production in T cells of multiple

myeloma-increased abnormalities with advancing stage. *Br. J. Haematol* 2004; 124: 315-24.

[35] Dianzani U, Pileri A, Boccadoro M, Palumbo A, Pioppo P, Bianchi A, Camponi A, Fossati G, Battaglio S, Massaia M. Activated idiotype-reactive cells in suppressor/cytotoxic subpopulations of monoclonal gammopathies: correlation with diagnosis and disease status. *Blood*. 1988; 72: 1064-8.

[36] Vacca A, Di Stefano R, Frassanito A, Iodice G, Dammacco F. A disturbance of the IL-2/IL-2 receptor system parallels the activity of multiple myeloma. *Clin. Exp. Immunol*. 1991; 84: 429-34.

[37] Frassanito MA, Silvestris F, Cafforio P, Dammacco F. CD8+/CD57 cells and apoptosis suppress T-cell functions in multiple myeloma. *Br. J. Haematol*. 1999; 100: 469-77.

[38] Frassanito MA, Cusmai A, Dammacco F. Frassanito MA, Cusmai A, Dammacco F. Deregulated cytokine network and defective Th1 immune response in multiple myeloma. *Clin. Exp. Immunol*. 2001; 125: 190-7.

[39] Sakaguchi S.Naturally arising Foxp3-expressing CD25+CD4+ regulatory T cells in immunological tolerance to self and non-self. *Nat. Immunol*. 2005; 6: 345-52.

[40] O'Garra A, Vieira P. Regulatory T cells and mechanisms of immune system control. *Nat. Med*. 2004; 10: 801-5.

[41] Nomura T, Sakaguchi S. Naturally arising CD25+CD4+ regulatory T cells in tumor immunity. *Curr. Top. Microbiol. Immunol*. 2005; 293: 287-302.

[42] von Boehmer H. Mechanisms of suppression by suppressor T cells. *Nat. Immunol*. 2005; 6: 338-44.

[43] Prabhala RH, Neri P, Bae JE, Tassone P, Shammas MA, Allam CK, Daley JF, Chauhan D, Blanchard E, Thatte HS, Anderson KC, Munshi NC. Dysfunctional T regulatory cells in multiple myeloma. *Blood*. 2006; 107: 301-4.

[44] Beyer M, Kochanek M, Giese T, Endl E, Weihrauch MR, Knolle PA, Classen S, Schultze JL. In vivo peripheral expansion of naive CD4+CD25high FoxP3+ regulatory T cells in patients with multiple myeloma. *Blood*. 2006; 107: 3940-9.

[45] Trześniewska W, Giannopoulos K, Dmoszyńska A. The estimation of subpopulation of peripheral blood dendritic cells and T-regulatory cells in patients with multiple myeloma-pilot study. *Acta Haemat. Pol.* 2007; 38:61-68.

[46] Brimnes MK, Svane IM, Johnsen HE. Impaired functionality and phenotypic profile of dendritic cells from patients with multiple myeloma. *Clin. Exp. Immunol*. 2006; 144: 76-84.

[47] Ratta M, Fagnoni F, Curti A, Vescovini R, Sansoni P, Oliviero B, Fogli M, Ferri E, Della Cuna GR, Tura S, Baccarani M, Lemoli RM Dendritic cells are functionally defective in multiple myeloma: the role of interleukin-6. *Blood.* 2002; 100: 230-7.

[48] Quach H, Ritchie D, Neeson P, Harrison S, Tai T, Tainton K, Lynch K, Prince M. Regulatory T Cells (Treg) Are Depressed in Patients with Relapsed/ Refractory Multiple Myeloma (MM) and Increases towards Normal Range in Responding Patients Treated with Lenalidomide (LEN). ASH 2008 abstract No 1696.

[49] Banerjee DK, Dhodapkar MV, Matayeva E, Steinman RM, Dhodapkar KM. Expansion of FOXP3high regulatory T cells by human dendritic cells (DCs) in vitro and after injection of cytokine-matured DCs in myeloma patients. *Blood.* 2006; 108: 2655-61.

[50] Klein B, Bataille R. Cytokine network in human multiple myeloma. *Hematol. Oncol. Clin. North Am*. 1992; 6: 273-84.

[51] Yang DH, Park JS, Jin CJ, Kang HK, Nam JH, Rhee JH, Kim YK, Chung SY, Choi SJ, Kim HJ, Chung IJ, Lee JJ. The dysfunction and abnormal signaling pathway of dendritic cells loaded by tumor antigen can be overcome by neutralizing VEGF in multiple myeloma. *Leuk Res*. 2009; 33: 665-70.

[52] Zhou L, Lopes JE, Chong MM, Ivanov II, Min R, Victora GD, Shen Y, Du J, Rubtsov YP, Rudensky AY, Ziegler SF, Littman DR. TGF-beta-induced Foxp3 inhibits T(H)17 cell differentiation by antagonizing RORgammat function. *Nature*. 2008; 453: 236-40.

[53] Annunziato F, Cosmi L, Santarlasci V, Maggi L, Liotta F, Mazzinghi B, Parente E, Filì L, Ferri S, Frosali F, Giudici F, Romagnani P, Parronchi P, Tonelli F, Maggi E, Romagnani S. Phenotypic and functional features of human Th17 cells. *J. Exp. Med*. 2007; 204: 1849-61.

[54] Kryczek I, Wei S, Zou L, Altuwaijri S, Szeliga W, Kolls J, Chang A, Zou W. Cutting edge: Th17 and regulatory T cell dynamics and the regulation by IL-2 in the tumor microenvironment. J Immunol. 2007; 178: 6730-3.

[55] Zhou L, Ivanov II, Spolski R, Min R, Shenderov K, Egawa T, Levy DE, Leonard WJ, Littman DR. IL-6 programs T(H)-17 cell differentiation by promoting sequential engagement of the IL-21 and IL-23 pathways. *Nat. Immunol*. 2007; 8: 967-74.

[56] Dhodapkar KM, Barbuto S, Matthews P, Kukreja A, Mazumder A, Vesole D, Jagannath S, Dhodapkar MV. Dendritic cells mediate the induction of polyfunctional human IL17-producing cells (Th17-1 cells) enriched in the bone marrow of patients with myeloma. *Blood*. 2008; 112: 2878-85.

[57] Alexandrakis MG, Pappa CA, Miyakis S, Sfiridaki A, Kafousi M, Alegakis A, Stathopoulos EN. Serum interleukin-17 and its relationship to angiogenic factors in multiple myeloma. *Eur. J. Intern. Med*. 2006; 17: 412-6.

[58] Sato K, Suematsu A, Okamoto K, Yamaguchi A, Morishita Y, Kadono Y, Tanaka S, Kodama T, Akira S, Iwakura Y, Cua DJ, Takayanagi H. Th17 functions as an osteoclastogenic helper T cell subset that links T cell activation and bone destruction. *J. Exp. Med*. 2006; 203: 2673-82.

[59] Kay NE, Oken MM, Kyle R, Van Ness B, Kalish L, Leong T, Greipp P. Sequential phenotyping of myeloma patients on chemotherapy: persistence of activated T-cells and natural killer cells. *Leuk Lymphoma*. 1995; 16: 351-4.

[60] Kay NE, Leong T, Bone N, Kyle RA, Greipp PR, Van Ness B, Oken MM. T-helper phenotypes in the blood of myeloma patients on ECOG phase III trials E9486/E3A93. *Br. J. Haematol*. 1998;100: 459-63.

[61] Laurenti L, Piccioni P, Piccirillo N, Sora' F, Chiusolo P, Garzia M, Reddiconto G, De Matteis S, Tarnani M, Leone G, Sica S. Immune recovery of lymphocyte subsets 6 years after autologous peripheral blood stem cell transplantation (PBSCT) for lymphoproliferative diseases. A comparison between NHL, HD and MM in group of 149 patients. *Leuk Lymphoma*. 2004; 45: 2063-70.

[62] Steingrimsdottir H, Gruber A, Björkholm M, Svensson A, Hansson M. Immune reconstitution after autologous hematopoietic stem cell transplantation in relation to

underlying disease, type of high-dose therapy and infectious complications. *Haematologica*. 2000; 85: 832-8.

[63] van der Velden AM, Claessen AM, van Velzen-Blad H, Biesma DH, Rijkers GT. Development of T cell-mediated immunity after autologous stem cell transplantation: prolonged impairment of antigen-stimulated production of gamma-interferon. *Bone Marrow Transplant.* 2007; 40: 261-6.

[64] Chanan-Khan A, Sonneveld P, Schuster MW, Stadtmauer EA, Facon T, Harousseau JL, Ben-Yehuda D, Lonial S, Goldschmidt H, Reece D, Neuwirth R, Anderson KC, Richardson PG. Analysis of herpes zoster events among bortezomib-treated patients in the phase III APEX study. *J.Clin. Oncol*. 2008; 26: 4784-90.

[65] Uy GL, Goyal SD, Fisher NM, Oza AY, Tomasson MH, Stockerl-Goldstein K, Dipersio JF, Vij R. Bortezomib administered pre-auto-SCT and as maintenance therapy post transplant for multiple myeloma: a single institution phase II study. *Bone Marrow Transplant*. 2008 (in press).

[66] Haslett PA, Hanekom WA, Muller G, Kaplan G. Thalidomide and a thalidomide analogue drug costimulate virus-specific CD8+ T cells in vitro. *J. Infect. Dis*. 2003;187: 946-55.

[67] Shannon EJ, Sandoval F. Thalidomide increases the synthesis of IL-2 in cultures of human mononuclear cells stimulated with Concanavalin-A, Staphylococcal enterotoxin A, and purified protein derivative. *Immunopharmacology*. 1995; 31: 109-16.

[68] McHugh SM, Rifkin IR, Deighton J, Wilson AB, Lachmann PJ, Lockwood CM, Ewan PW. The immunosuppressive drug thalidomide induces T helper cell type 2 (Th2) and concomitantly inhibits Th1 cytokine production in mitogen- and antigen-stimulated human peripheral blood mononuclear cell cultures. *Clin. Exp. Immunol*. 1995; 99: 160-7.

[69] Davies FE, Raje N, Hideshima T, Lentzsch S, Young G, Tai YT, Lin B, Podar K, Gupta D, Chauhan D, Treon SP, Richardson PG, Schlossman RL, Morgan GJ, Muller GW, Stirling DI, Anderson KC . Thalidomide and immunomodulatory derivatives augment natural killer cell cytotoxicity in multiple myeloma. *Blood*. 2001; 98: 210-6.

[70] Chang DH, Liu N, Klimek V, Hassoun H, Mazumder A, Nimer SD, Jagannath S, Dhodapkar MV. Enhancement of ligand-dependent activation of human natural killer T cells by lenalidomide: therapeutic implications. *Blood*. 2006; 108: 618-21.

[71] Dmoszynska A, Podhorecka M, Manko J, Bojarska-Junak A, Rolinski J, Skomra D. The influence of thalidomide therapy on cytokine secretion, immunophenotype, BCL-2 expression and microvessel density in patients with resistant or relapsed multiple myeloma. *Neoplasma*. 2005; 52: 175-81.

[72] Robertson JD, Nagesh K, Jowitt SN, Dougal M, Anderson H, Mutton K, Zambon M, Scarffe JH. Immunogenicity of vaccination against influenza, Streptococcus pneumoniae and Haemophilus influenzae type B in patients with multiple myeloma. *Br. J. Cancer*. 2000; 82: 1261-5.

In: Multiple Myeloma: Symptoms, Diagnosis and Treatment ISBN 978-1-60876-108-1
Editors: M. Georgiev and Ev. Bachev

Chapter 8

Surgical Options in the Treatment of Spinal Myeloma

M. Repko, R. Chaloupka, R. Grosman and M. Krbec
Department of Orthopaedic Surgery, Faculty Hospital Brno
Jihlavská 20, 625 00 Brno, Czech Republic, Europe

Abstract

Objective: Spinal myeloma is a disease requiring a multidisciplinary approach involving orthopaedic and oncology surgeons. Myeloma of the spine seriously affects spinal stability and can lead to compression of neural structures. The evaluation of security, possibilities, indications and efficiency of surgical management in patients with spinal myeloma are the main aim of our contribution.

Diagnostics: Imaging methods are essential for exact diagnostics as well as laboratory examinations. The techniques largely used are X-ray examinations, CT scanning and CT-myelography, MRI (magnetic resonance imaging), 99mTc-MIBI scintigraphy and FDG-PET (fluorodeoxyglucose positron emission tomography). We have to distinguish between solitary and multiple myeloma using all these diagnostic methods.

Therapeutic scheme: Instability of the spine, caused by pathological vertebral fracture without compression of the nerve structures, can be treated conservatively using an external orthosis. Surgery is indicated in patients whose survival prognosis is more than 3-6 month in a situation of existing or imminent spinal collapse or nerve damage. The primary aim of surgery is to stop the progress, improve or, in ideal case, prevent damage to the nerves. The surgery renews spinal stability and reduces or eliminates pain symptoms. We distinguish between posterior, anterior or combined surgical procedures.

Methods: We surgically managed 108 patients with spinal myeloma in the 1987-2008 period. Their average age was 58 years (range 28-78). There were 18 cervical, 59 thoracic and 31 lumbar spinal areas treated. We used the posterior approach in 47, anterior approach in 23, and combined surgery in 38 spines. The results, i.e. changes in neurological findings, were evaluated according to the Frankel grading system.

Results: In our group of surgically managed patients with spinal myeloma, 37 patients (38%) had improved neurological findings, 57 (58%) showed the same deficit, and only four patients (4%) had postoperative neurological deterioration.

Conclusions: Early diagnosis and urgent surgical decompression involving eventual stabilization of the spine can prevent irreversible damage to the nervous system due to pressure of the myeloma on the spine. Surgical treatment leads to complete consolidation in patients with solitary myeloma, and serves as a palliative treatment in patients with multiple myeloma.

Introduction

The spine is one of the body sites often affected by multiple myeloma. Since the spine provides strength, support and the facility of movement and protects neural structures, development of myeloma interferes with spinal stability and nerve functions of the whole body. With regard to the presence and nature of neurological complications as well as correct indications for surgical treatment, it is essential to distinguish whether the vertebral body or the vertebral arch and processes have been affected.

Any preoperative planning is based first of all on the use of imaging methods. The primary examination involves X-ray films of good quality in anteroposterior and lateral projections focused on the tumor-invaded spine segment, completed with methods visualizing conditions in the spinal canal. Former commonly used contrast perimyelography has recently been substituted with CT scanning or CT perimyelography [1]. The most thorough examination of the spinal canal is facilitated by magnetic resonance imaging (MRI) [2,3]. An accurate detection of the number of the segments affected is best achieved with MIBI scitingraphy [4,5]. Also fluorodeoxyglucose positron emission tomography (FDG-PET) can effectively contribute to the correct diagnosis of multiple myeloma and its differentiation from solitary plasmocytoma. The results of diagnostic examination then provide a basis for adequate surgical treatment.

In indicated cases, angiography is used in addition to imaging methods and, in the preoperative period, selective embolization to reduce intraoperative bleeding can be carried out. Neurological deficit is evaluated by the Frankel grading system, which is most widely used system (Table 1).

Table 1. Changes in Frankel´s scale

Frankel scale	
A	complete paralysis
B	sensory function only below the injury level
C	incomplete motor function below injury level
D	fair to good motor function below injury level
E	normal function

Conservative Treatment

The first sign of spinal myeloma is usually pain in the affected region. When neural structures are compressed, accompanying neurological signs are reported. Soon a pathological fracture of the vertebral body may occur, with subsequent compression or collapse of the vertebra. This development results in secondary spinal instability and progression of pain and neurological deficit. The first stage of disease is treated conservatively. A soft foam collar is applied to the unstable mid-cervical spine to immobilize the neck and alleviate pain during movements. A Philadelphia collar (Figure 1) is used for more extensive instability or when occipitocervical or cervicothoracic junctions are affected. This rigid orthosis provides more stable fixation.

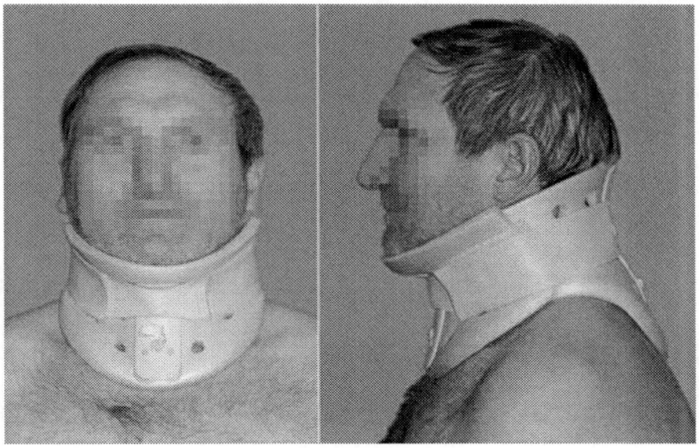

Figure 1. Philadelphia collar for cervical stabilization.

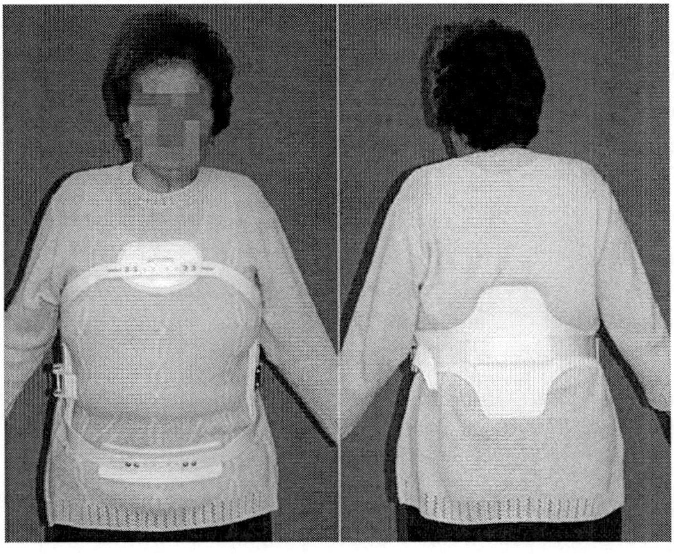

Figure 2. Jewett brace with three point stabilization.

The thoracic spine and thoracolumbar region are best immobilized in a Jewett brace, which is a three-point pressure system of orthosis (Figure 2). For the affected lumbar region, lower back belts with a varying degree of support are available (Figure 3). Orthotic devices are also used in postoperative rehabilitation for 3 to 6 months, or in patients with a poor disease prognosis to improve the quality of life and relieve pain.

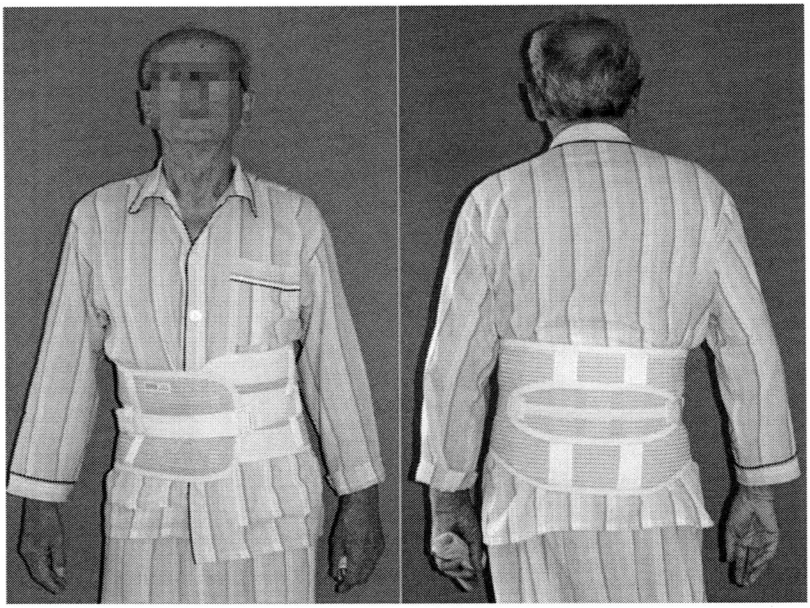

Figure 3. Lower back belts for lumbar spine stabilization.

Surgical Treatment

Surgical management is indicated in patients with the present or imminent vertebral collapse and/or neurological deficit, whose chances of survival are more than 3 to 6 months. The major goal of surgery is to arrest disease progression and improve neurological findings or, ideally, to prevent their development. Surgery aims at restoring spinal stability and at alleviation or complete elimination of painful symptoms [7]. If its outcome is good, the patient's life quality may improve considerably. However, operative management of spinal myeloma always only complements the comprehensive therapy of this disease.

In preoperative planning it is necessary to consider the degree of seriousness of the underlying disease and the consequent radicality of surgical intervention [8]. This is related to the degree of spinal decompression and secondary instability of the spine, which requires spinal instrumentation. The use of an operative technique is always based on the results of preoperative examination. If the results are ambiguous and the necessity of confirming the underlying disease arises, probatory biopsy can be performed and histopathological findings obtained [9].The procedure can involve either a needle aspiration biopsy, which is a CT-guided minimally invasive technique, or a major surgical biopsy permitting a more reliable tissue sample collection.

The surgical techniques include anterior, posterior and combined procedures. The choice of a method depends on the localization and extent of the lesion, prognosis of the underlying disease, the patient's age, their overall health status and anesthetic options.

The most frequent complications are intra- and postoperative bleeding, injury to the dural sac and neural structures, neurological deterioration, deep or superficial wound infection, urinary tract infection, pulmonary embolism, post-operative state of disorientation, late instability above the level of fusion, and possibly also death related to the surgical procedure. A worsening of neurological deficit owing to edema in the region operated on is the most feared early postoperative complication.

The patient undergoes all surgical procedures under general anesthesia, with peripheral and central venous cannulation, nasogastric tube insertion and urinary catheterization. After surgery the patients are placed in an intensive care unit or, if their condition is critical, in an acute care department. Stabilized patients wearing an orthosis immobilizing the treated region can start rehabilitation early with standing and walking.

Methods

Posterior Spine Surgery

The basic posterior procedure involves an isolated posterior lateral decompression of the spinal cord by removing posterior, tumor-invaded parts of the spine and neoplastic mass in the spinal canal. However, this treatment results in iatrogenic partial instability of the spine and is therefore used chiefly as a palliative therapy in patients with a prognosis for less than 6-months'survival, in whom lesions are not extensive and are usually localized in the cervical and lumbar lordosis areas [10]. Two to three segments can be decompressed without destabilizing the spine. When removal of intervertebral joints is not necessary, no big risk of spinal destabilization arises.

The operative time is 90 min. on average, and blood loss is about 600 ml. In patients with prognosis for a longer survival, the spine is stabilized by internal instrumentation with posterior lateral bony fusion. In posterior surgery, sublaminar wiring (chiefly for the cervical and thoracic spine, or transpedicular screw fixation are used (Figure4) [11,12]. This procedure requires 3 hours on average and blood loss is about 1500 ml.

Posterior procedures also include vertebroplasty and kyphoplasty, i.e., minimally invasive CT-guided techniques, by which bone cement is applied through a transcutaneous transpedicular approach [13]. Kyphoplasty can also be performed by an extra-articular approach and is done on one or both sides. It aims primarily at relieving or eliminating back pain, but can also treat osteolytic vertebral body lesions. However, it may be associated with some complications such as cement leakage into the spinal canal, with subsequent neurological deterioration. Vertebroplasty and/or kyphoplasty is indicated when one to three vertebrae are affected and no other technique can be used.

Anterior Spine Surgery

Access to the affected vertebra is gained from the anterior cervical, the thoracic or the retroperitoneal approach, and decompression of neural structures is carried out by somatectomy (removal of the vertebral body). Vertebral reconstruction is carried out with bone autograft or allograft, bone cement filling with Kirschner's wires inserted in the adjacent healthy vertebral bodies or a cage application. The cage is either rigid (Harms cage; Figure 5) or expandable (Synex implant; Figure 6) [14]. When decompression produces marked instability, vertebral reconstruction is completed with anterior stabilization. These procedures require between 4 and 5 hours of operative time, and blood loss is about 1 500 ml.

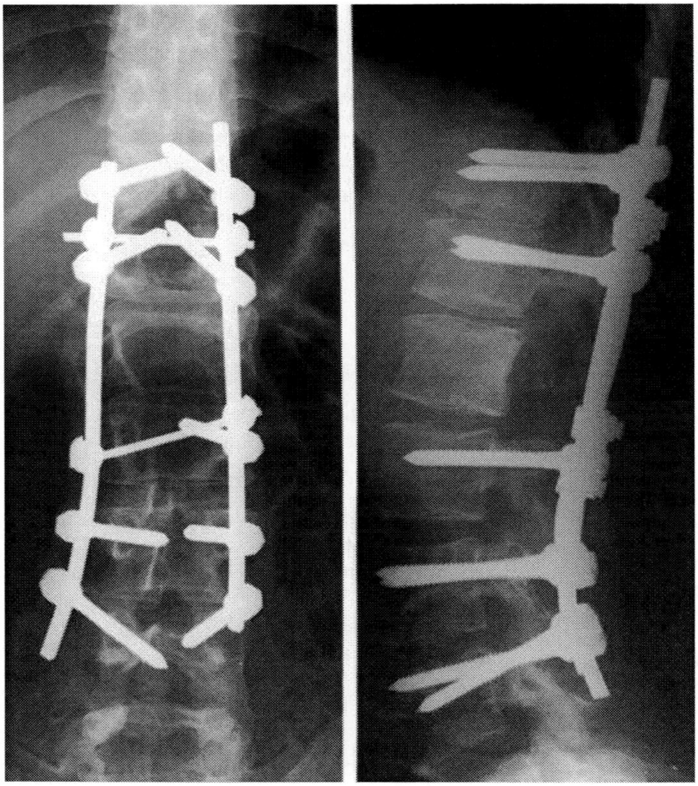

Figure 4. Transpedicular lumbar spine stabilization.

Combined Procedures

Spinal cord compression is most often caused by lesions in both anterior and posterior vertebral structures and therefore combined anteroposterior procedures are used. They include decompression by anterior somatectomy and vertebral reconstruction, followed by posterior decompression and stabilization (Figures 4,5,6). The surgery is carried out by two operating teams simultaneously as a single-stage procedure, at one stage with patient's position change, or at two stages a week or more apart, because blood loss was too high during the first operation. These procedures are very complex and, because of a long operative time (5 to 6 h) and large blood loss (up to 3 000 ml), they can only be performed on a patient in relatively good general health.

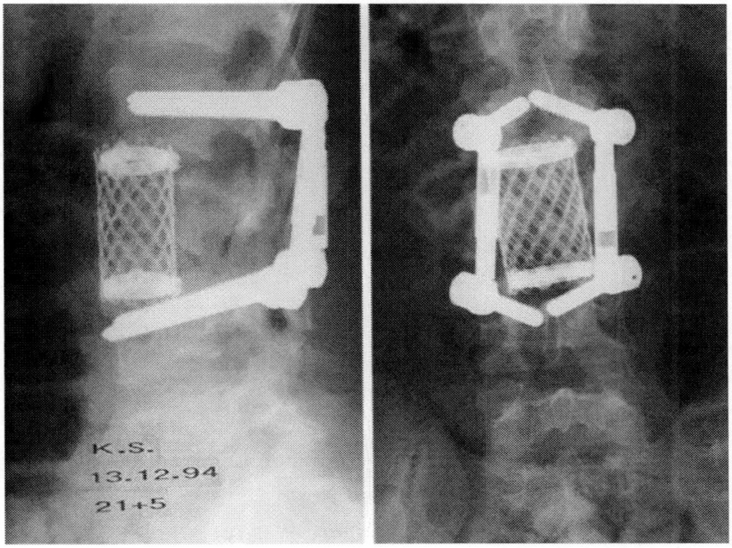

Figure 5 Reconstruction of the third vertebral body using the rigid Harms cage and transpedicular fixation.

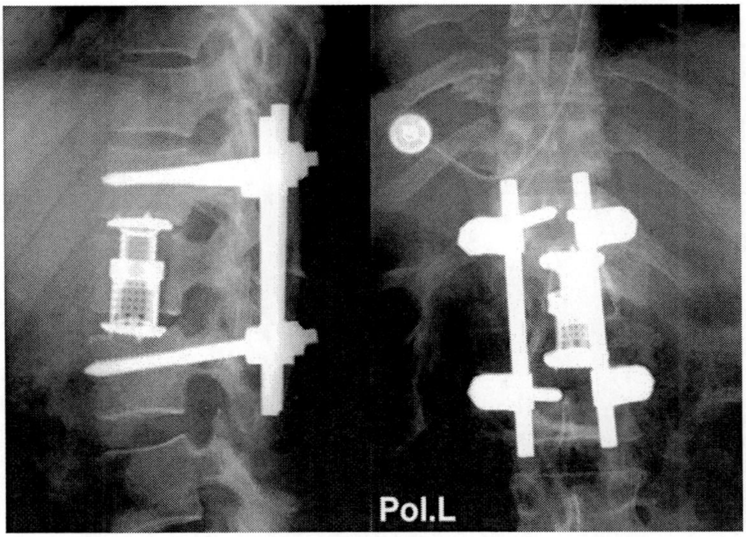

Figure 6. Reconstruction of the first lumbar vertebra using expandable Synex cage with transpedicular fixation.

Materials

Between 1987 and 2008, 108 patients with the underlying diagnosis of myeloma of the spine were surgically treated at the Department of Orthopaedic Surgery in Brno. The group comprised 50 (46 %) men and 58 (54 %) women, with an average age of 58 years and 6 months (range, 28 to 78 years). Of them, 99 had multiple myeloma and only nine had solitary plasma-cell myeloma. In terms of spinal regions, 18 cervical, 59 thoracic, 31 lumbar spines were operated on, using posterior surgery in 47, anterior surgery in 23 and combined procedures in 38 spines. The average operative time was 325 min and the average blood loss was 2 700 ml. The recurrence or deterioration of postoperative neurological findings required one revision surgery in 10 patients and two in four patients. One patient had to undergo three reoperations.

Results

The patients' neurological status was evaluated using the Frankel classification. The pre- and postoperative findings are presented in Table 2.

No change in neurological deficit after surgery was recorded in 67 (62 %) patients. An improvement was found in 37 (34 %) patients and, of these, by one Frankel grade in 35 patients and by two grades in two patients. Four patients (4 %) showed postoperative deterioration in neurological status, and this was from grade D to C in two patients and from grade D to B in one patient.

Table 2. Frankel´s scale

Frankel´s grade	A	B	C	D	E
preoperatively	4	5	27	34	38
postoperatively	3	10	14	32	49

Discussion

Surgical treatment for myeloma of the spine should be carried out in specialized departments whose surgeons have sufficient, long-time experience and full capacity to surgically manage malignant neoplasms and their potential complications. Economic issues also play a role because of high costs of this treatment, with the implants in particular. Good cooperation of the spinal surgeons with general medicine specialists who provide comprehensive care and treatment of the underlying myeloma diseases is also very important. When neurological deficit develops, it is necessary to begin anti-edema therapy immediately. Patients with progressive neurological deterioration should undergo urgent surgery. Operative intervention relieving pressure on neural structures must be carried out within 24 h of the onset of severe neurological findings. If this is not so, the deficit becomes permanent.

In patients with a good underlying disease prognosis, but progressive neurological deterioration, to postpone the treatment is a serious error. Surgical treatment of decompressed neural structures combined with a comprehensive therapy for the myeloma disease will result in prolonged survival and improved quality of life of the patients [15, 16].

Conclusions

In spinal myeloma the initial indication for surgical treatment is an imminent, existing or progressing neurological deficit. The benefits of surgical treatment include arrest of neurological deterioration, improvement of neurological deficit or its prevention, if this has not developed yet, as well as pain relief or its complete elimination. An early diagnosis and urgent surgery for spinal cord decompression, with spinal stabilization if needed, can prevent irreversible changes in the nervous system due to spinal myeloma. In patients with solitary myeloma, early operative intervention can lead to complete healing. Reliable cooperation of general medicine specialists, orthopedic surgeons, radiologists and neurologists will produce good outcomes, and such comprehensive care can only be provided by major medical centers.

References

[1] Horger M, Claussen CD, Bross-Bach U, Vonthein R, Trabold T, Heuschmid M, Pfannenberg C. Whole-body low-dose multidetector row-CT in the diagnosis of multiple myeloma: an alternative to conventional radiography. *Eur. J. Radiol.* 2005 May; 54(2): 289-97.

[2] Lecouvet FE, Vande Berg BC, Malghem J, Maldague BE. Magnetic resonance and computed tomography imaging in multiple myeloma. *Semin. Musculoskelet Radiol.* 2001;5(1):43-55.

[3] Scherer A, Wittsack HJ, Strupp C, Gattermann N, Haas R, Modder U. Vertebral fractures in multiple myeloma: first results of assessment of fracture risk using dynamic contrast-enhanced magnetic resonance imaging. *Ann. Hematol.* 2002 Sep; 81(9): 517-21. Epub 2002 Sep 14.

[4] Myslivecek M, Nekula J, Bacovsky J, Scudla V, Koranda P, Kaminek M. Multiple myeloma: predictive value of Tc-99m MIBI scintigraphy and MRI in its diagnosis and therapy. *Nucl. Med. Rev. Cent. East Eur.* 2008;11(1):12-6.

[5] Bačovský J, Ščudla V, Myslivеček M, Nekula J, Vytřasová M. Scintigraphy using ^{99m}Tc-MIBI (sestamibi), a sensitive parameter of activity of multiple myeloma. *Neoplasma* 2005; 52 (4): 302-306.

[6] Adam Z, Bolčák K, Staníček J, Pour L, Hájek R, Krejčí M, Prášek J, Neubauer J, Mareschova Y, Vorlíček J. The value of fluorodeoxyglucose positron emission tomography in multiple myeloma. *Vnitr. Lek.* 2006; 52(4): 436-442.

[7] Chaloupka R, Grosman R: The rules in surgical treatment of the malignant spinal tumors. *Acta spondylologica* 2002; 1(1): 39 – 41.

[8] Řehák S, Maisnar V, Málek V, Náhlovský J, Ryška P, Kaltofen K, et al. Indication and radicality of surgical treatment in spinal myeloma. *Acta Medica* (Hradec Kralove) Suppl. 2005; 48(1): 37-43.

[9] Togawa D, Lieberman IH, Bauer TW, Reinhardt MK, Kayanja MM. Histological evaluation of biopsies obtained from vertebral compression fractures: unsuspected myeloma and osteomalacia. *Spine*. 2005 Apr 1; 30(7): 781-6.

[10] Mazel C, Hoffmann E, Antonietti P, Grunenwald D, Henry M, Williams J. Posterior cervicothoracic instrumentation in spine tumors. *Spine* 2004 Jun 1; 29(11): 1246-53.

[11] Erdogan B, Sener L, Kilic D, Bolat F, Altinors N. Multiple myeloma of the thoracic spine developed at the previous trauma site: case report. *Eur. Spine J.* 2005 Sep; 14(7): 698-701. Epub 2005 Feb 4.

[12] Wegener B, Muller PE, Jansson V, Krodel A, Heinert G, Durr HR. Cervical spine metastasis of multiple myeloma: a case report with 16 years of follow-up. *Spine.* 2004 Sep 1; 29(17): E368-72.

[13] Bartolozzi B, Nozzoli C, Pandolfo C, Antonioli E, Guizzardi G, Morichi R, Bosi A. Percutaneous vertebroplasty and kyphoplasty in patients with multiple myeloma. *Eur. J. Haematol.* 2006 Feb; 76(2): 180-1.

[14] Krbec M, Štulík J, Tichý V. Replacement of the vertebral body with an expansion implant (Synex). *Acta Chir. orthop. Traum. čech*. 2002; 69: 158 – 62.

[15] Zeifang F, Zahlten-Hinguranage A, Goldschmidt H, Cremer F, Bernd L, Sabo D. Long-term survival after surgical intervention for bone disease in multiple myeloma. *Ann. Oncol.* 2005 Feb; 16(2): 222-7.

[16] Durr HR, Wegener B, Krodel A, Muller PE, Jansson V, Refior HJ. Multiple myeloma: surgery of the spine: retrospective analysis of 27 patients. *Spine* 2002 Feb 1; 27(3): 320-4; discussion 325-6.

In: Multiple Myeloma: Symptoms, Diagnosis and Treatment ISBN 978-1-60876-108-1
Editors: M. Georgiev and Ev. Bachev

Chapter 9

The Role of PBSC in Multiple Myeloma: From Biology to Treatment

Alessandro Corso**, *Patrizia Zappasodi and Marzia Varettoni
Division of Hematology, IRCCS Policlinico San Matteo,
University of Pavia, Italy

Abstract

Autologous peripheral blood stem cells (PBSCs) provide a rapid and effective hematopoietic recovery after the administration of chemotherapy alone or in combination with radiotherapy in patients with hematological malignancies, and guarantee a shorter time to engraftment and the lack of a need for surgical procedure necessary for bone marrow harvesting. For these reasons PBSCs have become the preferred source of stem cells for autologous transplantation in haematological and solid tumors. Multipotential and lineage-committed progenitor hemopoietic cells express the CD34 antigen, that represents the marker through which PBSCs are selected and collected. CD34+ PBSCs can be mobilized by the administration of G-CSF or GM-CSF alone or preceded by chemotherapy. The harvest of stem cells after mobilization can differ enormously inter-individually and for this reason several studies have been performed to identify those factors that can affect the yield of progenitors. Mobilized autologous peripheral blood stem cells have been increasingly used in the last decade within high-dose programs of therapy and represent by now the standard for many lymphoproliferative disease and in particular for multiple myeloma.

This comprehensive review tries to revisit the complex issue of the autologous peripheral blood stem cell transplantation in multiple myeloma patients focusing on all related aspect: biology of CD34+ stem cells, prognostic factor for mobilization, mobilizing regimens, high-dose approach of newly diagnosed patients, future perspective.

* Correspondence: Alessandro Corso, MD, Division of Hematology, Policlinico San Matteo, 27100, Pavia, Italy; Fax +0382.502250; E-mail: a.corso@smatteo.pv.it

Hematopoietic Stem Cells

Biology

Hematopoietic stem cells (HSCs) are a well characterised population of cells capable of self-renewal and multilineage differentiation [1]. The stem cell can undergo symmetric division, which results in the formation of two identical stem cells, or asymmetric division, leading to the formation of a stem cell and a more mature cell. During development there is a prevalence of symmetric divisions, resulting in an expansion of stem cell compartment. On the contrary, throughout life hematopoiesis is sustained by balanced asymmetric division which ensures a sufficient self-renewal and the maintenance of a pool of mature cells. During steady-state hematopoiesis, proliferating hematopoietic cells at various stages of differentiation are confined within specialized bone marrow niches, while mature cells leave the bone marrow and migrate into blood. A small proportion of morphologically unrecognizable primitive stem cells regularly escapes the bone marrow and circulates throughout life. The presence of stem/progenitors cells in the peripheral blood during steady-state hematopoiesis was firstly demonstrated in the 1960s in laboratory animals [2-3], and some years later was confirmed in man [4-5]. The amount of circulating progenitors during steady-state hematopoiesis, however, is usually low, with the exception of patients with myeloproliferative disorders [6].

An increased release of stem and progenitor cells from bone marrow into blood circulation physiologically occurs during inflammatory response, as a result of infection or injury-mediated release of stress signals. More importantly, the mobilization of haematopoietic stem and and progenitor cells to peripheral blood can be induced by treatment with chemotherapy alone or in association with cytokines. The mechanisms underlying this process are still incompletely understood, but new insights have emerged in the recent years from murine and human studies.

Mechanisms of Mobilisation

Stem and progenitor cells are anchorated to the bone marrow microenviroment by adhesion molecules. The molecules involved belong to the families of β1 and β2 integrin, selectin and superimmunoglobulins [7]. Corresponding ligands are expressed on endothelial cells and accessory marrow cells or form parts of extracellular matrix of the bone marrow microenviroment.

The relevance of some molecules for migration of hematopoietic stem cells into blood has been clarified by studies comparing the phenotype of mobilised progenitor cells with that of steady-state bone marrow cells. One of the most important differences regards the expression of very-late antigen 4 (VLA-4). VLA-4 is expressed on the surface of haematopoietic progenitors and binds to the vascular cell adhesion molecule-1 (VCAM-1) on endothelial cells as well as to the extracellular matrix protein fibronectin. Mobilised CD34+ cells express lower levels of VLA-4 when compared to bone marrow progenitors suggesting that the release of CD34+ cells and the ability to circulate relates to the expression levels of

VLA-4 [8]. Papayannopoulou demonstrated that treatment of primates and mice with monoclonal antibodies directed against VLA-4 antibodies resulted in a significant increase of circulating hematopoietic progenitor cells [9]. Furthermore, the analysis of functional state of VLA-4 by flow citometry demonstrated an inactivation of VLA-4 on G-CSF mobilized CD34+ cells in comparison to CD34+ cells from steady-state bone marrow [10].

Other adhesive molecules involved in the process of stem cell mobilization are the β-2 integrin leucocyte function-associated molecule-1 (LFA-1) and the corresponding ligands intercellular adhesion molecule (ICAM) 1 and 2, members of superimmunoglobulin family. Circulating CD34+ cells express LFA-1 at lower levels compared to bone marrow CD34+ cells, suggesting that LFA-1 expression is modulated during mobilization. This hypothesis is supported by the evidence that treatment with antibodies directed against LFA inhibits adhesion and migration of CD34+ through an endothelial layer [11]. Samely, it has been demonstrated that treatment of mice with anti CD-44 inhibits adhesion to bone marrow stroma and mobilize progenitor cells, suggesting that the disruption of adhesive interaction between CD44, which is highly expressed on hematopoietic progenitor cells, and hyaluronic acid and fibronectin secreted by the stromal cells is necessary for mobilization [12].

Besides adhesion molecules, some studies outlined the role of the alpha-chemokine stromal-derived factor-1 (SDF-1) in the process of mobilization. SDF-1 is constitutively produced by stromal cells and was isolated for the first time from a murine stromal cell line [13]. The natural ligand of SDF-1 is CXCR4, expressed on CD34+ cells. In steady-state hematopoiesis, the amount of SDF-1 produced by the microenvironment keeps hematopoietic precursors within the bone marrow. During mobilization, SDF-1 exerts its chemotactic function through the receptor CXCR4 expressed on CD34+ cells, which in turn promotes integrin-mediated adhesion and endothelial transmigration of hematopoietic stem cells, primitive hematopoietic precursors, long-term bone marrow culture initiating cells and cobblestone-area forming cells [14]. Other authors demonstrated that bone marrow ablation by irradiation or by other DNA-damaging agents, such as cyclophosphamide or 5-fluorouracil, induced an elevation of plasma levels of SDF-1 [15]. In the study of Heissig et al [16], 5-FU-induced SDF-1 secretion was followed by an up-regulation of the matrix metalloproteinase 9 (MMP-9) expression in bone marrow cells. Furthermore, MMP-9 was increased in bone marrow extracellular fluids of mice treated with G-CSF and cyclophosphamide [17]. This metalloproteinase acts by inducing the release of soluble KitL (sKitL) and consecutive recruitment of c-Kit+ stem/progenitors into circulation [16]. Moreover, plasma elevation of SDF-1 induced mobilization of hematopoietic progenitors and mature white blood cells in wild-type mice but not in MMP-9 mice [15], suggesting a key-role of this metalloproteinase for mobilization.

CD34: A Well Identified Marker

CD34 is a surface glycophosphoprotein expressed on developmentally early lymphohematopoietic stem and progenitor cells [18]. CD34+ cells represent only 1.5% of mononuclear cells in bone marrow aspirates from normal donors and less than 0.5% in peripheral blood [19]. Studies in primates and humans indicate that CD34+ cells purified from marrow can provide a durable donor-derived long-term host lymphohematopoietic reconstitution, demonstrating that the subset of CD34+ cells comprise precursors of all lymphohematopoietic lineages [20]. Immunoaffinity-purified CD34+ cells are 10- to 100-fold enriched in colony-forming units (CFUs) with respect to CD34- cell population. The CD34+ cells include CFU-macrophage (CFU-M), CFU-granulocyte (CFU-G), CFU-GM, burst-forming units-erythroid (BFU-E) and are particularly enriched in CFU-GEMM and CFU-blasts. The levels of CD34 expression, assessed by flow cytometric analysis, decrease from earliest hematopoietic progenitor cells to more mature cells, and reaches undetectable levels when cells lose the capacity to form colonies in vitro [21]. The $CD34^{bright}$ comprises the majority of immature hematopoietic progenitor cells, while the $CD34^{dim}$ population contains more lineage-committed progenitors. The discovery of CD34 as a marker of early hematopoietic stem/progenitor cells has important clinical applications in mobilization. Monoclonal antibodies directed to CD34 antigen are used to quantify stem/progenitor cells in peripheral blood and/or in the apheretic product and can be also used to purify normal stem/progenitor cells.

Stem Cells Mobilisation

In patients candidate to high dose therapy, the standard therapeutic approach includes several steps which go from the induction to the transplant procedure as shown in figure 1. It is known that CD34+ stem cells, normally homed in bone marrow, under a stimulus can mobilise in the peripheral circulation. After chemotherapy, during the growth factors stimulation, a daily monitoring of CD34+ cells number is performed through flow cytometric assay and when their number reach a count of at least 20/μl, stem cells are harvested with a continuous-flow blood cell separator Spectra generally processing a total volume per leukapheresis of 2-3 blood volumes. Daily leukaphereses are performed until a sufficient number of stem cells are harvested.

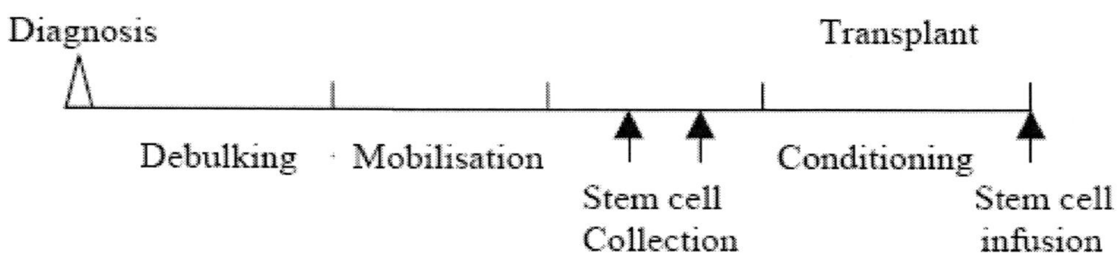

Figure 1. General outline of first line therapy of multiple myeloma patients eligible for transplant.

Mobilisation Schemes

Many different protocols have been investigated for stem cells mobilisation either containing chemotherapy, growth factors or both. The more frequently used growth factor is granulocyte growth factor (G-CSF), with different schedules and doses and variably associated to citotoxic agents.

Sheridan evaluated G-SCF at doses of 12 and 24 μg/kg/day and obtained better collections with the highest dose [22]. Zeller [23] demonstrated that the number of CD34+ cells collected with 24 μg/kg/day was significantly higher as compared to that obtained using G-CSF at the dose of 5 μg/kg/day. A similar dose-response effect has been showed even for GM-CSF [24], even though is less tolerated at the high doses. Other cytokines have demonstrated some activities as single mobilizing agents, including Erythropoetin (Epo) [25], IL-3 [26], IL-6 [27] and PIXY321, a fusion protein of GM-CSF and IL-3 [28]. These cytokines has been also investigated in combination. In a randomized study G-CSF + GM-CSF was not superior to G-CSF alone [29]. Stem cell factor (SCF) added to G-CSF demonstrated to allow a four-fold increase in CD34+ yield as compared to G-CSF alone in breast cancer patients [30]. More recently, PEG-filgrastim, a long half life form of G-CSF, given as a single subcutaneous injection in association with chemotherapy has been demonstrated effective for stem cell mobilization in lymphoma and myeloma patients [31-32].

Although G-CSF alone is effective in collecting CD34+ cells, the best combination to obtain high numbers of stem cells is with chemotherapy [33] and, therefore, this is considered the standard scheme to collect stem cells. The drug more widely used in mobilisation protocols is Cyclophosphamide administered at variable doses from 4 to 7 g/m^2 with the same efficacy but with more side effects for the higher dosages [34]. Samely, lower doses of cyclophosphamide have been indicated as equally effective in mobilising sufficient number of peripheral stem cells in not heavily pretreated patients. Cyclophosphamide 1.5 g/mq plus G-CSF 10 μg/mq given in outpatient manner obtains high number of CD34+ cells without significant toxicity [35]. Other studies report on polichemotherapic associations containing cyclophosphamide such as CHOP, d-TEC, platinum-based regimens like EDAP (Etoposide, Dexamethasone, Ara-C, Cysplatin), ESHAP, DCEP always in combination with growth factors. Experience with ESHAP protocol was tested as second line therapy in myeloma patients refractory to VAD cycles. It consists of a combination of Etoposide for four days, methylprednisolone for 5 days, Cytosine arabinoside in single dose, continuous infusion of cisplatin for 4 days and G-CSF. This regimen is tolerable with a good antitumor activity and good mobilising efficacy [36]. DCEP regimen, including high dose dexamethasone and 4 days infusion of cyclophosphamide, etoposide and cisplatin has proved to be as effective as high dose Cyclophosphamide in mobilising stem cells with a significant reduced hematological toxicity [37].

Stem cells Mobilisation: Factors Influencing the Harvest

The collection of an adequate amount of peripheral blood stem cells is mandatory to perform (safely) transplant safely. Several studies have tried to identify the optimal dose of stem cells, necessary to assure a rapid engraftment. However, the individual response to mobilizing therapy is highly variable and only partially predictable. Various factors have been correlated with a successful mobilisation, first of all the previous exposure to chemotherapy which is usually stem cell poison and can consequently affect the bone marrow cellularity [38]. In a series of 243 patients with a variety of malignancies, Bensinger et al demonstrated that patients receiving fewer cycles of chemotherapy or without a prior history of radiotherapy yield higher number of CD34+ cells [39]. Haas and collegues, in a cohort of malignant lymphoma non-irradiated patients, calculated a mean reduction of 0.2 X 10^6/kg CD34+ cells per each cycle of chemotherapy performed before mobilisation [40]. Some drugs however are more toxic than others, namely the alkylating agents (melphalan, busulfan) or the nitrosoureas (BCNU) [41]. In a study of Tricot et al on 225 multiple myeloma patients mobilized with high-dose cyclophosphamide and hematopoietic growth factors, the duration of exposure to alkylating agents inversely correlated with the likelihood to harvest adequate number of CD34+ stem cells [38].

In another retrospective study on 96 patients with refractory/relapsed Hodgkin's disease and non Hodgkin's lymphoma the use of Dexa-BEAM as salvage therapy adversely influencing collection [42] confirmed the negative impact on stem cell mobilization. These findings suggest that (drugs) potentially stem cell poison drugs should be avoided in the early phases of the treatment in patients candidates to transplant. The use of fludarabine, the number of previous cycles of chemotherapy or simply the duration of treatment before mobilisation have been identified as possible negative factors for mobilisation [43, 44, 39]. More than 70% of patients with a prior therapy lasting more than 24 months failed to mobilise adequately to ensure rapid platelet recovery [38].

In multiple myeloma, some authors reported (in multiple myeloma,) (elderly patients) a lower probability to collect adequate numbers of stem cells in elderly patients (than younger patients) even with limited pre-mobilization therapy. By contrast, in other studies age did not show any prognostic impact [40, 42, 45]. Bone marrow involvement was found to affect CD34+ cell harvests in some studies [39, 46, 47, 48], but not in others [40, 49, 44, 43]. In some studies, WBC and platelet count correlated significantly with the number of CD34+ cell harvested. Ketterer demonstrated that patients with a platelet count $\leq 150 \times 10^9$/L at mobilization are a higher risk of inadequate collection [46]. Krieger and (at) al demonstrated that collection of peripheral blood progenitor cells based on rising WBC and platelet count significantly increases the number of CD34+ cells [50]. A recent study identified an easy scoring system able to predict the probability of mobilising stem cells. Four parameters were indicated as negatively associated with the number of CD34+ cells collected: low platelets and WBC count, prior exposure to melphalan and an interval >6 months from the start of treatment. Patients scored as having 0, 1, 2, 3, 4 risks factors had a significantly lower median number of collected CD34+ cells if presented at mobilisation two or more risks factors [43].

Few authors have investigated the role of steady-state CD34+ cell count in peripheral blood and/or bone marrow as a predictive parameter for mobilization. Osma et al, in a retrospective study on 15 patients with hematologic and solid malignancies, found a strong correlation between peripheral blood CD34+ cell count during steady-state hematopoiesis and the CD34+ yield [51], whereas no correlation was found with bone marrow CD34+ cell count. On the contrary, in a study on 90 haematologic patients we found that a high-steady-state bone marrow CD34+ cell count was significantly correlated with adequate peripheral blood stem cell collections, particularly in multiple myeloma patients [52]. In this subset of patients, a bone marrow absolute number of CD34+ cells lower than 66/μL was associated with a higher probability of collecting less than $4x10^6$/kg CD34+ cells.

Stem Cells Mobilisation: Factors Influencing Engraftment

First condition for a successful transplant is the infusion of an adequate number of CD34+ cells. It is known that the engraftment mainly depends on the dose of CD34+ cells infused as rescue after conditioning treatment and there are several reports that suggest as safe a minimum number of 2 x 10^6/kg CD34+ cells to guarantee a good and rapid engraftment [53, 54, 55].

In particular, the number of CD34+ cells infused influences the platelet more than neutrophil recovery after transplantation [56]. Some authors reported a prolonged and incomplete engraftment of platelets, in patients receiving less than 2 x 10^6/kg CD34+ cells [57, 58, 59]. Under this threshold there is no more advantage of using PBPC instead of bone marrow. In a large single-center study on 243 patients, those receiving more than 2.5 x 10^6/kg CD34+ cells had a more rapid neutrophil and platelet recovery as compared to patients infused with less than 2.5 x 10^6/kg CD34+ cells [60]. However, patients treated for more than 12 months need more than 5 x 10^6/kg cells to obtain a rapid platelet recovery [38]. Also in the above mentioned study of Bensinger, higher doses (>5 x 10^6/kg) of CD34+ cells were found to shorten significantly the platelet recovery, while there was no significant influence on neutrophil kinetics over a limit of 2.5 x 10^6/kg CD34+ cells [39]. Other evidences confirmed the lack of advantages in using more than 5 x 10^6/kg stem cells [61].

An extensive use of alkylating agents or a chemotherapy lasting more than 24 months strongly interfere with a rapid hematopoietic recovery and in these conditions, a greater dose of CD34+ cells is mandatory in order to assure a prompt platelet reconstitution [38].

Several authors indicate the increasing age as responsible for a delayed platelet recovery post transplant; moreover in patients over the age of 70 years, the use of Melphalan 200 mg/m^2 was very toxic resulting in 16% deaths. For this reason an Italian group has planned three courses of intermediate dose of Melphalan (100 mg/m^2) supported by peripheral stem cells, obtaining, (without important toxicity) an improved response rate and EFS with respect to oral melphalan without important toxicity. Anyway, the advanced age by itself should not be an exclusion criterion for autologous transplantation, but dose adjustment is necessary to reduce toxicity.

Optimal Timing for Collection

The choice of the timing of PBPC collection is currently based on the daily evaluation of peripheral CD34+ cells by flow citometry [62, 63, 64]. At present there are two commercially available single platform tests for measuring CD34+ cells in blood (ProCount from Becton-Dickinson, Mt View, CA, and StemKit from Beckman-Coulter, Fullerton, CA). The optimal threshold of CD34+ cells in peripheral blood is still controversial. Siena et al recommended to begin apheresis when CD34+ first appear in the circulation during recovery from intensive chemotherapy-induced pancytopenia [62]. Haas et al reported that a peripheral CD34+ cell count of at least 50/μL was highly predictive for a yield greater than 2.5 x 10^6/kg in a single apheresis [40]. In a series of 95 patients treated with different mobilizing therapies for solid tumors or haematologic malignancies, a peripheral CD34+ cell count of 20/μL or greater was associated with collection of at least 2x10^6/kg CD34+ cells in 94% of apheresis [65].

The Management of Poor Mobilizers

Although the majority of patients achieve a good yield of CD34+ cells, for those who fail the mobilisation it is possible to increase the dose of G-CSF or to add different growth factors not routinely used as GM-CSF or stem cell factor (SCF) with the intent to improve stem cell collection [66]. When inadequate CD34+ cell number is achieved using growth factor alone, it is reasonable to undergo a new mobilisation with chemotherapy plus cytokines [67, 68]. The real challenge is the management of patients who fail an initial mobilization with chemotherapy plus growth factors. Remobilization strategies include chemotherapy plus cytokines [69, 70] or high-dose cytokine alone [71] or in combination [72]. In a series of 119 patients achieving less than 2.5 x 10^6/kg CD34+ cells with chemotherapy plus G-CSF or G-CSF alone, remobilisation with G-CSF was as effective as chemotherapy plus G-CSF and was associated with less morbidity [70]. In a study of Boeve et al, high-dose G-CSF (32 μg/kg/day) or the combination of G-CSF 10 μg/kg/day plus GM-CSF 5 μg/kg/day resulted equally effective to re-mobilize purpose in patients failing an initial procedure [72]. In a series of 48 patients collecting less than 2x10^6/kg with either chemotherapy plus G-CSF or G-CSF alone, the addition of recombinant human stem cell factor (rHuSCF) allowed successful remobilisation in 35% of patients [73] as a result of a synergistic effect in increasing the number of colonies; in fact, the administration of both stem cell factor and G-CSF was associated with a three fold greater chance of reaching 5x10^6/kg CD34+ cells in a single leucapheresis compared with patients mobilised with G-CSF alone [74].

Purging

For a long time relapse due to reinfused tumor cells has been considered the principal cause of treatment failure after autologous stem cell transplantation. Stem cell mobilization can result in tumor cell recruitment into peripheral blood [75] and more than a half of multiple myeloma patients have circulating malignant cells at the time of harvest [76, 77, 78]. Cremer et al reported that more than 90% of leukapheresis products contain cells belonging to the myeloma cell clone [79]. Many attempts have been made to eradicate tumor contamination from autologous harvests and different laboratory procedures have been performed with the CD34+ selection using magnetic beads or through high speed cell sorting, antibody-related techniques, drug and chemical techniques. However, removal of tumor cells does not seem to improve the serologic or molecular complete remission (CR) rate, event free survival (EFS), or overall survival (OS) of myeloma patients. In fact many authors, although described the feasibility of transplants with purged autografts, reported a lacking advantage in reaching higher percentages of CR or longer survivals [80, 81, 82] compared with patients receiving unmanipulated grafts [83]. Moreover, the purging of leukapheretic product determines a loss of CD34+ cells that should be compensated by increasing numbers of stem cells collected. Anyway, recent evidences belie that malignant plasma cells infusion could negatively affect the outcome of transplanted patients suggesting that in vivo residual tumor cells, rather than reinfused plasma cells are more likely to be responsible for relapse [84]. In conclusion, even though could be better to avoid tumor cell contamination in the apheresis, there is no evidence that infusion of mobilized tumor cells in the graft increase the incidence of relapse after autologous transplantation in multiple myeloma [84] non-Hodgkin's lymphoma [85], or breast cancer [86].

Autologous Transplantation

Conditioning Regimens

The most active drug in multiple myeloma is surely melphalan which gives the best results if employed at high doses. The high rates of complete remission obtained with this approach have induced to include, in the majority of conditioning protocols, high dose melphalan alone, with other chemotherapeutic agents or with radiotherapy followed by stem cell support (table 1). Melphalan has been combined at the dose of 140 mg/m^2 with radiotherapy given in four fractions at a variable total dose of 8 -14 Gy. This combination has produced high response rate but with a consistent toxicity. Barlogie reported a rising of TRM from 2% after the first transplant alone to 5% after the second whose conditioning regimen included melphalan and TBI [87]. Goldschmidt in a single-center experience demonstrated a higher extrahematological toxicity of the combination Melphalan + TBI with respect to melphalan alone [88]. High dose melphalan has also been associated in BEM regimen with Carmustine (BCNU) given i.v. at a dose of 600 mg/m^2, etoposide and cyclophosphamide [89]. Several studies have tried to define the optimal combination in terms of antineoplastic efficacy and toxicity. Some authors associate Busulfan to melphalan 60 mg/mq [90] or 140 mg/m^2 [91], others added also Idarubicin without registering an increase in TRM [92]. Other combinations like Busulfan, melphalan and thiotepa, or etoposide, melphalan and TBI did not show conclusive results. The efforts to improve the response rate have conducted some authors also to test escalating doses of melphalan: the conclusions of this study defined the maximum tolerated dose at 280 mg/m^2 [93]. Moreau et al selected high risk patients on the basis of high levels of $\beta 2$ microglobulin and on the presence of chromosome 13 deletion treating them with Melphalan 220 mg/m^2 at second transplant reporting good response rates without higher toxicity with respect to standard dose of 200 mg/m^2 administered at first transplant [94].

Recently, melphalan alone at 200 mg/m^2 has proved to be as effective as other protocols of combination with acceptable toxicity. Actually, Desikan retrospectively compared conditioning regimens for the second transplant of a planned tandem transplantation and determined better survival rates in patients who received Melphalan 200 mg/m^2 versus Melphalan 200 mg/m^2 associated to Cyclophosphamide or TBI [95]. Anyway, the more impressive results have been published by the IFM group who conducted the first prospective randomised study comparing the two most common regimens used for myeloma: Melphalan 200 mg/m^2 versus Melphalan 140 mg/m^2 plus total body irradiation 8 Gy. They showed that melphalan alone produced less severe toxic effects than the combined treatment Melphalan-TBI without significant differences in terms of response rate and EFS confirming melphalan at 200 mg/m^2 as the standard conditioning regimen for autologous transplant in myeloma patients [96].

Table 1. Autologous stem cell transplantation conditioning regimens (partially extracted from publication by Hahn and Collegues: 'The role of cytotoxic therapy with hematopoietic stem cell transplantation in the therapy of multiple myeloma: an evidenc-based review'. Biol of blood and marrow transplant 2003; 9: 4-37)

Reference	Conditioning regimen	TRM (%)	Median OS (months)	Median EFS (months)
Moreau et al	Mel 200 vs. Mel 140+TBI 800	0 4	NYR 43	20.5 21
Tribalto et al.	Bu 16 + Mel 60	3	57	21
Meloni et al.	Ida , Bu, Mel 60	0	NS	NS
Barlogie et al.	1st tx: Mel 200 2nd tx: Mel 200 vs. Mel 140 + TBI	 2 5	68	43
Goldshmidt et al.	Mel 200 vs. Mel 140 + TBI	0 4	NS	NS
Lahuerta et al.	Mel 200 Mel 140 + TBI Bu + Mel Bu + Cy	4 8 6 0	46 39 57 39	22 20 30 23
Desikan et al.	2nd tx: Mel 200 vs. Mel 200 + Cy vs. Mel 140 + TBI	0 0 8	76 39 25	61 27 15
Bensinger et al	Bu + Cy + vs. Bu + Cy + TBI vs. Bu + Mel 100 + Thiotepa	28 14 11	NS	NS

NYR: not yet reached.
NS: not stated in the original article.
Mel: Melphalan, Bu: Busulfan, Cy: Cyclophosphamide, Ida: Idarubicin.

One or Two Transplants?

The efficacy of high dose therapy over standard chemotherapy has been first demonstrated by the Intergroup Francophone du myelome (IFM) in 1996 [97]. The advantage has been showed in terms of response rate (81% with 22% of CR compared to 57% with 5% of CR in chemotherapy group), EFS (28% versus18%, Figure 2) and OS (57 versus 44 months) with an acceptable transplant related mortality (TRM) of less than 5%, not greater than that observed after chemotherapy.

Other studies demonstrated that the achievement of complete remission with negative immunofixation should be the main objective of the therapy because strictly related to the duration of survival [98]. The good results obtained with high dose therapy have been reproduced by others on larger cohorts [99].

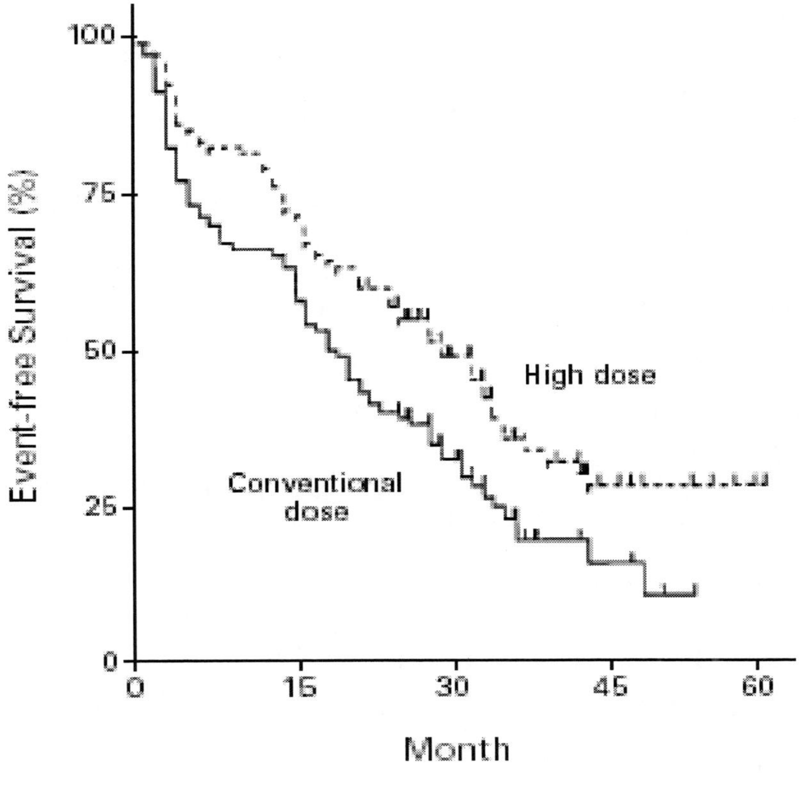

Figure 2. Event-free Survival According to Treatment Group. The numbers shown below the time points are probabilities of event-free survival (the percentages of patients surviving event-free) and 95 percent confidence intervals. From publication by Attal et al. (97).

A recent report of the English group has shown good long term results of a single autograft with high dose melphalan observing almost 30% of patients projected to be alive a decade after the transplant and a 16% disease free survival [100]. If one transplant increases CR rate to 20%, a further intensification with double transplant could allow a 40% of CR. This was the rationale of total therapy I designed by the Arkansas group who obtained encouraging EFS and OS results, respectively of 43 and 68 months and reported 15% of patients disease free after a follow up of 10 years [101]. The efficacy of double transplant has been investigated also by French group who randomly assigned one or two transplants in a population of 399 patients and reached a long follow up of more than 5 years. Although the program was completed in about 80% of patients in each arm, the double transplant was associated with a better outcome with a 7-year survival probability of 42% versus 21% in single transplant arm. Also the Italian randomised study, Bologna 96, concluded that double transplant is superior over single transplant, in terms of extended OS, EFS and time to progression (TTP) not only for patients who improved their response to at least a near CR after the second transplant, but also for patients with at least a PR at the end of the program [102]. With the same objective to improve the quality of response and to further ameliorate the results of double transplant, some groups intensified also the debulking chemotherapy in order to reduce as much as possible the tumor burden before high dose melphalan. A new intensive and complex approach, in fact, was planned by Arkansas group who, adding thalidomide before mobilisation, achieved an increase of CR rate to 66% and of 4-years EFS from 37% to 70%. The Bologna 2002 protocol is still evaluating the efficacy and the toxicity of combined thalidomide and dexamethasone for 4 months, followed by CD34+ cells mobilisation and two sequential courses of melphalan 200 mg/m^2. The preliminary results confirm the good tolerability of this induction regimen and its efficacy in improving the rate and the quality of response before transplant with respect to VAD chemotherapy. Besides evidences favouring the transplant, some authors suggest caution in promoting this procedure as first line approach. A randomised trial was designed to assess the optimal timing of high dose therapy in patients aged up to 56 years. The patients were randomised to receive early transplantation or as salvage therapy. No survival advantage was shown for early transplanted patients, while a better quality of life was observed in this setting [103]. Also the Spanish group is (are) evaluating the real need of an early transplant. They suggest that refractory patients after conventional therapy have little possibilities to respond to high dose melphalan. Therefore, they designed a trial investigating if responding patients to debulking treatment can have a benefit to be transplanted or to continue conventional chemotherapy. While significant better responses were reached in transplant arm, no significant survival advantage was shown between the two schemes [104]. By now, the transplant remains the standard approach for multiple myeloma patients, even though the previous observations induce to carefully reflect on its role. In fact, it is still difficult to identify an univocal effective therapy in a scenario in which a great variability in chemosensitivity, cytogenetic features, etc is present in patients with the same disease.

The Age in the Decision of the Best Therapy

Autologous transplantation has become the standard care of newly diagnosed multiple myeloma. Although there is not an univocal age cut-off for high dose therapy, the majority of hematology centers define 60 years, as upper limit and the older patients are usually treated with conventional chemotherapy. The median age of patients with this disease is approximately 65 years and, as a consequence, more than half of all myeloma population is not eligible for transplant. Some authors reported the feasibility of transplant procedure in elderly patients, demonstrating that age is not an absolute exclusion criteria for transplantation. An Italian group treated patients until 75 years of age with three courses of melphalan 100 mg/mq followed by stem cell support, reaching high response rates and low toxicity [105]. Also other experiences with autologous transplantation at different conditioning regimens in patients older than 60 years, registered no difference in CR, TRM,

EFS and OS with respect to younger group [106]. In other reports if a standard conditioning therapy is used, TRM was higher. In fact, with melphalan 200 mg/m^2 TRM was reported as 16%, while if melphalan is lowered to 140 mg/mq TRM decreases to 2% [107]. Anyway, a consideration is required: the older patients undergoing transplant represent a selected group of individuals with satisfactory organ function and good performance status; no data are available on the proportion of older myeloma patients ineligible to high dose therapy. Therefore, autologous transplantation, although safely adopted in selected cases, can not be considered, at the moment, the standard approach for elderly myeloma patients.

Future Perspectives

Despite impressive results in terms of remission rates and survival have been reported in literature with autologous transplantation, multiple myeloma remains an incurable disease. The more optimistic study report a 15% of long survivors with a percentage of patients who are in molecular remission after 10 years. However, the few cases of patients definitely cured are among those undergone to allogeneic transplantation.

More recently, new agents entered in the armamentarium of the hematologist in some cases by chance as thalidomide, sadly known because of its teratogenicity in the '60 and thean withdrawn from the market. This drug was found to be effective in multiple myeloma firstly as single agent in refractory/relapsed patients [108] till the more recent studies that have demonstrated its efficacy even when used upfront either in patients candidates to high dose therapy [109] either in elderly patients. In particular in this setting of patients, thalidomide in combination with melphalan and prednisone has proved to be more effective than the MEL 100 transplant adopted by Palumbo et al.[110].

On the contrary, other new agents are the result of biological studies that have shed lights on the pathogenetic mechanisms underlying the disease and have identified specific signalling pathways and some molecular target responsible for the survival of plasma cells, for the inhibition of apoptosis and for their resistance to chemotherapy. The most important among these emergent therapies are the ImiDS and the proteasome inhibitors. Among the first class Lenalidomide has produced the most striking results in refractory/relapsed patients but also preliminary results demonstrate its efficacy either as single agent or in combination with dexamethasone or chemotherapy [111]. Among proteasome inhibitors, Bortezomib is the most studied and for its efficacy is currently approved for the treatment of relapsed or primary resistant multiple myeloma. Studies evaluating bortezomib in earlier stages of myeloma, including first-line therapy, are under way. Preliminary data are encouraging either if used in combination with dexamethasone (response rate 87% with 17% of complete responses [112] either in association with chemotherapy in particular with doxorubicin producing response rates of 91% with 33% of complete response (PAD) [113].

Furthermore, the efficacy of bortezomib seems to overcome even the negative effect of the cytogenetic abnormalities as deletion of chromosome 13 [114].

These impressive results have prompted several new protocols evaluating all the possible combination between these new drugs and chemotherapy and then even if at the moment autologous transplant maintains its supremacy it is reasonably possible that in the near future these emerging drugs could call in question its primary role.

References

[1] Kondo M, Wagers AJ, Manz MG et al. Biology of hematopoietic stem cells and progenitors: implications for clinical application. *Annu. Rev. Immunol* 2003; 21: 759-806.

[2] Malinin TI, Perry VP, Donlan MF et al. Some observations on the histology of lethally irradiated guinea pigs protected with nucleated elements of homologous blood. *Blood* 1963; 22: 499-500 (Abst).

[3] Cavins JA, Scheer SC, Thomas ED, Ferrebee JW. The recovery of lethally irradiated dogs given infusions of autologous leucocytes preserved at –80°C. *Blood* 1964; 23: 38-42.

[4] Rubin SH, Cowan DH. Assay of granulocytic progenitor cells in human peripheral blood. *Exp. Hematol.* 1973; 1: 127-131.

[5] Barr RD, Whang-Peng J, Perry S. Hematopoietic stem cells in human peripheral blood. *Science* 1975; 190: 284-285.

[6] Hibbin JA, Njoku OS, Matutes E, Lewis Sm, Goldman JM. Myeloid progenitor cells in the circulation of patients with myelofibrosis and other myeloproliferative disorders. *Br. J. Haematol.* 1984; 57: 495-503.

[7] Soligo D, Schiro R, Luksch R et al. Expression of integrins in human bone marrow. *Br. J. Haematol.* 1990; 76: 323-332.

[8] Prosper F, Stroncekj D, McCarthy JB et al. Mobilization and homing of peripheral blood progenitors is related to reversible downregulation of alpha4 beta1 integrin expression and function. *J. Clin. Invest* 1998; 101: 2456-2467.

[9] Papayannopoulou, Nakamoto B. Peripheralization of CD34+ haematopoietic progenitors in primates treated with anti-VLA4 integrin. *Proc. Natl. Acad. Sci. USA* 1993; 90: 9374-9378.

[10] Lichterfeld M, Martin S, Burkly L et al. Mobilization of CD34+ haematopoietic stem cells is associated with a functional inactivation of the integrin very late antigen 4. *Br. J. Haematol.* 2000; 110: 71-81.

[11] Möhle R, Moore MA, Nachman Rl et al. Transendothelial migration of CD34+ and mature hematopoietic cells: an in vitro study using a human bone marrow endothelial cell line. *Blood* 1997; 89: 72-80.

[12] Oostendorp RA; Spitzer E, Brandl M et al. Evidence for differences in the mechanisms by which antibodies against CD44 promote adhesion of erythroid and granulopoietic progenitors to marrow stromal cells. *Br. J. Haematol.* 1998; 101: 436-445.

[13] Nagasawa T, Hirota S, Tachibana K, et al. Defects of B-cell lymphopoiesis and bone-marrow myelopoiesis in mice lacking the CXC chemokine PBSF/SDF-1. *Nature* 1996; 382: 635-638.

[14] Jo DY, Rafii S, Hamada T, et al. Chemotaxis of primitive hematopoietic cells in response to stromal cell-derived factor-1. *J. Clin. Investig* 2000; 105: 101-111.

[15] Hattori K, Heissig B, Tashiro K, et al. Plasma elevation of stromal cell-derived factor-1 induces mobilization of mature and immature hematopoietic progenitor and stem cells. *Blood* 2001; 97: 3354-3360.

[16] Heissig B, Hattori K, Dias S, et al. Recruitment of stem cells from the bone marrow niche requires MMP-9 mediated release of Kit-ligand. *Cell*, 2002; 139: 625-637.

[17] Petit I, Szyper-Kravitz M, Nagler A, et al. G-CSF induces stem cell mobilization by decreasing bone marrow SDF-1 and up-regulating CXCR4. *Nat. Immunol.*, 2002; 3: 687-694.

[18] Andrews RG, Singer JW, Bernstein ID: Monoclonal antibody 12-8 recognizes a 115-kd molecular present on both unipotent and multipotent hematopoietic colony-forming cells and their precursors. *Blood*, 1986; 67: 842-845.

[19] Loken MR, Shah Vo Dattilio KL et al. Flow cytometric analysis of human bone marrow. II. Normal B lymphocyte development. *Blood*, 1987; 70: 1316-1324.

[20] Wagermaker G, van Gils F, Bart-Baumeister J et al. Sustained engraftment of allogeneic CD34 positive hematopoietic stem cells in rhesus monkeys. *Exp. Hematol.* 1990; 18: 708-

[21] Strauss L, Rowley S, La Russa S et al. Antigenic analysis of hematopoiesis. V. Characterization of My-10 antigen expression by normal lymphohematopoietic progenitor cells. *Exp. Hematol.* 1986; 14: 878-886.

[22] Sheridan W, Begley G, Juttner C et al. Effect of different doses and schedules of filgrastim on mononuclear cell and PBPC collections and hematopoietic recovery after high dose chemotherapy and infusion of filgrastim mobilized PBPC without bone marrow. *ASH* 1992; 1315a.

[23] Zeller W, Cassens U, Stockschlader M et al. Higher dose of G-CSF increases yield of mobilized CD34+ cells. *Blood* 1994; 84 (suppl 1): 413a.

[24] Bishop MR, Anderson JR, Jackson JD et al. High-dose therapy and peripheral blood progenitor cell transplantation: effects of recombinant human granulocyte-macrophage colony-stimulating factor on the autograft. *Blood* 1994; 83: 610-616.

[25] Kessinger A, Bishop MR, Anderson LR et al. Erythropoietin for mobilization of circulating progenitor cells in patients with previously-treated relapsed malignancies. *Exp. Hematol.* 1995; 23: 609-612.

[26] Vose JM, Kessinger A, Bierman PJ et al. The use of rhIL-3 for mobilization of peripheral blood stem cells in previously treated patients with lymphoid malignancies. *Int. J. Cell Cloning* 1992; 10 (suppl 1): 62-64.

[27] Pettengel R, Luft T, de Wynter E et al. Effects of interleukin-6 on mobilization of primitive haemopoietic cells into the circulation. *Br. J. Haematol.* 1995; 89: 237-242.

[28] Bishop MR, Vose JM, Bierman PJ et al. Phase I trial of PIXY 321 for peripheral stem cell mobilization in patients with lymphoid malignancies. *Exp. Hematol.* 1994; 22: 369a.

[29] Spitzer G, Mathews M, Dunphy F et al. Are growth factors (GF) combinations superior to G-CSF alone for mobilization of peripheral blood stem cells (PBSC): a randomised study comparing G-CSF to G-CSF with GM-CSF for PBSC mobilization. *Blood* 1994; 84 (suppl 1): 415a.

[30] Shpall EJ, Wheeler CA, Turner SA, et al. A randomised phase 3 study of peripheral blood progenitor cell mobilization with stem cell factor and filgrastim in high-risk breast cancer patients. *Blood* 1999; 93: 2491-2501.

[31] Isidorins A, Tani M, Bonifazi F et al. Phase II study of a single pegfilgrastim injection as an adjunct to chemotherapy to mobilize stem cells into the peripheral blood of pretreated lymphoma patients. *Haematologica,* 2005; 90 (2): 225-231.

[32] Steidl U, Fenk R, Bruns I et al. Successful transplantation of peripheral blood stem cells mobilized by chemotherapy and a single dose of pegylated G-CSF in patients with multiple myeloma. *Bone Marrow Transplant*, 2005; 35 (1): 33-36.

[33] Koc ON, Gerson SL, Cooper BW et al. Randomized cross-over trial of progenitor-cell mobilization: high-dose cyclophosphamide plus granulocyte colony-stimulating factor (G-CSF) versus granulocyte-macrophage colony-stimulating factor plus G-CSF. *J. Clin. Oncol.* 2000; 18: 1824-1830.

[34] Fitoussi O, Perreau V, Boiron JM, et al. A comparison of toxicity following two different doses of cyclophosphamide for mobilization of peripheral blood progenitor cells in 116 multiple myeloma patients. *Bone Marrow Transplant* 2001; 27: 837-842.

[35] Lerro KA, Medoff E, Wu Y, et al. A simplified approach to stem cell mobilization in multiple myeloma patients not previously treated with alkylating agents. *Bone Marrow Transplant* 2003; 32: 1113-1117.

[36] D'SA S, Yong K, Kyriakou C, et al. Etoposide, methylprednisolone, cytarabine and cisplatin successfully cytoreduces resistant myeloma patients and mobilizes them for transplant without adverse effects. *Br. J. Haematol.* 2004; 125: 756-765.

[37] Corso A, Arcaini L, Caberlon S et al. A combination of dexamethasone, cyclophosphamide, etoposide, and cisplatin is less toxic and more effective than high-dose cyclophosphamide for peripheral stem cell mobilizaton in multiple myeloma. *Haematologica* 2002; 87 (10): 1041-1045.

[38] Tricot G, Jagannath S, Vesole D, et al. Peripheral blood stem cell transplants for multiple myeloma: identification of favourable variables for rapid engraftment in 225 patients. *Blood* 1995; 85: 588-596.

[39] Bensinger WI, Appelbaum F, Rowley S et al. Factors that influence collection and engraftment of autologous peripheral-blood stem cells. *J. Clin. Oncol.* 1995; 2547-2555.

[40] Haas R, Mohle R, Fruhauf S et al. Patient characteristics associated with successful mobilizing and autografting of peripheral blood progenitor cells in malignant lymphoma. *Blood* 1994; 83: 3787-3794.

[41] Neben S, Hemman S, Montgomery M, et al. Hematopoietic stem cell deficit of transplanted bone marrow previously exposed to cytotoxic agents. *Exp. Hematol.* 1993; 21: 156-162.

[42] Dreger P, Kloss M, Petersen B et al. Autologous progenitor cell transplantation: prior exposure to stem cell-toxic drugs determines yield and engrafment of peripheral blood progenitor cell but not of bone marrow grafts. *Blood* 1995; 86 (10): 3970-3978.

[43] Corso A, Caberlon S, Pagnucco G, et al. Blood stem cell collections in multiple myeloma: definition of a scoring system. *Bone Marrow Transplant* 2000; 26: 283-286.

[44] Goldschmidt H, Hegenbart U, Wallmeier M, et al. Factors influencing collection of peripheral blood progenitor cells following high dose cyclophosphamide and granulocyte-colony-stimulating factor in patients with multiple myeloma. *Br. J. Haematol.* 1997; 98: 736-744.

[45] Canales MA, Fernandez-Jimenez MC, Martin A et al. Identification of factors associated with poor peripheral blood progenitor cell mobilization in Hodgkin's disease. *Haematologica,* 2001: 86: 494-498.

[46] Ketterer N, Salles G, Moullet I, et al. Factors associated with successful mobilization of peripheral blood progenitor cells in 200 patients with lymphoid malignancies. *Br. J. Haematol.,* 1998; 103: 235-242.

[47] Perea G, Sureda A, Martino R, et al. Predictive factors for a successful mobilization of peripheral blood CD34+ cells in multiple myeloma. *Ann. Hematol.* 2001; 80: 592-597.

[48] Demirer T, Buckner CD, Gooley T et al. Factors influencing collection of peripheral blood stem cells in patients with multiple myeloma. *Bone Marrow Transplant*, 1996; 17: 937-941.

[49] Kotasek D, Shepherd KM, Sage RE et al. Factors affecting blood stem cell collections following high-dose cyclophosphamide mobilization in lymphoma, myeloma and solid tumors. *Bone Marrow Transplant* 1992; 9:11-17.

[50] Krieger MS; Schiller G, Berenson JR, et al. Collection of peripheral blood progenitor cells (PBPC) based on a rising WBC and platelet count significantly increases the number of CD34+ cells. *Bone Marrow Transplant* 1996; 18: 1-7.

[51] Osma MM, Ortũno F, de Arriba F et al. Bone marrow steady-state CD34+/CD71- cell content is a predictive value of rhG-CSF-mobilized CD34+ cells. *Blood* 1998; 21: 983-985.

[52] Corso A, Varettoni M, Mangiacavalli S, et al. Bone marrow CD34+ cell count is predictive for adequate peripheral progenitor cell collection. *Leukemia Research*, 2005; 29: 159-163.

[53] To LB, Haylock DN, Simmons PJ, Juttner CA. The biology and clinical uses of blood stem cells. *Blood* 1997; 89: 2223-2258.

[54] Catley L., Anderson K. Strategies to improve the outcome of stem cell transplantation in multiple myeloma. *The Haematology Journal* 2004; 5: 9-23.

[55] Mavroudis D, Read E, Cottler Fox M, et al. CD34 cell dose predicts survival, posttransplant morbidity, and rate of hematologic recovery after allogeneic marrow transplants for hematologic malignancies. *Blood* 1996: 88: 3223-3229.

[56] Shpall EJ, Champlin R, Glaspy JA. Effect of CD34+ peripheral blood progenitor cell dose on hematopoietic recovery. *Biol. Blood Marrow Transplant* 1998; 4: 84-92.

[57] Bensinger WI, Longin K, Appelbaum F et al. Peripheral blood stem cells (PBSCs) collected after recombinant granulocyte colony stimulating factor (rhG-CSF): an analysis of factors correlating with the tempo of engraftment after transplantation. *Br. J. Haematol.* 1994; 87: 825-831.

[58] Bender JG, To LB, Williams S et al. Defining a therapeutic dose of peripheral blood stem cells. *J. Hematotherapy*, 1992; 1: 329-341.

[59] Schiller G, Rosen L, Vescio R et al. Threshold dose of autologous CD34 positive peripheral blood progenitor cells required for engraftment after myeloablative treatment for multiple myeloma. *Blood* 1994; 84 (suppl 1): 813a.

[60] Weaver CH, Birch R, Schwartzberg L, et al. CD34 content of peripheral blood progenitor cells (PBPC) is the single most powerful predictor of recovery kinetics in patients receiving myeloablative high-dose chemotherapy and PBPC infusion. *Blood* 1994; 84 (suppl 1). 1388a.

[61] Lefrère F, Delarue R, Somme D, et al. High dose CD34+ cells are not clinically relevant in reducing cytopenia and blood component consumption following myeloablative therapy and peripheral blood progenitor cell transplantation as compared with standard dose. *Transfusion* 2002; 42: 443-450.

[62] Siena S, Bregni M, Brando B et al. Flow citometry for clinical estimation of circulating hematopoietic progenitors for autologous transplantation in cancer patients. *Blood* 1991; 77: 400-409.

[63] Bender JG, Williams SF, Myers S et al. Characterization of chemotherapy mobilized peripheral blood progenitor cells for use in autologous stem cell transplantation. *Bone Marrow Transplant* 1992; 10: 281-285.

[64] Passos-Coelho JL, Braine HG, Davis JM et al. Predictive factors for peripheral-blood progenitor-cell collections using a single large-volume leukapheresis after cyclophosphamide and granulocyte-macrophage colony-stimulating factor mobilization. *J. Clin. Oncol.* 1995; 13: 705-714.

[65] Armitage S, Hargreaves R, Samson D et al. CD34+ counts to predict the adequate collection of peripheral blood progenitor cells. *Bone Marrow Transplant*, 1997; 20 (7): 587-591.

[66] Lie AK, Hui CH, Rawling T, et al. Granulocyte colony stimulating factor (G-CSF) dose dependent efficacy in peripheral blood stem cell mobilization in patients who had failed initial mobilization with chemotherapy and G-CSF. *Bone marrow Transplant* 1998; 22: 853-857.

[67] Narayanasami U, Kanteti R, Morelli J et al. Randomized trial of filgrastim versus chemotherapy and filgrastim mobilization of haematopoietic progenitor cells for rescue in autologous transplantation. *Blood* 2001; 98: 2059-2064.

[68] Koc ON, Gerson SL, Cooper BW et al. Randomized cross-over trial of progenitor-cell mobilization: high-dose cyclophosphamide plus granulocyte colony-stimulating factor (G-CSF) versus granulocyte-macrophage colony-stimulating factor plus G-CSF. *J. Clin. Oncol* 2000; 18: 1824-1830.

[69] Watts MJ, Ings SJ, Flynn M et al. Remobilization of patients who fail to achieve a minimal progenitor threshold at the first attempt is clinically worthwhile. *Br. J. Haematol.* 2000; 111: 287-291.

[70] Weaver CH, Tauer K, Zhen B et al. Second attempts at mobilization of peripheral blood stem cells in patients with initial low CD34+ cell yields. *J. Hematother* 1998; 7: 241-249.

[71] Fraipoint V, Sautois B, Pereira M, et al. Successful mobilization of peripheral blood HPCs with G–CSF alone in patients failing to achieve sufficient numbers of CD34+

cells and/or CFU-GM with chemotherapy and G-CSF. *Transfusion*, 2000; 40(3): 339-347.

[72] Boeve S, Strupeck J, Creech S, et al. Analysis of remobilisation success in patients undergoing autologous stem cell transplants who fail an initial mobilization: risk factors, cytokine use and cost. *Bone Marrow Transplant*, 2004; 33 (10): 997-1003.

[73] Dawson MA, Schwarer AP, Muirhead JL et al. Successful mobilization of peripheral blood stem cells using recombinant human stem cell factor in heavily pretreated patients who have failed a previous attempt with a granulocyte colony-stimulating factor-based regimen. *Bone Marrow Transplant*, 2005; 36 (5): 389-396.

[74] Facon T, Harousseau JL, Maloisel F, et al. Stem cell factor in combination with filgrastim after chemotherapy improves peripheral blood progenitor cell yield and reduces apheresis requirements in multiple myeloma patients: a randomized control trial. *Blood* 1999; 94: 1218-1225.

[75] Ross AM, Cooper BW, Lazarus HM et al. Detection and viability of tumor cells in peripheral blood stem cell collections from breast cancer patients using immunocytochemical and clonogenic assay techniques. *Blood* 1993; 82: 2605-2610.

[76] Gibson J, Pope B, Petersen A et al. G-CSF stimulated PBSC harvests in myeloma contain immature malignant plasma cells. *Blood* 1994; 84 (suppl 1): 422a.

[77] Owen RG, Child JA, Rawson A et al. Detection of contaminating cells in PBPC harvests and the efficacy of CD34 selection in patients with multiple myeloma. *Blood* 1994; 84 (suppl 1): 1392a.

[78] Witzig TE, Gertz MA, Pineda AA et al. Detection of monoclonal plasma cells in the peripheral blood stem cell harvests of patients with multiple myeloma. *Blood* 1994; 84 (suppl 1): 1393a.

[79] Cremer FW, Kiel K, Wallmeier M, et al. A quantitative PCR assay for the detection of low amounts of malignant cells in multiple myeloma. *Annals Oncology* 1997; 8: 633-636.

[80] Bensinger WI. Should we purge? *Bone marrow Transplantation* 1998; 21: 113-115.

[81] Schiller G, Vescio R, Freytes C, et al. Autologous CD34-selected progenitor cell transplants for patients with advanced multiple myeloma. *Bone marrow transplant.* 1998; 21(2): 141-145.

[82] Lemoli RM, Martinelli G, Olivieri A, et al. Selection and transplantation of autologous CD34+ B lineage negative cells in advanced phase multiple myeloma patients: a pilot study. *Br. J. Haematol.* 1999; 107: 419-428.

[83] Barbui AM, Galli M, Dotti G, et al. Negative selection of peripheral blood stem cells to support a tandem autologous transplantation programme in multiple myeloma. *Br. J. Haematol.* 2002; 116: 202-210.

[84] Boccadoro M, Omedè P, Dominietto A, et al. Multiple myeloma: the number of reinfused plasma cells does not influence outcome of patients treated with intensified chemotherapy and PBPC support. *Bone Marrow Transplant* 2000; 25: 25-29.

[85] Kessinger A, Bierman PJ, Cowles MK, et al. Mobilized versus non-mobilized peripheral stem cell transplantation after high dose therapy for low grade non-Hodgkin lymphoma. *Cancer Res. Ther. Control.* 1998; 5: 113-119.

[86] Cooper BW, Moss TH, Ross AA et al. Occult tumor contamination of hematopoietic stem-cell products does not affect clinical outcome of autologous transplantation in patients with metastatic breast cancer. *J. Clin. Oncol* .1998; 16: 3509-3517.

[87] Barlogie B, Jagannath S, Desikan KR, et al. Total therapy with tandem transplants for newly diagnosed multiple myeloma. *Blood* 1999; 93: 55-65.

[88] Goldschmidt H, Cremer FW, Hagenbart U, et al. Comparison of 3 high dose regimens with autologous peripheral blood stem cell transplantation for multiple myeloma: a single center experience in 261 patients. *Proc. VIIth Int. Multiple Myeloma Workshop* 1999; 117a.

[89] Alessandrino EP, Bernasconi P, Colombo A, et al. Pulmonary toxicity following carmustine-based preparative regimens and autologous peripheral blood progenitor cell transplantation in hematological malignancies. *Bone Marrow Transpl* 2000; 25 (13):309-313.

[90] Tribalto M, Amadori S, Cudillo L, et al. Autologous peripheral blood stem cell transplantation as first line treatment of multiple myeloma: an Italian multicenter Study. *Haematologica* 2000; 85: 52-58.

[91] Alegre A, Lamana M, Arranz R, et al. Busulfan and melphalan as conditioning regimen for autologous peripheral blood stem cell transplantation in multiple myeloma. *Br. J. Haematol.* 1995 Oct;91(2):380-6.

[92] Meloni G, Capria S, Trasarti S, et al. High dose idarubicin, busulfan and melphalan as conditioning for autologous blood stem cell transplantation in multiple myeloma. A feasibility study. *Bone Marrow Transplant* 2000; 26: 1045-1049.

[93] Phillips GL, Meisenberg B, Reece DE, et al. Amifostine and autologous hematopoietic stem cell support of escalating-dose melphalan: a phase I study. *Biol Blood Marrow Transplant* 2004; 10: 473-483.

[94] Moreau P, Hullin C, Frederic G, et al. Tandem autologous stem cell transplantation in high risk de novo multiple myeloma: final results of the prospective and randomized IFM 99-04 protocol. *Blood* 2005 prepublished online.

[95] Desikan KR, Tricot G, Dhodapkar M, et al. Melphalan plus total body irradiation (MEL-TBI) or Cyclophosphamide (MEL-CY) as a conditioning regimen with second autotransplant in responding patients with myeloma is inferior compared to historical controls receiving tandem transplants with melphalan alone. *Bone Marrow Transplant* 2000; 25: 483-487.

[96] Moreau P, Facon T, Attal M, et al. Comparison of 200 mg/mq melphalan and 8 Gy total body irradiation plus 140 mg/mq melphalan as conditioning regimens for peripheral stem cell transplantation in patients with newly diagnosed multiple myeloma: final analysis of the Intergroupe Francophone du Myelome 9505 randomized trial. *Blood* 2002; 99. 731-735.

[97] Attal M, Harousseau JL, Stoppa AM, et al. A prospective, randomised trial of autologous bone marrow transplantation and chemotherapy in multiple myeloma. Intergroupe Francais du Myelome. *NEJM* 1996; 335 (2): 91-97.

[98] Barlogie B, Shaughnessy J, Tricot G, et al. Treatment of multiple myeloma. *Blood* 2004; 103: 20-32.

[99] Child JA, Morgan GJ, Davies FE, et al. High dose chemotherapy with hematopoietic stem cell rescue for multiple myeloma. *N. Engl. J. Med.* 2003; 348: 1875-1883.

[100] Sirohi B, Powles R, Mehta J, et al. An elective single autograft with high-dose melphalan: single-center study of 451 patients. *Bone Marrow Transplant* 2005; 1-6.

[101] Barlogie B, Jagannath S, Desikan KR, et al. Total therapy with tandem transplant for newly diagnosed multiple myeloma. *Blood* 1999; 93: 55-65.

[102] Cavo M, Cellini C, Zamagni E, et al. Update on high dose therapy-Italian studies. The *Hematology Journal* 2005: 90(s1): 39.

[103] Fermand JP, Ravaud P, Chevret S, et al. High dose therapy and autologous peripheral blood stem cell transplantation in multiple myeloma: up front or rescue treatment? Results of a multicenter sequential randomised clinical trial. *Blood* 1998; 92: 3131-3136.

[104] Bladé J, Rosinol L, Sureda A, et al. High-dose therapy intensification versus continued standard chemotherapy in multiple myeloma patients responding to the initial chemotherapy: long term results from a prospective randomized trial from the Spanish cooperative group PETHEMA. *Blood* 2005; Aug 16 (Epub ahead).

[105] Palumbo A, Triolo S, Argentino C, et al. Dose-intensive melphalan with stem cell support (MEL 100) is superior to standard treatment in elderly myeloma patients. *Blood* 1999; 94: 1248-1253.

[106] Reece DE, Bredeson C, Pérez WS, et al. Autologous stem cell transplantation in multiple myeloma patients<60 vs ≥60 years of age. *Bone Marrow Transplant* 2003; 32: 1135-1143.

[107] Badros A, Barlogie B, Siegel E, et al. Autologous stem cell transplantation in elderly multiple myeloma patients over the age of 70 years. *Br. J. Haematol.* 2001; 114: 600-607.

[108] Singhal S, Metha J, Desikan R. Antitumor activity of thalidomide in refractory multiple myeloma. *N. Engl. J. Med*,1999; 341:1565-71.

[109] 109)Cavo M, Zamagni E, Tosi P, et al. Superiority of thalidomide and dexamethason eover vincristine-doxorubicin-dexamethasone (VAD) as primary therapy in preparation for autologous transplantation for multiple myeloma. *Blood* 2005; 106: 35-39.

[110] Palumbo A, Bertola A, Musto P, et al. Oral melphalan, prednisone, and thalidomide for newly diagnosed patients with myeloma. *Cancer*. 2005 Oct 1;104(7):1428-33.

[111] Weber DM, Chen C, Niesvizky R, et al. A multicenter randomized parallel group double-blind placebo-controlled study of lenalidomide plus dexamethasone versus dexamethasone alone in previously treated subjects with multiple myeloma. *Haematologica* 2005; suppl 1: 155.

[112] Harousseau JL, Attal M, Leleu X, et al. Bortezomib plus dexamethasone as induction treatment prior to autologous transplantation in patients with newly diagnosed multiple myeloma: preliminary results of an IFM pfase II study. *Haematologica* 2005; 90(suppl 1): 148 (Abstract PO. 724).

[113] Kervee HE, Popat R, Curry N, et al. PAD combination therapy (PS-341/bortezomib, doxorubicin and dexamethasone) for previously untreated patients with multiple myeloma. *Br. J. Haematol.* 2005 Jun;129(6):755-62.

[114] Wu KL, van Wieringen, Vellenga E, et al. Analysis of the efficacy and toxicity of bortezomib for treatment of relapsed or resistant multiple myeloma in community practice. *Haematologica* 2005; 90: 996-997.

In: Multiple Myeloma: Symptoms, Diagnosis and Treatment ISBN 978-1-60876-108-1
Editors: M. Georgiev and Ev. Bachev

Chapter 10

Autologous and Allogeneic Stem Cell Transplantation for Multiple Myeloma

***Evangelos Terpos*[1,2] *and John Meletis*[3]**
[1]Department of Haematology and Medical Research,
General Airforce Hospital, Athens, Greece
[2]Department of Haematology,
Faculty of Medicine Imperial College London, London, UK
[3]First Department of Internal Medicine,
University of Athens School of Medicine,
Laikon General Hospital, Athens, Greece

Abstract

Multiple myeloma (MM) is an incurable plasma cell malignancy. Despite the use of conventional therapy or high dose chemotherapy with autologous stem cell support (ASCT) patients continue to relapse at constant rate. A small minority of patients are cured by allogeneic transplantation. Up to now, ASCT has been the treatment of choice for eligible myeloma patients aged below 65 years of age. Melphalan at a dose of 200 mg/m^2 is considered the standard conditioning regimen for ASCT in MM. Early ASCT seems to be beneficial. A planned double ASCT gives better results than a single ASCT, especially in cases who have not achieved a complete response (CR) after the first ASCT. ASCT is also a suitable procedure for myeloma patients with renal failure.

Allogeneic bone marrow transplantation is too risky to be considered for most patients but the possibility of a potentially curable graft-versus-myeloma (GVM) effect, which has been demonstrated in MM, gives this procedure the best chance for long-term disease control and may be considered as a possible treatment option for patients aged less than 50 years with an HLA-identical sibling. Registry data show that in patients who have undergone allogeneic matched sibling-donor transplantation, the long-term survival is around 25%. However, the median survival is comparable with patients who receive ASCT, mainly due to the high TRM rate of between 20%-40%, which seems to be higher in male patients. Allogeneic transplantations with matched unrelated donors have an even higher TRM and may be considered only in exceptional cases. Chronic graft-versus-host disease (GVHD) correlates with CR in allotransplant patients and provides evidence of an allogeneic GVM effect. In order to harness the GVM effect, current research is focused on allogeneic transplantation from HLA identical sibling after conditioning with a non-myeloablative or reduced intensity conditioning (RIC) regimens followed by DLI to eradicate residual tumour. In a significant proportion of patients disease response is preceded by GVHD, suggesting a clear relationship between GVHD and GVM.

However, many questions regarding the management of myeloma patients remain unanswered. How safe is ASCT in elderly patients? Is there a role for non-myeloablative allogeneic transplantation in MM and in which subgroup of patients? What is the role of novel agents, such as thalidomide, its analogues, and bortezomib, in maintenance therapy post ASCT or allogeneic SCT? This chapter will summarize all available data for the role of SCT in MM.

Introduction

Definition and Epidemiology

Multiple myeloma (MM) is a B-cell malignancy characterized by a monoclonal expansion and accumulation of abnormal plasma cells in the bone marrow compartment. The clinical manifestations of myeloma are heterogeneous, and include bone complications, symptoms of impaired haemopoiesis and hyperviscosity, renal dysfunction, infections, peripheral neuropathy and extramedullary disease. MM comprises 1% of all cancers, and accounts for approximately 10% of haematological malignancies. Myeloma has an annual incidence in the United Kingdom (U.K.) of 60 per million per annum; at any one time there will be 10 - 15,000 patients with the condition. The median age at diagnosis is 60 - 65 years; fewer than 2% of myeloma patients are under 40 years old at diagnosis [1]. There are various theories about the age at onset and these include: (a) a reduction in ability of immune system of the elderly to eliminate potential myeloma precursors; (b) the cumulative impact of environmental exposures with age; and (c) hormonal effects of aging. However, recent statistics indicate that myeloma is increasing in incidence and occurring more frequently in individuals aged below 55 years. Myeloma seems to be more common in men than women. The reasons for this are unclear but may include both hormonal effects and job-related exposure. Myeloma has a higher incidence in Afro-Caribbean ethnic groups compared to Caucasians in the U.K., while in the U.S.A. the incidence also varies by race: from about 1/100,000 population/year for Asians, to about 4/100,000 population/year for Caucasians and to 8-10/100,000 population/year for Afro-Americans. A variety of genetic and environmental factors have been proposed to explain the increased incidence in individuals of African descent. Differences in hormone receptors, immune reactivity and toxin metabolism have been evaluated. The diversity of possible exposures and genetic susceptibility factors make proof difficult. Although there is a tendency for myeloma to occur in families (3-5%), the likelihood of inheritance is low and no inherited genes have been identified [2].

Pathogenesis

The precise stage at which malignant change occurs in myeloma cells has not yet been clarified. Current evidence suggests, however, that myeloma cell is a long-lived plasma cell, which has been exposed to antigen having undergone the B-cell maturation processes (Figure 1).

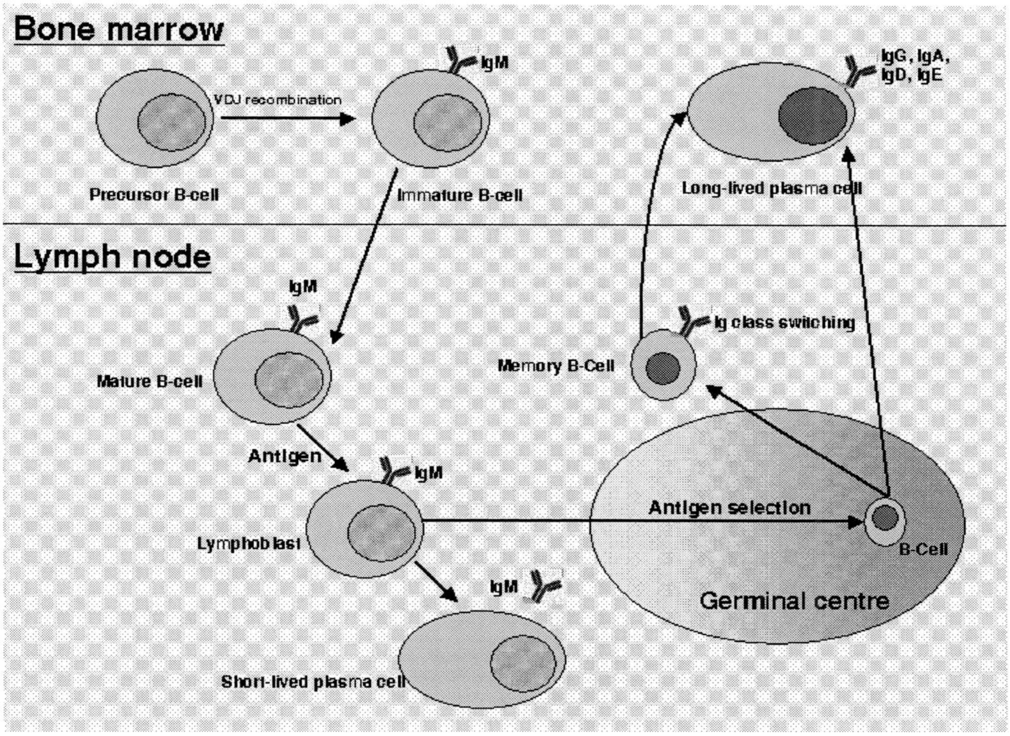

Figure 1. Maturation of normal B-cell precursors to mature plasma cells involves rearrangement of the Ig genes with subsequent somatic mutation of the variable (V) region. The myeloma cell is a post-germinal centre plasma cell, which has undergone immunoglobulin gene recombination, class-switching, and somatic hypermutation, and homes to the bone marrow.

The myeloma cell is a post-germinal centre plasma cell, which has undergone immunoglobulin gene recombination, class-switching, and somatic hypermutation, and homes to the bone marrow. Myeloma cells proliferate at a low rate. The plasma-cell labelling index typically detects less than 1% of tumour cells that are actively synthesising DNA until late in the course of the disease, and is a better prognostic indicator than plasma-cell infiltration of the bone marrow. Plasma cells may be identified by high CD38, high CD138 and low CD45 expression by flow cytometry. Myeloma cells are also $CD19^-$ or $CD19^+/CD56^+$, whereas normal plasma cells are consistently $CD19^+/CD56^-$. In myeloma, the proliferative cells usually express CD45 and the level of expression of this gene is higher than that observed in the non-proliferative compartment. Better clarification of the myeloma cell compartments will help to better understand the biology of the disease [3-6].

Table 1. Structural chromosomal abnormalities and involved oncogenes in myeloma

	Chromosomal abnormality	Genetical location	Incidence of cytogenetic abnormalities detected by conventional cytogenetics or FISH ( )	Involved oncogene	Function
High risk- Unfavourable cytogenetic abnormalities	13q deletion	usually 13q14	15% (50%)	RB-1	Cell cycle regulator
	t(4;14)	4p16.3 14q32	Undetected (15%)	1)FGFR3 2)MMSET 3)TACC3 4)CYCLIN D2	1)Growth factor receptor tyrosine kinase 2) Regulator of transcription 3)Unknown 4)Cell cycle regulator
	t(6;14)(p21;q32)	6p2114q32	(3-4%)	Cyclin D3	Cell cycle regulator
	t(6 ;14)(p25;q32)	6p25 14q32	(5%)	MUM/IRF4	Transcriptional regulator of IFN
	t(14;16)	14q32 16q23	(2-10%)	1)c-MAF 2)WWOX	1)Transcription factor 2)Unknown
	t(8;14)(q24 ;q32)	8q24 14q32	4-5%	c-myc	Cell cycle regulator
	t(14;20)	14q32 20q12	Recently defined	b-MAF	Transcription factor
	t(14;18)	14q32.33 18q21.3	(5%)	BCL-2	Apoptosis inhibitor
	17 p deletion	17p13	5% (10-15%)	P53	Cell cycle regulator; DNA repair replication
	Chromosome 1 abnormalities		20%	K-ras, N-ras gene mutations	Signal tranduction regulator; Cell cycle regulator
Low risk- favourable cytogenetic abnormalities	t(11;14)	14q32	5% (15-20%)	1)Cyclin D1 2)MYEOV	1)Cell cycle regulator 2)Unknown

Increasing evidence suggests that the development of myeloma is a multi-step process that includes the progressive occurrence of multiple structural chromosomal changes. Karyotypes of myeloma are more similar to those of epithelial tumours and the blast phase of chronic myeloid leukaemia than to those of other haemopoietic malignancies [7].

Monosomy 13, translocations into the switch regions of the IgH genes involving a large array of chromosomal partners (switch translocations), chromosome 8q (c-myc oncogene) abnormalities and other numerical chromosomal changes (monosomy, trisomy) are detected in up to 80%-90% of myeloma cases (Table 1).

Several studies have demonstrated that monosomy 13, detected by conventional cytogenetics, is a predictor for survival. However, the high incidence of this cytogenetic abnormality in MGUS patients and its co-existence in many cases with a large variety of other chromosomal aberrations, revealed by molecular cytogenetics, makes the prognostic value of monosomy 13 alone more difficult to ascertain. Conventional karyotyping has also demonstrated a poor prognosis associated with chromosome 11q translocations, including t(11;14) and reciprocal translocations with chromosomes 8, 9, and 12. However, this was not confirmed by molecular cytogenetics and the possibility that conventional karyotyping technique has selected out cases, which are hyperproliferative must be considered. Gene expression profile from microarray technology may provide a more accurate and comprehensive assessment of molecular changes in myeloma, and is currently used to characterize myeloma at a molecular level and correlate gene-expression with response rates in current trials of novel agents [8-12].

The pathogenesis of multiple myeloma is very complex and includes mutual interactions that affect the number and function of both malignant cells and normal bone marrow stromal cells (BMSCs). Bone marrow microenvironment includes the extracellular matrix, and at least five types of stromal cells: fibroblasts, osteoblasts, osteoclasts, vascular endothelial cells and lymphocytes. Reciprocal positive and negative interactions among these cells are mediated by a variety of cytokines and adhesion molecules. The homing of myeloma cells to the bone marrow seems to involve selective adhesion to bone marrow endothelial cells, transendothelial migration and adhesion to stromal cells through the production of stromal-derived factor 1 (SDF-1) and insulin-like growth factor 1 (IGF-1), which are secreted by bone marrow endothelial and stromal cells and have a chemoattractant effect on myeloma cells. Adhesion of myeloma cells to BMSCs, through the $\alpha 4\beta 1$ integrin/vascular cell-adhesion molecule 1 (VCAM-1) interaction, induces the paracrine secretion of cytokines such as interleukin-6 (IL-6), IL-1β, IL-11, tumour necrosis factors (TNFs), transforming growth factor-beta (TGF-β), macrophage inflammatory protein-1 alpha (MIP-1α) and receptor activator of nuclear factor-kappa B ligand (RANKL) by BMSCs (Figure 2). The production of IL-6 by BMSCs, which is *via* activation of the nuclear factor-kappa B (NF-κB), triggers the proliferation of myeloma cells, and protects them against dexamethasone-induced apoptosis. The activation of NF-κB, which is a transcriptional factor, is responsible for the production of other growth factors and adhesion molecules, such as vascular endothelial growth factor (VEGF), VCAM-1 and E-selectin, by the BMSCs and myeloma cells. Angiogenesis is also increased in some cases of myeloma and correlates with disease activity and survival. Secreted VEGF from myeloma cells interacts with receptors on endothelial cells to enhance their migration and proliferation. Additional factors, such as the basic fibroblast growth factor (bFGF), produced by either myeloma or stromal cells, also induce angiogenesis. Most of these cytokines (RANKL, IL-6, IL-1b, IL-11, MIP-1α, VEGF, bFGF, etc.) are potent osteoclast activators and lead to bone lytic disease, a major feature of MM. In myeloma, there is also an inhibition of T-lymphocyte function through mechanisms, which are not clear but may include production of inhibitory molecules, such as interferon-alpha (IFN-α) at high concentrations and reduction of interferon-gamma (IFN-γ) [13-23].

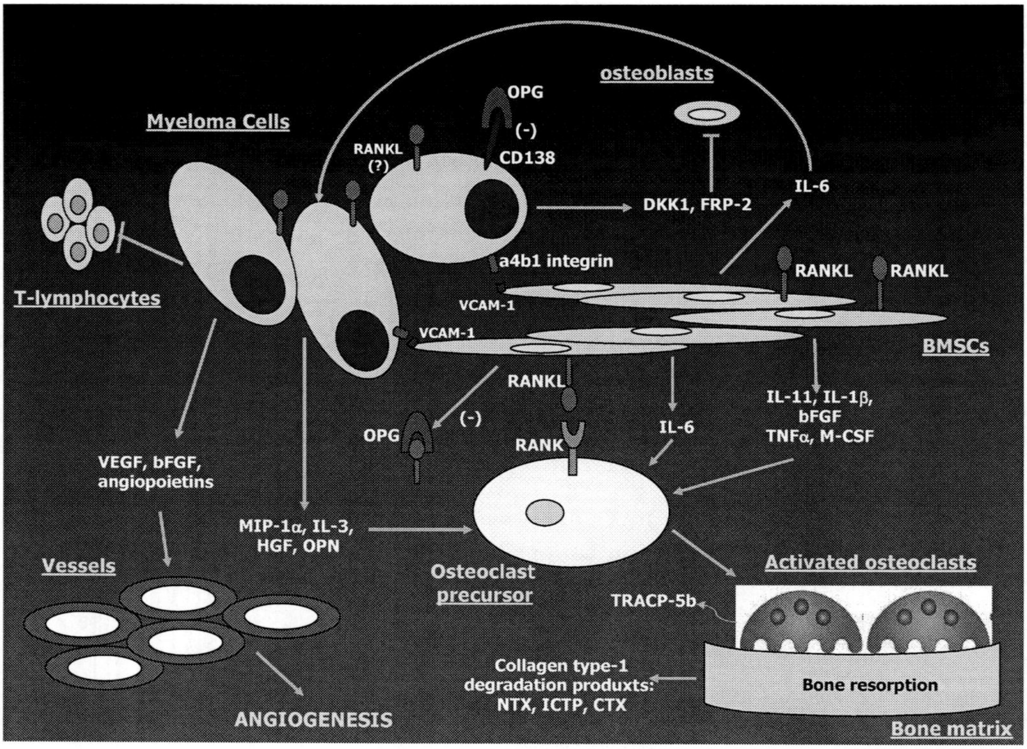

Figure 2. The bone marrow microenvironment in multiple myeloma. The multiple interactions between myeloma, stromal, endothelial cells, and osteoclasts reflect the vital role of the bone marrow microenvironment in the biology of the disease. The production of different cytokines by both stromal and myeloma cells enhances myeloma proliferation and growth, osteoclast activation, and vessel formation. Furthermore, the inhibition of T-lymphocytes, through mechanisms, which are unclear, increases the immunodeficiency in myeloma, while the suppression of osteoblasts in combination with osteoclast activation leads to bone loss.

Clinical Features

Plasma cell infiltration of bone marrow results in bone marrow failure and bone lesions. Patients, therefore, present with symptoms due to bone disease, hypercalcaemia, impaired haemopoiesis, immune paresis and renal failure.

Bone pain is the most common symptom and results from osteolytic lesions and pathological fractures. A large proportion of patients with multiple myeloma has reduced serum levels of normal immunoglobulins. In some of these patient, the immune paresis is severe enough to make them susceptible to bacterial infections and levels of immunoglobulin rarely return to normal levels following chemotherapy even if the disease has responded well and paraprotein levels have fallen. Immune paresis, renal failure, neutropenia and anti-myeloma therapy can combine to cause severe immuno-deficiency and infections are a major cause of death in these patients.

Table 2. Criteria for the diagnosis of multiple myeloma, indolent myeloma, and MGUS

A	Multiple myeloma		
	Major criteria	I	Plasmacytoma on tissue biopsy
		II	Bone marrow infiltration with > 30% of plasma cells
		III	Monoclonal globulin spike (paraprotein) on serum electrophoresis (IgG>35 g/L, IgA> 20 g/L), or on concentrated urine electrophoresis (>1g/24h of κ or λ light chains)
	Minor criteria	a	Bone marrow infiltration with 10 to 30% of plasma cells
		b	Paraprotein less than the level defined above
		c	Lytic bone lesions
		d	Normal IgM <0.5 g/L, IgA <1 g/L, or IgG <6 g/L
B	Indolent (or asymptomatic) multiple myeloma		
	Same as multiple myeloma except : No bone lesions or one asymptomatic lytic lesion (X-ray survey) Paraprotein level: IgG <70 g/L and IgA <50 g/L No symptoms : - haemoglobin > 10 g/dL - serum calcium normal - serum creatinine <170 μmol/L - no infections		
C	MGUS		
	Paraprotein present, but at levels:		IgG <35 g/L, IgA<20 g/L, urinary light chains <1g/24h
	Furthermore: Normal level of residual polyclonal immunoglobulins Bone marrow plasma cells <10% (and without cytological abnormalities) No bone lesions; No symptoms No evidence of other B-cell proliferative disorder		

Normochromic, normocytic anaemia is a common finding in myeloma and symptoms related to this may be a presenting feature at diagnosis. Anaemia may be due to the infiltration of the bone marrow by myeloma cells, due to chronic inflammation or the use of cytotoxic drugs. Neurological abnormalities are mainly caused by tumour growth compressing the spinal cord or cranial nerves. Peripheral neuropathy is frequently due to perineuronal amyloid deposition. Polyneuropathy may also be observed as a part of POEMS syndrome (polyneuropathy, organomegaly, endocrinopathy, monoclonal gammopathy, and skin changes). Plasma-cell leukaemia may involve the meninges, while intracerebral mass lesions are very rare. Hyperviscosity occurs in less than 10% of patients and usually associated with an IgA paraprotein. Coagulopathy in MM is well documented but is rarely a clinical problem. Amyloidosis results from the abnormal extracellular deposition and accumulation of protein and protein derivatives and is clinically evident in around 5% of patients with MM. In a minority of patients plasma cell infiltration of soft tissues is seen at presentation. Plasmacytomas may spread extradurally or may cause spinal cord compression. High serum paraprotein may result in hyperviscosity and high levels of light chains (Bence-Jones protein) in the urine may result in renal failure [2].

Staging and Diagnosis

Table 2 summarizes the diagnostic criteria for MM, while tables 3 and 4 depict the Durie- Salmon and International Staging System, respectively [2,24].

Table 3. The Durie – Salmon staging system

Stage I
All of the following
Haemoglobin >10.5 g/dL
Serum calcium normal
X-rays show normal bone structure or solitary bone plasmacytoma only
Low paraprotein levels:
IgG <50 g/L
IgA <30 g/L
Urinary light chain <4g/24h
Stage II
Fitting neither stage I nor stage III
Stage III
One or more of the following
Haemoglobin <8.5 g/dL
Serum calcium > 3mmol/L
Advanced lytic bone lesions (>3 lytic lesions)
High paraprotein levels:
IgG >70 g/L
IgA >50 g/L
Urinary light chain >12 g/24h

Subclassification (either A or B):
A: serum creatinine <170μmol/L
B: serum creatinine ≥170μmol/L

Treatment of Multiple Myeloma

Myeloma remains an incurable neoplasia. The median survival is less than 3 years and the prospects for survival at ten years are poor with conventional chemotherapy (CC). Autologous stem cell transplantation (ASCT) after high-dose melphalan conditioning has substantially increased the frequency of remission and has prolonged progression-free survival (PFS) and overall survival (OS) compared with CC [25]. However, patients inevitably relapse and salvage chemotherapy is usually ineffective.

Table 4. International Prognostic Index for multiple myeloma

Staging	Parameters	No of patients	Median survival (months)
STAGE 1	$\beta_2M < 3.5$ ALB ≥ 35	2401	62
STAGE 2	$\beta_2M < 3.5$ ALB < 35 or β_2M 3.5-5.5	3278	44
STAGE 3	$\beta_2M > 5.5$	2770	29

β2M: serum β2-microglobulin in mg/L
ALB: serum albumin in g/L
Factors that predicting for lower risk:
Age < 60 + β2M < 3.5 mg/L + ALB > 35 g/L
Factors that predicting for higher risk: β2M > 10 mg/L + ALB < 35 g/L low platelet count.
Cytogenetics do influence outcome; however, chromosome 13 deletion and complex chromosome abnormalities do not seem to add to the impact of age, β2M and ALB.

Treatment of Asymptomatic/Indolent Multiple Myeloma

Patients with paraprotein level in the serum of ≥30 g/L and/or bone marrow clonal plasma cells of ≥10%, with no symptoms, and no myeloma-related organ or tissue impairment, who have asymptomatic or smouldering myeloma, according to the International Myeloma Working Group [1], may remain stable for a long time without any chemotherapy. These patients account for about 15-20% of myeloma patients, and have a median time to disease progression of between 2-3 years. The survival is similar when CC is administered just after diagnosis or at disease progression [26]. However, there are no data for the effect of ASCT on eligible stage I patients in terms of PFS. In these patients, disease needs to be evaluated at regular intervals (every 2-3 months) to separate the stable, asymptomatic patients, from patients with progressive, symptomatic disease. Signs of disease progression, such as rising paraprotein levels, falling haemoglobin levels, radiological evidence of bone disease, or an increase in bone marrow infiltration, are indications to start treatment. Asymptomatic patients with at least one lytic lesion in X-rays have a median time to progression of 8 months; therefore, they should be treated at diagnosis. Moreover, abnormal marrow appearance on magnetic resonance imaging (MRI) is also associated with higher risk of disease progression [27,28]. Further studies are needed to clarify if these patients need to start treatment earlier.

Treatment of Symptomatic Multiple Myeloma

Conventional chemotherapy has been the gold standard for myeloma therapy since 1960's. The classical anti-myeloma regimen of melphalan plus prednisolone (MP) induces partial remission (PR), in approximately 50% patients, while CR is very rare [29]. The combination of vincristine and adriamycin administered by continuous 4 days infusion with the addition of high-dose oral dexamethasone (VAD) is the most frequently used first-line chemotherapy regimen for myeloma. This regimen produces quick and high response rates (up to 80%) with a CR rate of 10-25% [30,31]. Several other combined chemotherapeutic regimens have been used for the management of myeloma patients (Table 5).

Table 5. Conventional chemotherapy regimens for the treatment of multiple myeloma

Drug Regimen	Dose	Days
MP (many variations) M = Melphalan P = Prednisolone	 7mg/m^2/day p.o. 60mg/day p.o.	 1-5 1-5
Cyclophosphamide Prednisolone	400mg/m^2 p.o. 60mg p.o. alternate days for 6 weeks	Once a week for 12 weeks Alternate days
VAD regimen (28-day cycle) V = Vincristine A = Doxorubicin (adriamycin) D = Dexamethasone	 0.4mg/day c.i.v. 9mg/m^2/day c.i.v. 40mg/day p.o.	 1-4 1-4 1-4 (and 9-12, 17-20 in the first cycle)
VAMP (28 day cycle) V= Vincristine A = Doxorubicin (adriamycin) MP = Methylprednisolone	 0.4mg/day c.i.v. 9mg/m^2/day c.i.v. Methylprednisolone 1.5g i.v./p.o.	 1-4 1-4 1-5
C-VAMP (28 day cycle) C = Cyclophosphamide V= Vincristine A = Doxorubicin (adriamycin) MP = Methylprednisolone	 Cyclophosphamide 500mg i.v 0.4mg/day c.i.v. 9mg/m^2/day c.i.v. Methylprednisolone 1.5g i.v./p.o.	 1, 8, 15 1-4 1-4 1-5
Z-Dex (21-day cycle) Z = Idarubicin (Zavedos) Dex = Dexamethasone	 10mg/m^2/day p.o. 40mg/day p.o.	1-4 1-4(and 8-11, 15-18 in the first cycle
VMCP (21-day cycle) V = Vincristine M = Melphalan C = Cyclophosphamide P = Prednisolone	 1mg i.v. 5mg/m^2/day p.o. 110mg/m^2/day p.o. 60mg/m^2/day p.o.	 1 1-4 1-4 1-4

Drug Regimen	Dose	Days
ABCM (28-day cycle) A = Doxorubicin B = BCNU C = Cyclophosphamide M = Melphalan	 30mg/m^2 i.v. 30mg/m^2 i.v. 100mg/m^2/day p.o. 6mg/m^2/day p.o.	 1 1 22-25 22-25
Thalidomide	100mg-600mg/day p.o.	Daily
CTD (21-day cycle) C = Cyclophosphamide T = Thalidomide D = Dexamethasone	 500mg p.o. 100-200mg/day p.o. 40mg/day p.o.	 1, 8, 15 Daily 1-4 and 12-15
CVAD (21-day cycle) C = Cyclophosphamide V = Vincristine A = Doxorubicin (adriamycin) D = Dexamethasone	 500mg p.o. or i.v. 0.4mg/day c.i.v. 9mg/m^2/day c.i.v. 40mg/day p.o.	 1, 8, 15 1-4 1-4 1-4 and 12-15
Thal/ Dex (28-day cycle) (many variations) Thal = Thalidomide Dex = Dexamethasone	 100-200mg/day p.o. 40mg/day p.o.	 daily 1-4 (and 14-18) or once a week
TCED (28-day cycle) T = Thalidomide C = Cyclophosphamide E = Etoposide D = Dexamethasone	 400mg/day p.o. 400mg/m^2/day c.i.v. 40mg/m^2/day c.i.v. 40mg/day p.o.	 Daily 1-4 1-4 1-4
Bortezomib (21-day cycle x 8 then 35-day cycle x 3) with or without Dex	Bortezomib: 1.3mg/m^2 i.v Dex: as in VAD	1,4,8,11 (in the 21 day cycle) 1,8,15,22 (in the 35-day cycle)
Lenalidomide plus Dex (28-day cycle x 9)	Len: 25 mg/d p.o. Dex: as in VAD	D1-21

c.i.v = continuous intravenous infusion.

A meta-analysis of 6,633 patients from 27 randomised trials comparing combination chemotherapy with MP showed that response rates were higher in combination regimens than in MP (60% *vs.* 53.2%; p<0.00001). However, outcome after treatment with combined regimens is very similar and they offer no advantage over MP [32]. Nevertheless, MP must be avoided in patients who are going to be treated with ASCT due to its toxicity to bone marrow stem cells.

The role of interferon-alpha (IFN-α) as part of induction therapy in MM has been controversial for several years. Two large meta-analyses studies of 4802 patients showed a slight benefit in both PFS and OS (6 and 2 months, respectively) in patients treated with chemotherapy plus IFN-α [33,34]. However, the Nordic Myeloma Study Group has shown no benefit in survival in patients treated with IFN-α during induction chemotherapy, while there is a significant reduction in quality of life for patients receiving IFN-α during the first year of treatment [35,36]. Therefore, it seems that there is no role for IFN-α in induction treatment.

Autologous stem cell transplantation for Myeloma

In the absence of any significant progress in CC, HDT with ASCT has become the treatment of choice for symptomatic eligible patients with MM. It is usually given after initial cytoreduction with VAD-related regimens. The median overall survival (OS) from diagnosis for patients who underwent ASCT is approximately 6 years [37-40].

Asct versus Conventional Chemotherapy

Several randomized trials have demonstrated the superiority of ASCT against CC in terms of increasing CR rate, median PFS and OS. The first was conducted by the Intergroupe Francophone du Myélome (IFM) in 200 previously untreated patients under the age of 65 years with stage II/III myeloma. Patients received four to six cycles of VMCP/BVAP induction followed by randomisation to additional CC for a total of 18 cycles or high-dose melphalan and total body irradiation (TBI) followed by ASCT. The response rate among the patients who received ASCT was 81% (including CR in 22% and very good PR (vgPR) in 16%), whereas it was 57% (CR in 5% and vgPR in 9%) in the group treated with CC ($p<0.001$). The probability of event-free survival (EFS) for five years was 28% in the ASCT group and 10% in the conventional-dose group ($p=0.01$); the overall estimated rate of survival for five years was 52% in the high-dose group and 12% in the CC group ($p=0.03$). Treatment-related mortality was similar in the two groups [41]. This result was confirmed by a large MRC trial in which 407 patients with previously untreated myeloma who were younger than 65 years of age received either CC alone or CC followed by HDT and ASCT. Among the 401 patients who could be evaluated, the rates of CR were higher in the ASCT group than in the standard-therapy group (44% *vs.* 8%, $p<0.001$), while the rates of PR were similar (42% and 40%, respectively), and the rates of minimal response were lower in ASCT group than in the standard-therapy group (3% vs. 18%, $p<0.001$). Intention-to-treat analysis showed a higher rate of OS ($p=0.04$) and PFS ($p<0.001$) in the ASCT group than in the standard-therapy group. As compared with standard therapy, HDT+ASCT increased median OS by almost 12 months (54.1 months vs. 42.3 months). There was a trend toward a greater survival benefit in the group of patients with a poor prognosis, as defined by a high beta2-microglobulin level (more than 8 mg/L) [42].

However, other trials have not confirmed the superiority of ASCT in terms of OS, although most of them have shown a better CR rate and a longer median PFS. Fermand *et al* evaluated the impact of HDT with ASCT in 190 patients with symptomatic MM aged between 55 and 65 years. These patients were randomly assigned to receive either CC (monthly courses of a regimen of vincristine, melphalan, cyclophosphamide, and prednisone) or HDT and ASCT (using either melphalan alone 200 mg/m^2, iv, or melphalan 140 mg/m^2, iv, plus busulfan 16 mg/kg orally as pre-transplantation cytoreduction. Within a median follow-up of 120 months, median EFS times were 25 and 19 months in the HDT and CC groups, respectively. Median OS time was 47.8 months in the HDT group compared with 47.6 months in the CC group. A trend to better EFS ($p=0.07$) was observed in favour of HDT, whereas OS curves were not statistically different. The period of time without symptoms, treatment, and treatment toxicity (TwiSTT) was significantly longer for the HDT patients than for the CC patients (p=0.03) [43]. These controversial results led three North American cooperative groups to launch a prospective randomized trial in 1993 comparing HDT (melphalan 140 mg/m^2 plus total-body irradiation 12 Gy) with CC using the vincristine, carmustine, melphalan, cyclophosphamide, and prednisone regimen. The results were published recently. Responders on both arms were randomly assigned to IFN-α or no maintenance treatment. With a median follow-up time of 76 months, no differences were observed in response rates between the two study arms (HDT, n = 261 patients; CC, n = 255 patients). Similarly, PFS and OS durations did not differ between the HDT and CC arms, with 7-year estimates of PFS of 17% and 16%, respectively, and OS of 37% and 42%, respectively. Of 242 patients achieving at least 75% tumour reduction, no difference was observed in PFS or OS among the 121 patients randomly assigned to IFN-α and the 121 patients randomly assigned to no maintenance therapy. Among 157 patients relapsing on SDT, 87 received a salvage ASCT; their median survival time of 30 months was only slightly better than the survival time of the remaining patients who were managed with further CC (23 months; p=0.13) [44].

In all studies, transplant related mortality (TRM) was <5% and not greater than that observed with CC. From this large experience we conclude that HDT supported by ASCT is the standard treatment for patients with newly diagnosed MM, at least up to the age of 65, as it increases response rates and quality of life and at least in some of them OS and PFS. Larger trials are needed to clarify the group of patients who have the major advantage from this procedure.

What is the best Conditioning Regimen?

A randomised controlled trial compared two widely used conditioning regimens before ASCT in newly diagnosed MM patients younger than 65 years old: 8 Gy total body irradiation plus 140 mg/m^2 melphalan (arm A) *versus* 200 mg/m^2 melphalan (arm B). A total of 282 evaluable patients were compared: 140 in arm A and 142 in arm B. Baseline characteristics and disease response to 4 cycles of the VAD regimen performed before randomization and ASCT were identical in the two treatment arms. In arm B, haematologic recovery was significantly faster for both the duration of neutropenia and thrombocytopenia, transfusion requirements were also significantly lower, and the median duration of hospitalization was significantly shorter. In arm A, the incidence of severe mucositis was significantly increased. The median duration of EFS was similar in both arms (21 *vs.* 20.5 months), but the 45-month OS was 65.8% in arm B *vs.* 45.5% in arm A (p=0.05) [45]. Therefore, 200 mg/m^2 melphalan is considered the standard conditioning regimen for ASCT in MM.

What is the best Time for ASCT Following MM Diagnosis?

One randomised trial enrolling 202 patients that compared early *versus* late ASCT showed that there were similar rates of deaths in both groups with no significant different OS. However, early ASCT was associated with shorter period of chemotherapy administration and lower toxicity [46]. In a retrospective analysis based on 211 myeloma patients who underwent an ASCT in Hammersmith Hospital, we also found no difference in OS between patients who were transplanted within 6, 9 or 12 months following initial diagnosis [40]. Based on available data we propose early ASCT. One strategy could be to perform early ASCT but to store before hand stem cells for another ASCT at relapse.

Is Purging of Autologous Stem Cells Beneficial?

A randomised, multicentre trial, compared patients who received an autograft of CD34-selected or unselected peripheral blood stem cells (PBSC). The median time to recovery of normal cell count, number of transfusions required, hospitalisation days, TRM, PFS, and OS were similar between the two transplant groups. This trial showed that although CD34 selection reduces myeloma cell contamination in PBSC collections, no improvement in survival was achieved [47].

Factors that Predict for Survival Post ASCT

High levels of β_2-microglobulin, C-reactive protein or lactate dehydrogenase and low levels of albumin at diagnosis have been associated with poorer OS [48,49]. The achievement of CR post ASCT correlates with better prognosis [37,40,50]. Genetic abnormalities, such as hypodiploidy, chromosome 13 deletions, t(4;14) translocation and myelodysplastic-type abnormalities, evaluated by conventional cytogenetics or FISH techniques, are also associated with poor prognosis post ASCT [51-54]. Furthermore, the combination of standard biochemical markers, such as high β_2-microglobulin, and cytogenetic abnormalities (hypodiploidy and/or chromosome 13 deletions) have revealed groups of patients with very poor prognosis, even with tandem transplants, for whom novel treatment strategies are needed [55,56]. Other biological parameters, such as the dose of infused lymphocytes in the autograft and the levels of VEGF pre-ASCT, directly correlate with clinical outcome after ASCT [57,58]. Finally, gene expression profiling of CD138-enriched plasma cells from untreated myeloma patients has recently allowed the identification of myeloma patients with poor outcome and seems to be in near future the method of choice for the identification of patients who need specific/targeted treatment regimens [59].

Single versus Double Autologous Transplantation

A randomised IFM trial (IFM94) compared single *versus* double ASCT in 399 previously untreated MM patients. Patients who received a tandem double transplantation had a better probability of 7-year PFS (23% *vs.* 13%, respectively; $p<0.01$) and 7-year OS (42% *vs.* 21%, respectively; $p=0.01$). There was no difference in terms of haematopoietic reconstitution and TRM between the two studied groups. Unfortunately, the patients in the single transplant group received HDT with 140mg/m^2 melphalan and 8Gy total body [60]. This combination has already been shown to result in inferior survival when compared with HDT of 200mg/m^2 melphalan alone [45]. Therefore, the same group evaluated the effect of HDT and double tandem ASCT in high risk myeloma patients, as assessed by the combination of high levels of β_2-microglobulin and chromosome 13 deletion. In this cohort of patients, the impact of a murine anti-IL-6 monoclonal antibody (BE-8) was also evaluated as part of the second conditioning regimen. Conditioning for the first ASCT was accomplished with melphalan 200 mg/m^2 and for the second one with melphalan 220 mg/m^2 plus dexamethasone with or without BE-8 infusion. This trial included 219 patients, of whom 166 were randomized, 85 without BE-8 (arm A) and 81 with BE-8 (arm B). The median OS and EFS times of the whole group of patients were 41 and 30 months, respectively. Response rates, OS, and EFS were not different between the 2 arms of the trial. OS at 54 months was 46% in arm A and 51% in arm B; median EFS was 35 months in arm A and 31 in arm B. The authors concluded that in high-risk patients the dose intensity of melphalan at 420 mg/m^2 led to encouraging results, but the addition of anti-IL-6 monoclonal antibody to the second conditioning regimen did not improve either OS, nor EFS [61].

The "Bologna 96" trial confirmed the beneficial effect of tandem ASCT in terms of EFS, but not in terms of OS, in 288 previously untreated symptomatic MM patients. The comparison was between one single 200 mg/m^2 melphalan and a tandem ASCT (the first was a 200 mg/m^2 ASCT followed 3-6 months later by a melphalan 120 mg/m^2 plus busulfan 12 mg/kg ASCT). The authors concluded that double transplantation prolonged both EFS and PFS and was of particular benefit for patients who failed to achieve at least near CR post first ASCT [62]. Two other studies, using different doses of melphalan plus TBI as conditioning regimens, showed also no superiority of tandem transplants in terms of OS, although there was a trend in favour of double ASCT in terms of EFS [63,64]. A recent meta-analysis, based on 7452 patients of the EBMT registry showed that the median survival from transplantation is 60 months for the planned second ASCT, compared with 51 months for the remainder group. A time-dependent multivariate Cox analysis showed that, taking patients without a second transplantation as a reference group, those receiving a second transplantation in first remission (i.e. before relapse) showed an increased probability of TRM, especially if the transplantation is performed more than 12 months after the first, and the reduction of the risk of relapse is less than when the transplantation is performed earlier. Performing a second transplantation after relapse did not seem to prolong survival, though a second transplantation before relapse is associated with a higher probability of mortality [65]. Therefore, to improve survival of tandem ASCT in MM, the second transplantation should preferably be performed before relapse and within 6 to 12 months of the first transplantation.

Finally, a recent study from Arkansas group showed that a planned third ASCT can achieve a meaningful survival (median 10 months post 3rd ASCT) in approximately 50% of patients who have derived survival from the 2nd ASCT of at least 3 years and have a preserved albumin concentration as an indication of their overall performance status [66].

Is Autologous Transplantation Suitable For The Elderly?

The role of ASCT in older MM patients is unclear. A recent pair-matched analysis compared the outcome of 110 patients ≥60 years, who underwent ASCT with that of 382 patients <60 years. The one-year TRM was 9% in patients <60 years, compared with 8% in patients ≥60 years. The relapse rate, PFS and OS in the two groups were also similar [67]. Our group has also shown that age was not an important prognostic factor for OS post ASCT at a cut-off value of 55, 60 or 65 years [37,40]. Palumbo *et al* studied 194 myeloma patients who were randomized to receive at diagnosis either CC (6 courses of MP) or intermediate-dose therapy (2 courses of melphalan at 100 mg/m^2) with ASCT. Response rate was higher after ASCT. Near-complete remission (nCR) was 6% after MP and 25% after ASCT (p=0.0002). At 3 years, ASCT increased EFS from 16% to 37% and OS from 62% to 77% (p<0.001). Similar results were observed in patients aged 65 to 70: nCR was 8% after MP and 25% after ASCT (p=0 .05); at 3 years, ASCT improved EFS from 18% to 31% (p =0.01) and OS from 58% to 73% (p=0 .01). Patients aged 65 to 70 had a median OS of 37.2 months (MP) *versus* 58 months (ASCT) [68]. The results of these and other studies indicate that ASCT can be safely performed in selected older patients with good performance status.

Is ASCT a Suitable Procedure for Myeloma Patients with Renal Failure?

HDT with ASCT may also be carried out in patients with renal failure if they are otherwise fit. Renal failure did not affect the quality of stem cell collections or engraftment [69]. The TRM for patients with renal impairment is around 6% and the probability of survival at three years is 55% [69], while the probability of OS at five years is 35% in dialysis-dependent patients [70]. The Spanish registry reported that response to HDT was independent of renal function. In this study, 43% of patients with renal failure both at diagnosis and pre-ASCT (group 2) showed an improvement in renal function (creatinine < 2 mg/dL) after transplant. The three-year overall survival from transplantation was 56, 49 and 61% for patients with renal failure only at diagnosis, for patients of group 2, and for patients without renal failure (control group), respectively, with a statistically significant difference favouring control group (p<0.01). According to these results, ASCT is an attractive alternative for MM patients with renal insufficiency, and it should not constitute a criterion for exclusion from transplant unless patients display poor performance status and very high creatinine levels (>5 mg/dL) [71]. The suggested dose of melphalan as conditioning regimen is 140 mg/m^2.

Can Maintenance Therapy Prolong the Beneficial Effect Of ASCT?

Several studies tries to answer this critical question, as most myeloma patients develop recurrent disease after undergoing transplantation and new treatment approaches are needed. The use of CC post-ASCT has not produced promising results as only half of the patients could tolerate it [72]. The use of novel agents, such as thalidomide, bortezomib and lenalidomide has led to the administration of such agents post-ASCT. There is only one published, retrospective, study in 112 patients with MM: 54 patients had received busulfan, cyclophosphamide, and etoposide (Bu/Cy/VP-16), and 58 patients received high-dose melphalan (200 mg/m^2) followed by ASCT. After transplantation, 36 patients received thalidomide for maintenance or salvage therapy, and 76 patients received no post-transplantation thalidomide. At a median follow-up of 58 months, the median survival was 54 months. There was no statistically significant difference noted with regard to response to conditioning regimen, PFS, or OS between the Bu/Cy/VP-16 and ASCT cohorts. Patients who received thalidomide after transplantation had improved median survival (65.5 months) compared with patients who did not receive thalidomide (44.5 months). More importantly, patients who received thalidomide as maintenance had improved OS compared with patients who received thalidomide as salvage (65 months *vs.* 54 months) [73]. The post-ASCT use of thalidomide seems to improve the survival of patients compared with historical controls from the prethalidomide era. However, the prospective trials that are underway will show the benefit (if any) of thalidomide in the post-transplantation setting.

A Canadian group conducted a phase II pilot study with 28 post-ASCT myeloma patients treated with a sequential, cycling maintenance regimen. The regimen was designed to include a variety of active myeloma agents chosen for ease of administration to enhance patient compliance and scheduled sequentially to minimize toxicity. The 12-month cycling schedule included dexamethasone (months 1-3); melphalan and prednisone (months 4, 5); cyclophosphamide and prednisone (months 6, 7); alpha-interferon (months 8-10); followed by a drug holiday (months 11, 12). The regimen was generally well tolerated with five patients developing reversible grade III-IV toxicity (diabetes-induced hyperglycemia in four, neutropenia in one). There was one toxic death on study due to non-neutropenic pneumonia and sepsis. Median EFS from transplant was 36.9 months with median OS not yet reached at a median follow-up of 44 months [74]. This concept of cycling, sequential maintenance with various agents, perhaps including newer biological, targeted agents, seems to warrant further investigation in multiple myeloma.

ASCT in Refractory/Relapsed Patients

ASCT has been also used for the management of relapsed and refractory myeloma. Patients with alkylating agent- or VAD-refractory disease may still respond to high dose melphalan followed by ASCT [75]. In a study conducted in 130 consecutive myeloma patients eligible for HDT, a second ASCT was offered in case of relapse or progression after the first ASCT. A total of 107 (82%) patients completed the first ASCT. Relapse or progression occurred in 70 patients; 26 received a second ASCT (with a median time of 20.4

months from first ASCT). An objective response (CR+PR) was obtained in 69% of these patients. Median OS and EFS after the second ASCT were 38.1 and 14.8 months. TRM was 1.9% after the first ASCT but no deaths occurred after the second [76]. This study suggests that a second ASCT after relapse or progression is a safe and effective global strategy to treat MM patients.

In a recent study, 26 patients with advanced-stage relapsed/refractory myeloma were treated with melphalan 50 mg/m^2 and bortezomib 1.3 mg/m^2 on days -6 and -3 in association with thalidomide 200 mg and dexamethasone 20 mg on days -6 through -3, followed by ASCT on day 0. Non-haematologic toxicities included pneumonia, febrile neutropenia, and peripheral neuropathy. All patients had undergone ASCT at diagnosis, and 13 patients (50%) underwent an additional transplantation at relapse. Responses occurred in 17 of 26 patients (65%), including 1 CR, 3 nCR (12%), and 2 vgPR (8%). Response rate was higher than that induced by the previous line of treatment in 12 patients (46%) [77]. This study shows that the combination of novel agents with ASCT produces encouraging antimyeloma activity in patients with refractory and relapsed disease and warrants further evaluation.

Allogeneic Stem Cell Transplantation

Standard Allogeneic Transplantation

Allogeneic bone marrow transplantation is too risky to be considered for most patients but the possibility of a potentially curable graft-versus-myeloma (GVM) effect, which has been demonstrated in MM [78], gives this procedure the best chance for long-term disease control and may be considered as a possible treatment option for patients aged less than 50 years with an HLA-identical sibling. Registry data show that in patients who have undergone allogeneic matched sibling-donor transplantation, the long-term survival is around 25% [79]. However, the median survival is comparable with patients who receive ASCT (especially ASCT shows better short-term OS than allo-transplantation), mainly due to the high TRM rate of between 20%-40%, which seems to be higher in male patients [50,80,81]. Allogeneic transplantations with matched unrelated donors have an even higher TRM and may be considered only in exceptional cases and carried out at specialized centres in the context of a clinical trial [82]. Patients who survive the procedure have a 60% chance of achieving a CR and a 50% possibility of achieving molecular remission compared with 7% of patients who have a molecular remission after ASCT [83]. However, only around 20% of allografted patients are in continued CR five or more years post transplant [84]. Chronic graft-versus-host disease (GVHD) correlates with CR in allotransplant patients and provides further evidence of an allogeneic GVM effect [85]. There are a number of small studies in the literature showing a direct GVM effect of donor lymphocyte infusions (DLI). The GVM effect of DLI is often accompanied by severe GVHD [86]. The response to DLI is related to GVHD, suggesting that in MM, targets for GVH and GVM are possibly identical or that antitumour activity is related to GVHD [78].

We conclude that allogeneic transplantation may be an alternative for patients below the age of 50 years with adverse prognostic factors (i.e. chromosome 13 deletions), who have an available HLA-identical sibling and have relapsed after tandem autologous transplantation.

Reduced-Intensity Allogeneic Transplantation

In order to harness the GVM effect, current research is focused on allogeneic transplantation from HLA identical sibling after conditioning with a non-myeloablative or reduced intensity conditioning (RIC) regimens followed by DLI to eradicate residual tumour. These "mini-transplants" have the theoretical advantage of low TRM and may be proposed to older patients (up to 65 years of age), while maintaining the GVM effect. In a significant proportion of patients disease response is preceded by GVHD, suggesting a clear relationship between GVHD and GVM. Nevertheless these patients are at risk of developing life threatening complications and, on the contrary, some patients who reach disease control after GVHD and respond to GVHD therapy may finally relapse [87]. RIC transplantation has also been used in an attempt to improve the results of ASCT. Two groups have published their preliminary experience using RIC transplantation following ASCT [88,89]. The median age of myeloma patients was 52 years in both studies. ASCT was performed after 200 mg/m^2 melphalan conditioning and RIC transplantation followed low dose TBI [88] or the combination of fludarabine, melphalan and antithymocyte globulin [89] as conditioning regimens. The CR rate was near 50-55%, the 3-year probability of EFS was 54% and OS was 70%. The 100-day TRM was 2-6%, while the one-year TRM was 15%. However, there is no evidence of *plateau* with RIC-transplantation and this procedure is unlikely to be a curable approach. Furthermore, Kroger *et al* have shown that RIC-transplantation produces poor outcome in patients with deletions of chromosome 13 at diagnosis [90]. Prospective multicentre trials comparing tandem ASCT and tandem ASCT/RIC transplantation are ongoing to fully evaluate this procedure.

Conclusion

The use of HDT and ASCT has improved quality of life and survival and is now considered the standard therapy for eligible patients after initial chemotherapy with VAD or VAD-related regimen. For patients not suitable for ASCT, MP remains the treatment of choice. Unfortunately, most patients die from their disease and strategies to improve the outcome of ASCT such as tandem transplantation and manipulation of the graft have not been helpful. Allogeneic SCT may be curative in a proportion of patients and should be considered in younger patients with HLA compatible siblings. Current transplantation trials involve "debulking" the disease with an ASCT followed by reduced intensity conditioned allogeneic sibling transplant. This strategy is aimed at harnessing the GVM of the donor graft while maintaining a low TRM.

Thalidomide and bortezomib have managed to improve response rates and survival in patients with refractory/relapsed myeloma and may also be useful for newly diagnosed patients. However, their effect in combination with ASCT remains to be revealed. Furthermore, the use of multi-combination strategies (chemotherapy + bortezomib + thalidomide + ASCT) in newly diagnosed patients that aim to maximise and accelerate tumour mass reduction in an effort to overcome the negative consequences of cytogenetic abnormalities may provide a better policy in the management of myeloma.

The use of gene microarray and proteomic studies from patients treated on clinical trial may allow us to define group of patients who are going to benefit from a specific treatment, resulting in the development of more selective, and less toxic targeted therapies. The near future seems to include many exciting developments in the drug therapy of myeloma which will result in better management of myeloma patients.

References

[1] The International Myeloma Working Group. Criteria for the classification of monoclonal gammopathies, multiple myeloma and related disorders: a report of the International Myeloma Working Group. *Br. J. Haematol.* 2003;121:749-57.

[2] Terpos E, Rahemtulla A. Myeloma. In: Hoffbrand V, Catovsky D, Tuddenham EGD, (eds), *Postgraduate Haematology*, Fifth Edition, Blackwell Publishing, London, 2005, pp. 681-702.

[3] Kuehl WM, Bergsagel PL. Multiple myeloma: evolving genetic events and host interactions. *Nature Rev. Cancer* 2002;2:175-87.

[4] Rawstron AC, Davies FE, DasGupta R, et al. Flow cytometric disease monitoring in multiple myeloma: the relationship between normal and neoplastic plasma cells predicts outcome after transplantation. *Blood* 2002;100:3095-100.

[5] Hideshima T, Bergsagel PL, Kuehl WM, Anderson KC. Advances in biology of multiple myeloma: clinical applications. *Blood* 2004;104:607-18.

[6] Bergsagel PL, Kuehl WM. Molecular pathogenesis and a consequent classification of multiple myeloma. *J. Clin. Oncol.* 2005;23:6333-8.

[7] Pellat-Deceunynck C.Tumour-associated antigens in multiple myeloma. *Br. J. haematol* 2003;120:3-9.

[8] Zandecki M, Lai Jean-Luc, Facon T. Multiple myeloma: almost all patients are cytogenetically abnormal. *Br. J. Hematol.* 1996;94:217-27.

[9] Tricot G, Sawyer JR, Jagannath S, et al. Unique role of cytogenetics in the prognosis of patients with myeloma receiving high-dose therapy and autotransplants. *J. Clin. Oncol.* 1997;15:2659-66.

[10] Seong C, Delasalle K, Hayes K, et al. Prognostic value of cytogenetics in multiple myeloma. *Br. J. Haematol.* 1998;101:189-94.

[11] Stewart AK, Fonseca R. Prognostic and therapeutic significance of myeloma genetics and gene expression profiling. *J. Clin. Oncol.* 2005;23:6339-44.

[12] Terpos E, Eleutherakis-Papaiakovou V, Dimopoulos MA. Clinical implications of chromosomal abnormalities in multiple myeloma. *Leuk Lymphoma* 2006;47:803-14.

[13] Alsina M, Boyce B, Devlin RD, et al. Development of an in vivo model of human multiple myeloma bone disease. *Blood* 1996; 87:1495-501.

[14] Donovan KA, Lacy MQ, Gertz MA, Lust JA. IL-1beta expression in IgM monoclonal gammopathy and its relationship to multiple myeloma. *Leukemia* 2002;16:382-5.

[15] Terpos E, Szydlo R, Apperley JF, et al. Soluble receptor activator of nuclear factor {kappa}B ligand (RANKL)/osteoprotegerin (OPG) ratio predicts survival in multiple myeloma. Proposal for a novel prognostic index. *Blood* 2003;102:1064-9.

[16] Terpos E, Politou M, Szydlo R, et al. Serum levels of macrophage inflammatory protein-1 alpha (MIP-1α) correlate with the extent of bone disease and survival in patients with Multiple Myeloma. *Br. J. Haematol.* 2003;123:106-9.

[17] Tian E, Zhan F, Walker R et al. The role of the Wnt-signaling antagonist DKK1 in the development of osteolytic lesions in multiple myeloma. *N. Engl. J. Med.* 2003;349:2483-94.

[18] Terpos E, Politou M, Rahemtulla A. New insights into the pathophysiology and management of bone disease in multiple myeloma. *Br. J. Haematol.* 2003;123:758-69.

[19] Lee JW, Chung HY, Ehrlich LA, et al. IL-3 expression by myeloma cells increases both osteoclast formation and growth of myeloma cells. *Blood* 2004;103:2308-15.

[20] Politou M, Terpos E, Anagnostopoulos A, et al. Role of receptor activator of nuclear factor-kappa B ligand (RANKL), osteoprotegerin and macrophage protein 1-alpha (MIP-1α) in monoclonal gammopathy of undetermined significance (MGUS). *Br. J. Haematol.* 2004;126:686-9.

[21] Terpos E, Dimopoulos MA. Myeloma bone disease: pathophysiology and management. *Ann. Oncol.* 2005;16:1223-31.

[22] Vacca A, Ribatti D. Bone marrow angiogenesis in multiple myeloma. *Leukemia* 2006;20:193-9.

[23] Gunn WG, Conley A, Deininger L, et al. A crosstalk between myeloma cells and marrow stromal cells stimulates production of DKK1 and interleukin-6: a potential role in the development of lytic bone disease and tumor progression in multiple myeloma. *Stem Cells* 2006;24:986-91.

[24] Greipp PR, San Miguel J, Durie BG, et al. International staging system for multiple myeloma. *J. Clin. Oncol.* 2005;23:3412-20.

[25] Blade J, Vesole DH, Gertz M. High-dose therapy in multiple myeloma. *Blood* 2003;102:3469-70.

[26] He Y, Wheatley K, Clark O, et al. Early versus deferred treatment for early stage multiple myeloma. *Cochrane Database Syst. Rev.* 2003;1:CD004023.

[27] Weber DM, Dimopoulos MA, Moulopoulos LA, et al. Prognostic features of asymptomatic multiple myeloma. *Br. J. Haematol.* 1997;97:810-4.

[28] Mariette X, Zagdanski AM, Guermazi A, et al. Prognostic value of vertebral lesions detected by magnetic resonance imaging in patients with stage I multiple myeloma. *Br. J. Haematol.* 1999;104:723-9.

[29] Alexanian R, Haut A, Khan AU, et al. Treatment of multiple myeloma. Combination chemotherapy with different melphalan dose regimens. *JAMA* 1969;208:1680-5.

[30] Alexanian R, Dimopoulos M. The treatment of multiple myeloma. *N Engl J Med* 1994;330:484-9.

[31] Dimopoulos MA, Pouli A, Zervas K, et al. Prospective randomized comparison of vincristine, doxorubicin and dexamethasone (VAD) administered as intravenous bolus

injection and VAD with liposomal doxorubicin as first-line treatment in multiple myeloma. *Ann. Oncol.* 2003;14:1039-44.

[32] The Myeloma Trialists' Collaborative Group. Combination chemotherapy vs. melphalan plus prednisone as treatment for multiple myeloma: an overview of 6,633 patients from 27 randomized trials. *J. Clin. Oncol.* 1998;16:3832-42.

[33] The Myeloma Trialists' Collaborative Group. Interferon as therapy for multiple myeloma: an individual patient data overview of 24 randomized trials and 4012 patients. *Br. J. Haematol.* 2001;113:1020-34.

[34] Fritz E, Ludwig H. Interferon-alpha treatment in multiple myeloma: meta-analysis of 30 randomised trials among 3948 patients. *Ann. Oncol.* 2000;11:1427-36.

[35] Wisloff F, Hjorth M, Kaasa S, Westin J. Effect of interferon on the health-related quality of life of multiple myeloma patients: results of a Nordic randomized trial comparing melphalan-prednisone to melphalan-prednisone + alpha-interferon. The Nordic Myeloma Study Group. *Br. J. Haematol.* 1996;94:324-32.

[36] Wisloff F, Gulbrandsen N. Health-related quality of life and patients' perceptions in interferon-treated multiple myeloma patients. Nordic Myeloma Study Group. *Acta Oncol.* 2000;39:809-13.

[37] Terpos E, Apperley JF, Samson D, et al. Autologous stem cell transplantation in multiple myeloma: improved survival in nonsecretory multiple myeloma but lack of influence of age, status at transplant, previous treatment and conditioning regimen. A single-centre experience in 127 patients. *Bone Marrow Transplant* 2003;31:163-70.

[38] Gahrton G, Iacobelli S, Bjorkstrand B, et al. Role of stem cell transplantation in myeloma. *Hematology* 2005;10 Suppl 1:127-8.

[39] Terpos E, Rahemtulla A, Dimopoulos MA. Current treatment options for myeloma. *Expert Opin. Pharmacother* 2005;6:1127-42.

[40] O'shea D, Giles C, Terpos E, et al. Predictive factors for survival in myeloma patients who undergo autologous stem cell transplantation: a single-centre experience in 211 patients. *Bone Marrow Transplant* 2006;37:731-7.

[41] Attal M, Harousseau JL, Stoppa AM, et al. A prospective, randomised trial of autologous bone marrow transplantation and chemotherapy in multiple myeloma. Intergroupe Francais du Myelome. *N. Engl. J. Med.* 1996;335:91-7.

[42] Child JA, Morgan GJ, Davies FE, et al. High-dose chemotherapy with hematopoietic stem-cell rescue for multiple myeloma. *N. Engl. J. Med.* 2003;348:1875-83.

[43] Fermand JP, Katsahian S, Divine M, et al. High-dose therapy and autologous blood stem-cell transplantation compared with conventional treatment in myeloma patients aged 55 to 65 years: long-term results of a randomized control trial from the Group Myelome-Autogreffe. *J. Clin. Oncol.* 2005;23:9227-33.

[44] Barlogie B, Kyle RA, Anderson KC, et al. Standard chemotherapy compared with high-dose chemoradiotherapy for multiple myeloma: final results of phase III US Intergroup Trial S9321. *J Clin Oncol* 2006;24:929-36.

[45] Moreau P, Facon T, Attal M, et al. Comparison of 200 mg/m^2 melphalan and 8 Gy total body irradiation plus 140 mg/m^2 melphalan as conditioning regimens for peripheral blood stem cell transplantation in patients with newly diagnosed multiple myeloma:

final analysis of the Intregroupe Francophone du Myelome 9502 randomized trial. *Blood* 2002;99:731-5.

[46] Fermand JP, Ravaud P, Chevret S, et al. High-dose therapy and autologous peripheral blood stem cell transplantation in multiple myeloma: up-front or rescue treatment? Results of a multicenter sequential randomised clinical trial. *Blood* 1998;92:3131-6.

[47] Stewart AK, Vescio R, Schiller G, et al. Purging of autologous peripheral-blood stem cells using CD34 selection does not improve overall or progression-free survival after high-dose chemotherapy for multiple myeloma: results of a multicenter randomized controlled trial. *J. Clin. Oncol.* 2001;19:3771-9.

[48] Alegre A, Diaz-Mediavilla J, San-Miguel J, et al. Autologous peripheral blood stem cell transplantation for multiple myeloma: a report of 259 cases from the Spanish Registry. Spanish Registry for Transplant in MM and PETHEMA. *Bone Marrow Transplant* 1998;21:133-40.

[49] Majolino I, Vignetti M, Meloni G, et al. Autologous transplantation in multiple myeloma: a GITMO retrospective analysis on 290 patients. *Haematologica* 1999;84:844-52.

[50] Barlogie B, Shaughnessy J, Tricot G, et al. Treatment of multiple myeloma. *Blood* 2004;103:20-32.

[51] Fassas AB, Spencer T, Sawyer J, et al. Both hypodiploidy and deletion of chromosome 13 independently confer poor prognosis in multiple myeloma. *Br. J. Haematol.* 2002; 118:1041-7.

[52] Shaughnessy J, Jacobson J, Sawyer J, et al. Continuous absence of metaphase-defined cytogenetic abnormalities, especially of chromosome 13 and hypodiploidy ensure long term survival in myeloma treated with Total Therapy I: interpretation in the context of global gene expression. *Blood* 2003;101:3849-56.

[53] Jacobson J, Barlogie B, Shaughnessy J, et al. MDS-type abnormalities with myeloma signature karyotype: only 13% 1-year survival despite tandem transplants. *Br. J. Haematol.* 2003;122:430-40.

[54] Cavo M, Terragna C, Renzulli M, et al. Poor outcome with front-line autologous transplantation in t(4;14) multiple myeloma: low complete remission rate and short duration of remission. *J. Clin. Oncol.* 2006;24:e4-5 [letter].

[55] Facon T, Avet-Loiseau H, Guillerm G, et al. Chromosome 13 abnormalities identified by FISH analysis and serum β2-microglobulin produce a powerful myeloma staging system for patients receiving high-dose therapy. *Blood* 2001;97:1566-71.

[56] Shaughnessy J, Tian E, Sawyer J, et al. Prognostic impact of cytogenetic and interphase fluorescence in situ hybridization defined chromosome 13 deletion in multiple myeloma: early results of Total Therapy II. *Br. J. Haematol.* 2003;120:44-52.

[57] Porrata LF, Gertz MA, Geyer SM, et al. The dose of infused lymphocytes in the autograft directly correlates with clinical outcome after autologous peripheral blood hematopoietic stem cell transplantation in multiple myeloma. *Leukemia* 2004;18:1085-92.

[58] Politou M, Terpos E, Crawley D, et al. Pre-transplant VEGF levels in multiple myeloma are predictive for progression free survival. *Hematol. J.* 2004;5(Suppl 2):S13 [abstract].

[59] Harousseau JL, Shaughnessy J Jr, Richardson P. Multiple Myeloma. *Hematology*. (Am. Soc. Hematol. Educ. Program) 2004:237-56.

[60] Attal M, Harousseau JL, Facon T, et al. Single versus double autologous stem cell transplantation for multiple myeloma. *N. Engl. J. Med.* 2003;349:2495-502.

[61] Moreau P, Hullin C, Garban F, et al. Tandem autologous stem cell transplantation in high-risk de novo multiple myeloma: final results of the prospective and randomized IFM 99-04 protocol. *Blood* 2006;107:397-403.

[62] Cavo M, Cellini C, Zamagni E, et al. Superiority of double over single autologous stem cell transplantation as first-line therapy for multiple myeloma. *Blood* 2004;104:155a-156a [abstract].

[63] Sonneveld P, van der Holt B, Segeren C, et al. Intensive versus double intensive therapy in untreated multiple myeloma: updated analysis of the randomized phase III study Hovon 24 MM. *Blood* 2004;104:271a-272a [abstract].

[64] Fermand JP, Alberti C, Marolleau JP. Single versus double high dose therapy supported with autologous blood stem cell transplantation using unselected or CD34 enriched ABSC: results of a two by two designed randomized trial in 230 young patients with multiple myeloma. *Hematol. J.* 2003; 4 (Suppl 1): S59 [abstract].

[65] Morris C, Iacobelli S, Brand R et al. Benefit and timing of second transplantations in multiple myeloma: clinical findings and methodological limitations in a European Group for Blood and Marrow Transplantation registry study. *J. Clin. Oncol.* 2004;22:1674-81.

[66] Lee CK, Barlogie B, Fassas A, et al. Third autotransplant for the management of 98 patients among 1358 who had received prior tandem autotransplants: benefit apparent when 2nd to 3rd transplant interval exceeds 3 years. *Blood* 2004;104:157a [abstract].

[67] Reece DE, Bredeson C, Perez WS, et al. Autologous stem cell transplantation in multiple myeloma patients <60 vs. ≥ 60 years of age. *Bone Marrow Transplant* 2003;32:1135-43.

[68] Palumbo A, Bringhen S, Petrucci MT, et al. Intermediate-dose melphalan improves survival of myeloma patients aged 50 to 70: results of a randomized controlled trial. *Blood* 2004;104:3052-7.

[69] Badros A, Barlogie B, Siegel E, et al. Results of autologous stem cell transplant in multiple myeloma patients with renal failure. *Br. J. Haematol.* 2001;114:822-9.

[70] Lee CK, Zangari M, Barlogie B, et al. Dialysis-dependent renal failure in patients with myeloma can be reversed by high-dose myeloablative therapy and autotransplant. *Bone Marrow Transplant* 2004;33:823-828.

[71] San Miguel JF, Lahuerta JJ, Garcia-Sanz R, et al. Are myeloma patients with renal failure candidates for autologous stem cell transplantation? *Hematol. J.* 2000;1:28-36.

[72] Gojo I, Meisenberg B, Guo C, et al. Autologous stem cell transplantation followed by consolidation chemotherapy for patients with multiple myeloma. *Bone Marrow Transplant* 2006;37:65-72.

[73] Brinker BT, Waller EK, Leong T, et al. Maintenance therapy with thalidomide improves overall survival after autologous hematopoietic progenitor cell transplantation for multiple myeloma. *Cancer* 2006;106:2171-80.

[74] Chen CI, Nanji S, Prabhu A, et al. Sequential, cycling maintenance therapy for post transplant multiple myeloma. *Bone Marrow Transplant* 2006;37:89-94.

[75] Rajkumar SV, Fonseca R, Lacy MQ, et al. Autologous stem cell transplantation for relapsed and primary refractory myeloma. *Bone Marrow Transplant* 1999;23:1267-72.

[76] Elice F, Raimondi R, Tosetto A, et al. Prolonged overall survival with second on-demand autologous transplant in multiple myeloma. *Am. J. Hematol.* 2006;81:426-31.

[77] Palumbo A, Avonto I, Bruno B, et al. Intermediate-dose melphalan (100 mg/m2)/bortezomib/thalidomide/dexamethasone and stem cell support in patients with refractory or relapsed myeloma. *Clin. Lymphoma Myeloma* 2006;6:475-7.

[78] Lokhorst HM, Wu K, Verdonck LF, et al. The occurrence of graft-versus host disease is the major predictive factor for response to donor lymphocyte infusions in multiple myeloma. *Blood* 2004;103:4362-4.

[79] Gahrton G, Svensson H, Cavo M, et al. Progress in allogenic bone marrow and peripheral blood stem cell transplantation for multiple myeloma: a comparison between transplants performed 1983-93 and 1994-8 at European Group for Blood and Marrow Transplantation centres. *Br. J. Haematol.* 2001;113:209-16.

[80] Bjorkstrand B, Ljungman P, Svensson H, et al. Allogenic bone marrow transplantation versus autologous stem cell transplantation in multiple myeloma: a retrospective case-matched study from the European Group fro Blood and Marrow Transplantation. *Blood* 1996;88:4711–8.

[81] Alyea E, Weller E, Schlossman R, et al. Outcome after autologous and allogeneic stem cell transplantation for patients with multiple myeloma: impact of graft-versus-myeloma effect. *Bone Marrow Transplant* 2003;32:1145-51.

[82] The UK Myeloma Forum Guidelines Working Group. Guidelines on the diagnosis and management of multiple myeloma. *Br. J. Haematol.* 2001;115:522-40.

[83] Corradini P, Voena C, Tarella C, et al. Molecular and clinical remissions in multiple myeloma: role of autologous and allogeneic transplantation of hematopoietic cells. *J. Clin. Oncol.* 1999;17:208-215.

[84] Durie BG, Kyle RA, Belch A et al. Myeloma management guidelines: a consensus report from the Scientific Advisors of the International Myeloma Foundation. *Haematol. J.* 2003;4:379-98.

[85] Le Blanc R, Montminy-Metivier S, Belanger R, et al. Allogeneic transplantation for multiple myeloma: further evidence for a GVHD-associated graft-versus-myeloma effect. *Bone Marrow Transplant* 2001;28:841-8.

[86] Alyea E, Weller E, Schlossman R, et al. T-cell-depleted allogeneic bone marrow transplantation followed by donor lymphocyte infusion in patients with multiple myeloma: induction of graft-versus-myeloma effect. *Blood* 2001;98:934-9.

[87] Perez-Simon J, Caballero D, Mateos M, Miguel JS. Graft vs. Host Disease and Graft vs. Myeloma effect after non-myeloablative allogeneic transplantation. *Leuk Lymphoma* 2004;45:1725-9.

[88] Kroger N, Schwerdtfeger R, Kiehl M, et al. Autologous stem cell transplantation followed by a dose-reduced allograft induces high complete remission rate in multiple myeloma. *Blood* 2002;100:755-60.

[89] Maloney DG, Molina AJ, Sahebi F, et al. Allografting with non myeloabaltive conditioning following cytoreductive autograft for the treatment of patients with multiple myeloma. *Blood* 2003;102:3447-54.

[90] Kroger N, Schilling G, Einsele H, et al. Deletion of chromosome band 13q14 as detected by fluorescence in situ hybridization is a prognostic factor in patients with multiple myeloma who are receiving allogeneic dose-reduced stem cell transplantation. *Blood* 2004;103:4056-61.

Chapter Sources

The following chapters have been previously published:

Chapter 9 was also published in *Bone Marrow Transplantation: New Research*, edited by Dale F. Davidson, published by Nova Science Publishers. It was submitted for appropriate modifications in an effort to encourage wider dissemination of research.

Chapter 10 was also published in *Stem Cells and Cancer*, edited by Devon W. Parsons, published by Nova Science Publishers. It was submitted for appropriate modifications in an effort to encourage wider dissemination of research.

Index

B

C

D

E

F

I

J

K

L

M

N

O

P

P

Q

R

S

T

U

V

W

X

Y

Z